Health and Human Values:

An Ecological Approach

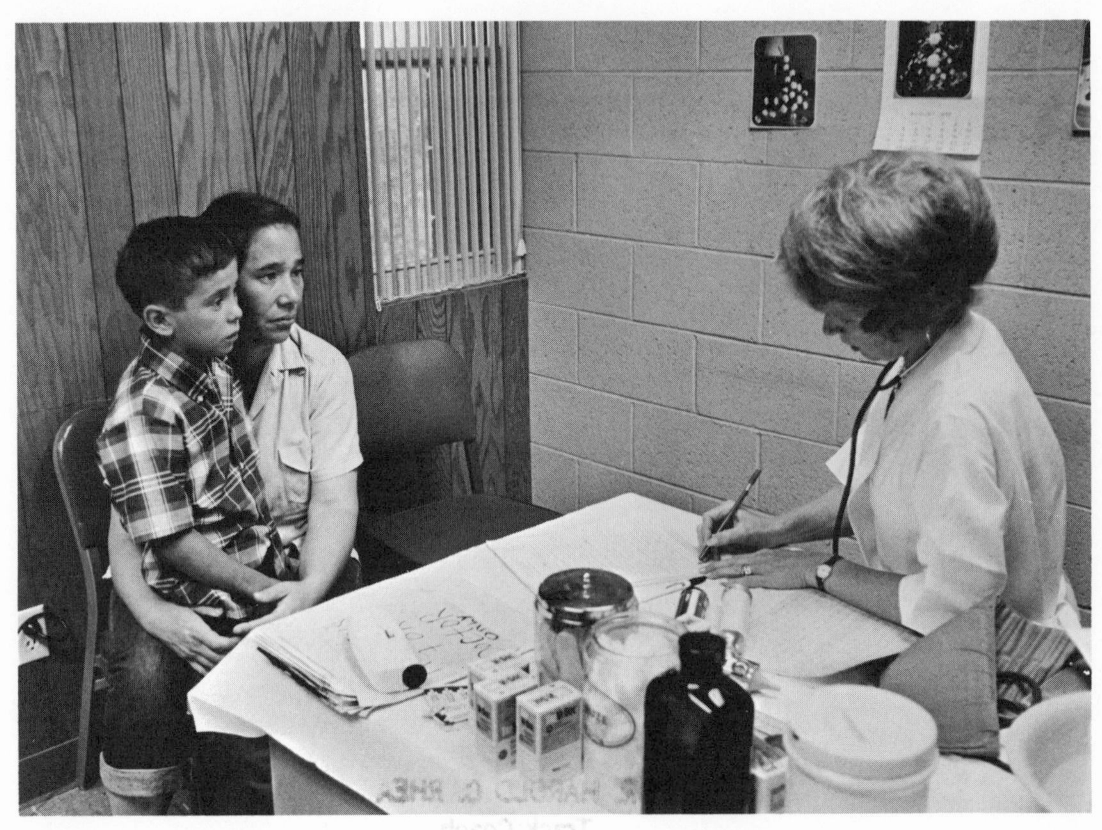

Health and Human Values
An Ecological Approach

by Allure Jefcoat

Diablo Valley College

John Wiley & Sons, Inc.

New York London Sydney Toronto

PHOTO CREDITS

Units I & II: Stanford University News Service

Units III, IV, V, & Frontispiece: Phiz Mezey

Library of Congress Catalog Card Number: 70-37934

ISBN 0-471-44100-7

Printed in the United States of America.

10 9 8 7 6 5 4 3 2 1

to

Colleen

Steve

and Cindy

Preface

In a book of this size I can merely present a sampling of the discussion and research concerning a few selected areas of major importance to human health. I have chosen areas I believe to be relevant for the present times and to have a far-reaching impact on the health of people young or old. Many of the topics are controversial, and in spite of their daily importance to our lives, many of those topics are not presented at all in most college texts.

I believe the most effective use of this book of readings would be as the common base from which the class would discuss the ideas presented, give group or individual presentations of varying viewpoints, and do related projects. An understanding of the personal value systems of people in the class is of the utmost importance.

I am very grateful to several of my colleagues for their contributions that have led to this finished book, particularly to Dan Clancy with whom I compiled the first book of readings several years ago that we used in place of any texts then available, and to Marje Smith who has contributed articles and ideas which helped shape some important understandings concerning health in general and the book in particular. Munroe Pastermack, Harry Byrne, Dianne Bruckmeir, Eric Yoeman, and Karen Taylor have also contributed significant ideas or articles. I am grateful to Cheryl La Fleur for typing the manuscript and to my daughter, Colleen, and my brother, Terry, for helpful criticisms of my own writings in the book, and to Bob Martincich for his very helpful criticism of the entire manuscript.

I appreciate permission granted by the various authors and publishers of the articles, particularly Dr. Calvin J. Frederick who wrote the article on suicide specifically for the readers of this book.

Allure Jefcoat
Walnut Creek, California

Contents

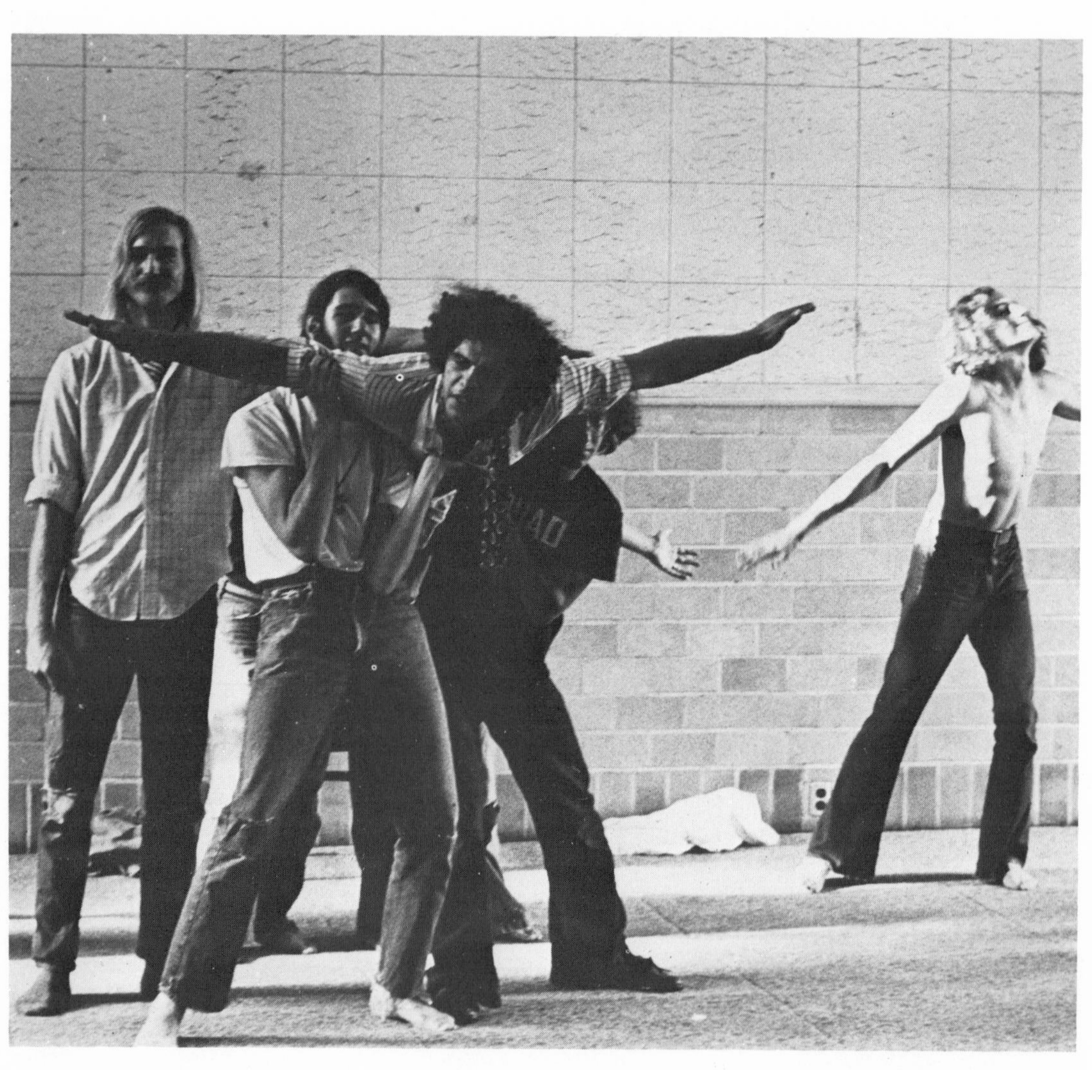

UNIT 1
The Human Potential

Unlike the turn of the twentieth century, it is no longer the plague, nor diptheria, nor death due to any other virulent strain of germ that carries us off in droves. It has a good chance of being the case in the future if by design or by accident we release some of the germs we are cultivating in our biological warfare labs, or if our people become weakened and susceptible to a natural germ in the aftermath of over-population or nuclear war. However, today it is diseases originating in or associated with the mind that carry most of us off.

More than half of all the people who die each year in the United States do so as a result of hardening of the arteries, which causes heart attack, stroke, and other vascular diseases. Automobile accidents are the greatest killers of college age people and the fourth largest killer of the total population. Suicide ranks second in numbers of deaths of college age people, and is the tenth greatest killer of all ages.

An extremely important factor involved in deaths due to hardening of the arteries, accidents, and suicides is *mental stress*. Only in recent years have there been extensive studies and the identification of the cause-effect relationship of psychological problems and their physiological consequences. A great amount of research has been done on what has come to be known as the "pituitary-adrenal stress syndrome." This syndrome, beginning with psycogenic stress, leads through complex biochemical reactions in the body, to non-adaptive behavior and hardening of the arteries, and finally to stroke and other such consequences.

The use of alcohol is involved in over 50% of the 53,000 annual automobile accident deaths and another million serious injuries. This is a nation with 6,000,000 alcoholics. Alcoholism is a symptom of deep-rooted psychological problems.

Dr. Frederick reviews the psychological implications of the suicides in the first article of this unit. In addition to the deaths due to ills of the psyche, over 50% of all prescriptions filled annually are for mind-altering drugs. Essentially all of us suffer mentally to a degree ranging from total debility with life committment to a mental institution through a constant mild free floating anxiety to simply a failure to realize our full human potential.

By the time we reach adulthood most of us are weighted down with tensions, anxieties, and fears. We are afraid we engage in dull conversations, aren't pleasing our neighbor with the condition of the lawn or the appearance of the company who visit our homes, or our style of dress. We fear different social or ethnic groups, homosexuality, atheism, or communism. We are afraid our breath is offensive, our teeth aren't bright and straight enough, we have underarm odor, or—a new one presently being created by advertisements—we need the new "feminine hygiene" deoderant!

We have accepted fear and conformity imposed on us (1) by Madison Avenue in its desire to sell us products we don't need; (2) by our various institutions which have often forgotten that their purpose is to help develop the human potential and now aim at keeping us unchanged and easily manageable; or (3) by our own parents in their mistaken belief that they are protecting us for our own good when in reality they are motivated by a desire for stability for themselves—an attempt to hang on to a world that no longer exists. Too many of us are panic stricken and don't know how to handle a world where change occurs at an exponential rate, whose complexity is incomprehensible to most or all of us with the general loss of value systems that many still cherish though they no longer make sense in today's new world.

I like the encouraging optimistic statement of Raza Gustaitis: "The turned-on person recognizes that continuous change is the nature of the universe. Everything is part of a constantly flowing pattern of particles. Nothing stands still or is ever repeated. All systems are temporary. There is nothing to cling to. We, as part of it all, change and shift, move and evolve, level beyond level . . . The only way of life that makes sense builds on acceptance of change . . . "

A sign of health, though frightening to many due to the lack of understanding, is an expanding search for new values which enhance the human potential and make more sense in today's world. Multitudes of people are now conscious that something is missing in their lives and are attempting to shed the ego defense mechanisms, the barriers and filters to total perception, that cloud their perception and evaluation of each incoming stimulus and prevent their making the decisions that best meet their total needs.

People are attempting to arrive at these ends over a variety of pathways, the effectiveness of each varying for the individual. Esalen Institute at Big Sur, California near Monterey was the first of well over 50 institutes now offering Gestalt, sensitivity awareness, encounter, meditation, yoga and other workshops whose intent is to expand awareness and break entrapping mind-sets. They all emphasize self-actualization and the development of the human potential. Over 100,000 individuals, mostly rather "square" middle class white Americans, have enrolled in Esalen Institute alone since its opening in 1962. The soul-searching is obviously there!

Who are all these people in the process of self-actualization? We are all unique individuals, but in misguided attempts to meet the needs of other unhealthy individuals we have been lumped and stereotyped into "they" groups—people to play the contrived "male-female" roles, the "Indian" "Nigger," "Wop," "Jew," "Queer," "Commie," "Dumb Female," "Mr. Sick," "Hippie," "Town Stud," and "Intellectual" roles. "They" have cast us in the roles; and "we" have accepted the parts and played them well! It is always our choice to accept or refuse the part. Frequently the choice is very difficult to see, as when there is a unanimous decision among the people who control the jobs that people of a certain color or sex "haven't the ability" to handle that job, or when "everyone" agrees a certain look or behavior is "right" it doesn't occur to us to question it.

More than in any preceding generation Americans are knocking down barriers of repression and non-working entrapping value systems. A few are achieving this by changing existing institutions; more are building new institutions such as Esalen; and many others feel they are able to achieve it better by rejecting most or all institutions.

This movement has been more effective for some roles than for others. Young people, particularly college students, and black people have made a fair start. Chicanos and women have just begun. We've heard just a whisper from American Indians who are trapped in poverty, whose total life is controlled by the Bureau of Indian Affairs so that they have no voice.

The elderly in America cry out to us but we can't hear them. In general we shut them off to lie in a bed or sit in front of a television set at convalescent hospitals and homes for the aged. We use our ego defense mechanisms to keep us from sensing their boredom, loneliness and feelings of worthlessness.

We put those same ego defense mechanisms to work to keep from learning the information and becoming aware that 6.5 million black men work full time for less than poverty wages; then we use the same defense mechanisms to castigate them when they don't stay and "support" their families and to brand them "lazy, satisfied with their lot!"

We use these defense mechanisms to accept that people with long hair or unfashionable clothing may not draw unemployment insurance money in Sacramento County because they do not accept the value system of the boss on the job, and we lay the "fault" on them for not conforming!

We use these defense mechanisms to accept the natural inferiority of women as the reason that the average salary of women working full time in 1969 was $4,979 per year as compared with an average salary for men of $8,227 per year. Thirty-seven percent of all women worked full time outside the home. Nearly half of these were the heads of households and only 2% earned over $10,000 per year. Women have accepted the role and they, even more than blacks and Chicanos, have a low self-image, low motivation and very little concept of how to plan for and cope with change. Women play the role well!

We let ourselves believe that prisoners are "so lacking in penitence or even common decency that punishment seems to be the only thing left." (Dr. Karl Menninger) We accept that prisons are "reformatory" and cut down on crime, yet we aren't able to hear the charges of their inhumanity and ineffectiveness.

Cutting across all roles, we obediently plunge ourselves into debt at exorbitant finance charges buying the new high-powered automobiles that advertisers assure us will make us "sexy," feel guilt as we are told we should when we try to act out the "sex" and obediently drink our way to alcoholism as every third billboard along the freeway tells us in attempt to ease the pain of our financial burden, guilt feelings, and the empty realization that we aren't any "sexier" than we were at the beginning!

Some of us can see that such role assigning and role playing is mentally and physically unhealthy. A lot of us can now accept that the person who practices prejudice and the one against whom it is practiced are both made less healthy by the prejudice. A lot of us want to stop the role playing and be individuals.

What are the masses of people who attend the institutes and try out different life styles searching for? What would the profile of the mentally healthy person look like at the end of his searching therapy?

As Dr. Carl Rogers describes, a healthy person, though an integrated unity, has three facets: (1) This person would be open to his experience. He has no need for his ego defense mechanisms." . . . he no longer needs to fear what experience may hold, but welcomes it freely as part of his changing and developing self . . . every stimulus, whether originating within the organism or in the environment, would be freely relayed through the nervous system without being distorted by any defense mechanism." (2) "The person would live in an existential fashion . . . our hypothetical person would realize that 'what I will be in the next moment, and what I will do, grows out of that moment, and cannot be predicted in advance either by me or by others' . . . the self and personality would emerge from experience, rather than that the experience is being truncated or twisted to fit a preconceived self-structure." (3) "This person would find his organism a trustworthy means of arriving at the most satisfying behavior in each existential situation. He would do what "felt right" in this immediate moment and would find this in general to be a competent and trustworthy guide to his behavior."

The health (both *mental* and *physical*) of each individual and of the nation will be vastly improved when mind-entrapping stereotyping and role playing is rejected to allow the rich human potential to more fully emerge. Our health will improve when we are able to accept ourselves and all other humans as *unique, valuable individuals* with the right to our own value systems.

This unit takes a look at some of the pressures which have been applied against various segments of the society to block the attainment of the human potential, and it takes a look at some old but seldom considered prospects and some new ones for attaining the full human potential.

New Light on the Human Potential 1

by Herbert A. Otto

William James once estimated that the healthy human being is functioning at less than 10 percent of his capacity. It took more than half a century before this idea found acceptance among a small proportion of behavioral scientists. In 1954, the highly respected and widely known psychologist Gardner Murphy published his pioneering volume *Human Potentialities.* The early Sixties saw the beginnings of the human potentialities research project at the University of Utah and the organization of Esalen Institute in California, the first of a series of "Growth Centers" that were later to be referred to as the Human Potentialities Movement.

Today, many well-known scientists such as Abraham Maslow, Margaret Mead, Gardner Murphy, O. Spurgeon English, and Carl Rogers subscribe to the hypothesis that man is using a very small fraction of his capacities. Margaret Mead quotes a 6 per cent figure, and my own estimate is 5 per cent or less. Commitment to the hypothesis is not restricted to the United States. Scientists in the U.S.S.R. and other countries are also at work. Surprisingly, the so-called human potentialities hypothesis is still largely unknown.

What are the dimensions of the human potential? The knowledge we do have about man is minimal and has not as yet been brought together with the human potentialities hypothesis as an organizing

SOURCE: Reprinted with permission from: *Saturday Review*, December 20, 1969.

force and synthesizing element. Of course, we know more about man today than we did fifty years ago, but this is like the very small part of the iceberg we see above the water. Man essentially remains a mystery. From the depths of this mystery there are numerous indicators of the human potential.

Certain indicators of man's potential are revealed to us in childhood. They become "lost" or submerged as we succumb to the imprinting of the cultural mold in the "growing up" process. Do you remember when you were a child and it rained after a dry spell and there was a very particular, intensive earthy smell in the air? Do you remember how people smelled when they hugged you? Do you recall the brilliant colors of leaves, flowers, grass, and even brick surfaces and lighted signs that you experienced as a child? Furthermore, do you recall that when father and mother stepped into the room you knew how they felt about themselves, about life, and about you—at that moment.

Today we know that man's sense of smell, one of the most powerful and primitive senses, is highly developed. In the average man this capacity has been suppressed except for very occasional use. Some scientists claim that man's sense of smell is almost as keen as a hunting dog's. Some connoisseurs of wines, for example, can tell by the bouquet not only the type of grape and locality where they were grown but even the vintage year and vineyard. Perfume mixers can often detect fantastically minute amounts in mixed essences; finally there are considerable data on odor discrimination from the laboratory. It is also clear that, since the air has become an overcrowded garbage dump for industrial wastes and the internal combustion engine, it is easier to turn off our sense of smell than to keep it functioning. The capacity to experience the environment more fully through our olfactory organs remains a potential.

It is possible to regain these capacities through training. In a similar manner, sensory and other capacities, including visual, kinesthetic, and tactile abilities, have become stunted and dulled. We perceive less clearly, and as a result we feel less—we use our dulled senses to close ourselves off from both our physical and interpersonal environment. Today we also dull our perceptions of how other people feel and we consistently shut off awareness of our own feelings. For many who put their senses to sleep it is a sleep that lasts until death. Again, through sensory and other training the doors of perception can be cleansed (to use Blake's words) and our capacities reawakened. Anthropological research abounds with reports of primitive tribes that have developed exceptional sensory and perceptive abilities as a result of training. Utilization of these capacities by modern man for life enrichment purposes awaits the future.

Neurological research has shed new light on man's potential. Work at the UCLA Brain Research Institute points to enormous abilities latent in everyone by suggesting an incredible hypothesis: The ultimate creative capacity of the human brain may be, for all practical purposes, infinite. To use the computer analogy, man is a vast storehouse of data, but we have not learned how to program ourselves to utilize these data for problem-solving purposes. Recall of experiential data is extremely spotty and selective for most adults. My own research has convinced me that the recall of experiences can be vastly improved by use of certain simple training techniques, provided sufficient motivation is present.

Under emergency conditions, man is capable of prodigious feats of physical strength. For example, a middle-aged California woman with various ailments lifted a car just enough to let her son roll out from under it after it had collapsed on him. According to newspaper reports the car weighed in excess of 2,000 pounds. There are numerous similar accounts indicating that every person has vast physical reserve capacities that can be tapped. Similarly, the extraordinary feats of athletes and acrobats—involving the conscious and specialized development of certain parts of the human organism as a result of consistent application and a high degree of motivation—point to the fantastic plasticity and capabilities of the human being.

Until World War II, the field of hypnosis was not regarded as respectable by many scientists and was associated with stage performances and charlatanism. Since that time hypnosis has attained a measure of scientific respectability. Medical and therapeutic applications of hypnosis include the use of this technique in surgery and anesthesiology (hypnoanesthesia for major and minor surgery), gynecology (infertility, frigidity, menopausal conditions), pediatrics (enuresis, tics, asthma in children, etc.), and in dentistry. Scores of texts on medical and dental hypnosis are available. Dr. William S. Kroger, one of the specialists in the field and author of the well-known text *Clinical and Experimental Hypnosis*, writes that hypnotherapy is "directed to the patient's needs and is a methodology to tap the 'forgotten assets' of the hidden potentials of behavior and response that so often lead to new learnings and understanding." (My italics.) As far as we know now, the possibilities opened by hypnosis for the potential functioning of the human organism are not brought about by the hypnotist. Changes are induced by the subject, utilizing his belief-structure, with the hypnotist operating as an "enabler," making it possible for the subject to tape some of his unrealized potential.

The whole area of parapsychology that deals with extrasensory perception (ESP), "mental telepathy," and other paranormal phenomena, and that owes much of its development to the work of J.B. Rhine and others is still regarded by much of the scientific establishment with the same measure of suspicion accorded hypnosis in the pre-World War II days. It is of interest that a number of laboratories in the U.S.S.R. are devoted to the study of telepathy as a physical phenomenon, with research conducted under the heading, "cerebral radio-communication" and "bioelectronics." The work is supported by the Soviet government. The reluctance to accept findings from this field of research is perhaps best summarized by an observation of Carl C. Jung's in 1958:

> [Some] people deny the findings of parapsychology outright, either for philosophical reasons or from intellectual laziness. This can hardly be considered a scientifically responsible attitude, even though it is a popular way out of quite extraordinary intellectual difficulty.

Although the intensive study of creativity had its beginnings in fairly recent times, much of value has been discovered about man's creative potential. There is evidence that every person has creative abilities that can be developed. A considerable number of studies indicate that much in our educational system—including conformity pressures exerted by teachers, emphasis on memory development, and rote learning, plus the overcrowding of classrooms—militates against the development of creative capacities. Research has established that children between the ages of two and three can learn to read, tape record a story, and type it as it is played back. Hundreds of children between the ages of four and six have been taught by the Japanese pedagogue Suzuki to play violin concertos. Japanese research with infants and small children also suggests the value of early "maximum input" (music, color, verbal, tactile stimuli) in the personality development of infants. My own observations tend to confirm this. We have consistently underestimated the child's capacity to learn and his ability to realize his potential while enjoying both the play elements and the discipline involved in this process.

In contrast to the Japanese work, much recent Russian research appears to be concentrated in the area of mentation, with special emphasis on extending and enlarging man's mental processes and his capacity for learning. As early as 1964 the following appeared in *Soviet Life Today*, a U. S. S. R. English language magazine:

> The latest findings in anthropology, psychology, logic, and physiology show that the potential of the human mind is very great indeed. "As soon as modern science gave us some understanding of the structure and work of the human brain, we were struck with its enormous reserve capacity," writes Yefremov (Ivan Yefremov, eminent Soviet scholar and writer.) "Man under average conditions of work and life, uses only a small part of his thinking equipment . . . If we were able to force our brain to work at only half its capacity, we could, without any difficulty whatever, learn forty languages, memorize the large Soviet Encyclopedia from cover to cover, and complete the required courses of dozens of colleges." The statement is hardly an exaggeration. It is the generally accepted theoretical view of man's mental potentialities. How can we tap this gigantic potential? It is a big and very complex problem with many ramifications.

Another signpost of man's potential is what I have come to call the "Grandma Moses effect." This artist's experience indicates that artistic talents can be discovered and brought to full flowering in the latter part of the life cycle. In every retirement community there can be found similar examples of residents who did not use latent artistic abilities or other talents until after retirement. In many instances the presence of a talent is suspected or known but allowed to remain fallow for the best part of a lifetime.

Reasons why well-functioning mature adults do not use specific abilities are complex. Studies conducted at the University of Utah as a part of the Human Potentialities Research Project revealed that unconscious blocks are often present. In a number of instances a person with definite evidence that he has a specific talent (let's say he won a state-wide contest in sculpture while in high school) may not wish to realize this talent at a later time because he fears this would introduce a change in life-style. Sometimes fear of the passion of creation is another roadblock in self-actualization. On the basis of work at Utah it became clear that persons who live close to their capacity, who continue to activate their potential, have a pronounced sense of wellbeing and considerable energy and see themselves as leading purposeful and creative lives.

Most people are unaware of their strengths and potentialities. If a person with some college background is handed a form and asked to write out his personality strengths, he will list, on an average, five or six strengths. Asked to do the same thing for his weaknesses, the list will be two to three times as long. There are a number of reasons for this low self-assessment. Many participants in my classes and marathon group weekends have pointed out that "listing your strengths feels like bragging about yourself. It's something that just isn't done." Paradoxically, in a group, people feel more comfortable about sharing problem areas and hang-ups than they do about personality resources and latent abilities. This is traceable to the fact that we are members of a pathology-oriented culture. Psychological and psychiatric jargon dealing with emotional dysfunction and mental illness has become the parlance of the man in the street. In addition, from early childhood in our educational system we learn largely by our mistakes—by having them pointed out to us repeatedly. All this results in early "negative conditioning" and influences our attitude and perception of ourselves and other people. An attitudinal climate has become established which is continually fed and reinforced.

As a part of this negative conditioning there is a heavy emphasis by communications media on violence in television programs and motion pictures. The current American news format of radio, television, and newspapers—the widely prevalent ideas of what constitutes news—results from a narrow, brutalizing concept thirty or forty years behind the times and is inimical to the development of human potential.

The news media give much time and prominent space to violence and consistently underplay "good" news. This gives the consumer the impression that important things that happen are various types of destructive activities. Consistent and repeated emphasis on bad news not only creates anxiety and tension but instills the belief that there is little except violence, disasters, accidents, and mayhem abroad in the world. As a consequence, the consumer of such news gradually experiences a shift in his outlook about the world leading to the formation of feelings of alienation and separation. The world is increasingly perceived as a threat, as the viewer becomes anxious that violence and mayhem may be perpetrated on him from somewhere out of the strange and unpredictable environment in which he lives. There slowly grows a conviction that it is safer to withdraw from such a world, to isolate himself from its struggles, and to let others make the decisions and become involved.

As a result of the steady diet of violence in the media, an even more fundamental and insidious erosion in man's self-system takes place. The erosion affects what I call the "trust factor." If we have been given a certain amount of affection, love, and understanding in our formative years, we are able to place a certain amount of trust in our fellow man. Trust is one of the most important elements in today's society although we tend to minimize its importance. We basically trust people. For example, we place an enormous amount of trust in our fellow man when driving on a freeway or in an express lane. We trust those with whom we are associated to fulfill their obligations and responsibilities. The element of trust is the basic rule in human relations. When we distrust people, they usually sense our attitude and reciprocate in kind.

The consistent emphasis in the news on criminal violence, burglarizing, and assault makes slow but pervasive inroads into our reservoir of trust. As we hear and read much about the acts of violence and injury men perpetrate upon one another, year after year, with so little emphasis placed on the loving, caring, and humanitarian acts of man, we begin to trust our fellow man less, and we thereby diminish ourselves. It is my conclusion the media's excessive emphasis on violence, like the drop of water on the stone, erodes and wears away the trust factor in man. By undermining the trust factor in man, media contribute to man's estrangement from man and prevent the full flourishing and deeper development of a sense of community and communion with all men.

Our self-concept, how we feel about ourselves and our fellow man and the world, is determined to a considerable extent by the inputs from the physical and interpersonal environment to which we are exposed. In the physical environment, there are the irritants in the air, i.e., air pollution plus the ugliness and noise of megapolis. Our interpersonal environment is characterized by estrangement and distance from others (and self), and by the artificiality and superficiality of our social encounters and the resultant violation of authenticity. Existing in a setting that provides as consistent inputs multiple irritants, ugliness and violence, and lack of close and meaningful relationships, man is in danger of becoming increasingly irritated, ugly, and violent.

As work in the area of human potentialities progressed, it has become ever clearer that personality, to a much greater degree than previously suspected, functions in response to the environment. This is additional confirmation of what field theorists and proponents of the holistic approach to the study of man have long suspected.

Perhaps the most important task facing us today is the regeneration of our environment and institutional structures such as school, government, church, etc. With increasing sophistication has come the recognition that institutions are not sacrosanct and that they have but one purpose and function—to serve as a framework for the actualization of human potential. It is possible to evaluate both the institution and the contribution of the institution by asking this question: "To what extent does the function of the institution foster the realization of human potential?"

Experimental groups consistently have found that the more a person's environment can be involved in the process of realizing potential, the greater the gains. It is understandable why scientists concerned with the study of personality have been reluctant to consider the importance of here-and-now inputs in relation to personality functioning. To do so would open a Pandora's box of possibilities and complex forces that until fairly recently were considered to be the exclusive domain of the social scientist. Many scientists and professionals, particularly psychotherapists, feel they have acquired a certain familiarity with the topography of "intrapsychic forces" and are reluctant to admit the reality of additional complex factors in the functioning of the personality.

It is significant that an increasing number of psychologists, psychiatrists, and social workers now realize that over and beyond keeping up with developments in their respective fields, the best way to acquire additional professional competence is through group experiences designed for personal growth and that focus on the unfolding of individual possibilities. From this group of aware professionals and others came much of the initial support and interest in Esalen Institute and similar "Growth Centers" later referred to as the Human Potentialities Movement.

Esalen Institute in Big Sur, California, was organized in 1962 by Michael Murphy and his partner, Dick Price. Under their imaginative management the institute experienced a phenomenal growth, established a branch in San Francisco, and is now famous for its seminars and weekend experiences offered by pioneering professionals. Since 1962 more than 100,000 persons have enrolled for one of these activities.

The past three years have seen a rapid mushrooming of Growth Centers. There are more than fifty such organizations ranging from Esalen and Kairos Institutes in California to Oasis in Chicago and Aureon Institute in New York. The experiences offered at these Growth Centers are based on several hypotheses: (1) that the average healthy person functions at a fraction of his capacity; (2) that man's most exciting life-long adventure is actualizing his potential; (3) that the group environment is one of the best settings in which to achieve growth; and (4) that personality growth can be achieved by anyone willing to invest himself in this process.

Human potentialities is rapidly emerging as a discrete field of scientific inquiry. Exploring the human potential can become the meeting ground for a wide range of disciplines, offering a dynamic synthesis for seemingly divergent areas of research. It is possible that the field of human potentialities offers an answer to the long search for a synthesizing and organizing principle which will unify the sciences. The explosive growth of the Human Potentialities Movement is indicative of a growing public interest. Although there exist a considerable number of methods—all designed to tap human potential—work on assessment or evaluation of these methods has in most instances not progressed beyond field testing and informal feedback of results. The need for research in the area of human potentialities has never been more pressing. The National Center for the Exploration of Human Potential in La Jolla, California, has recently been organized for this purpose. A nonprofit organization, the center will act as a clearing house of information for current and past approaches that have been successful in fostering personal growth. One of the main purposes of the center will be to conduct and coordinate basic and applied research concerning the expansion of human potential.

Among the many fascinating questions posed by researchers are some of the following: What is the relationship of body-rhythms, biorhythms, and the expansion of sensory awareness to the uncovering of human potential? What are the applications of methods and approaches from other cultures such as yoga techniques, Sufi methods, types of meditation, etc.? What is the role of ecstasy and play vis-a-vis the realizing of human possibilities? The exploration of these and similar questions can help us create a society truly devoted to the full development of human capacities—particularly the capacities for love, joy, creativity, spiritual experiencing. This is the challenge and promise of our lifetime.

2 The Wave of the Future—Brain Waves

by David M. Rorvik

Psychedelic drugs may soon give way to the electronic high, a new brain-wave mastery over mind and body.

In the soaring sixties, we'd get it on with acid, trip the lysergic light fantastic, groove, turn on, tune in, drop out, blow our minds and occasionally crash, whimpering, "Oh, wow!!! Often we didn't know where we'd been or where we were going the next time. We'd sit like zombies watching the movies in our minds, never quite able to control the content, volume or focus.

Yet unsatisfactory, unpredictable and unsafe as all this was, it was a start. In considerable numbers, we began to engage the mind, the consciousness, the inner man directly, to measure quantites that the behaviorists had declared unknowable. Still, some of the more thoughtful heads were worried; if LSD were really the answer to everything, a chemical shortcut to Nirvana, why were so few Zen adepts abdicating meditation for acid? Could it be that they had something better? As guru stock skyrocketed, it became clear that that "something" was conscious control over one's internal states of feeling and being, rather than mindless submission to them.

SOURCE: Published by permission of the author, David M. Rorvik. Originally published in LOOK magazine, October 6, 1970.

Skeptical behaviorist-bombarded Western man began to sit up and take note when science declared that many dedicated Zen and Yogi meditators were indeed capable of asserting mind over matter. Researchers wired them to electroencephalogram (EEG) machines and found that meditators could, by sheer force of will beefed up by years of training, produce on command profound trance states, raise and lower blood pressure, reduce body temperature, slow heart rates, and, in general, tap into physiological functions thought to be forever beyond the reach of conscious control.

Now, with the dawning of the biocybernetic seventies, it is not too surprising that LSD is about to be eclipsed, in a sense, by an electronic successor: BFT. Bio-Feedback Training, or "electronic Yoga" as it has been called, puts you in touch with inner space just as LSD does but, unlike acid, leaves you in full control of your senses. And, unlike meditation, it doesn't take years of sitting on the mountaintops to master. It gives strong indication of being safe and predictable and promises to revolutionize psychology and medicine. Bio-feedback pioneers say that BFT could, among other things, completely replace many drugs, help people overcome anxiety, overwhelm numerous psychosomatic ills, facilitate learning, enhance memory, alleviate heart and circulatory diseases, illuminate the many processes of the mind and even provide access to previously unimagined experiences, thus not only defining the dimensions of inner man but also extending those dimensions in the process.

"I may be an optimist," concedes Dr. Joseph Kamiya, reflecting on this latter possibility, "but I do believe that the next step in man's evolution will be in the experiential domain." Dr. Kamiya, a research specialist with Langley Porter Neuropsychiatric Institute in San Francisco and a lecturer in medical psychology at the University of California School of Medicine, is one of the foremost explorers in that domain. His experiments in 1958, as much as anything else, set the stage for the current explosion in BFT research.

Explaining that early work, Dr. Kamiya notes that the brain produces electrical activity that can be visualized—with the help of an EEG machine—in the form of constantly changing wave patterns. Electrical signals, picked up by electrodes attached to the scalp with a special conductive glue, are translated onto graph paper by the EEG machine, revealing brain waves of varying frequencies and amplitudes. Four primary brain-wave patterns have been identified using this technique—delta, theta, alpha and beta, all contained within a total energy spectrum of about 0 to 40 cycles per second.

Alpha, which moves at a frequency of eight to twelve cycles per second, happens to be the most prominent type of brain-wave activity, and, because it can be traced so easily by EEG, Dr. Kamiya seized upon it when he decided to see whether a subject could be taught awareness of an internal state. Nearly all of us slip in and out of alpha from five to thirty times a minute without ever knowing it.

Dr. Kamiya and his associates, then at the University of Chicago, wired a subject for EEG, placed him in a darkened room and then monitored his brain waves from an adjacent cubicle. The subject was instructed to close his eyes and guess whether he was in "state A" (alpha) or "state B" (non-alpha) whenever a bell rang. He was told after each guess whether he was right or wrong. Given this sort of feedback, the subject quickly learned to discriminate between the two states. He went from 50 per cent accuracy (no better than chance) on the first day to 100 per cent accuracy on the fourth day, making the correct guess 400 times in a row. Other subjects were tested with similar results. And once the subjects had learned to discriminate between the two states, it developed that they could switch either state on or off at will, on command from the experimenters!

Since moving to Langley Porter, Dr. Kamiya has altered his experimental procedure somewhat. He now trains subjects in only four or five hours to sustain or repress alpha, through the sounding of an audio feedback tone.

"All of this is very important to us," Dr. Kamiya says, "because it shows that man is capable of achieving and controlling various states of consciousness that he is normally only vaguely aware of, if at all; states ordinarily so elusive that he is unable to graph them." Then, too, there are the therapeutic possibilities. When they try to explain how they learn to sustain alpha, subjects typically observe that they begin to associate with the sounding of the tone a feeling of serenity, detachment, drifting, but at the same time a feeling of alertness so that the state is unlike drowsiness. Some find it highly pleasurable and even begin to talk of getting an "alpha high." ("It used to be that I had to pay subjects to come in for experiments," Dr. Kamiya says. "Now I've got more volunteers than I know what to do with.") Most important, an almost complete lack of anxiety seems to accompany the alpha state, suggesting that it might become a useful tranquilizer, liberating thousands from chemical sedatives, hypnotics and soporifics, and from the damaging and sometimes addicting side effects that accompany them.

But as for alpha becoming a substitute for euphoriant drugs or deep meditation, Dr. Kamiya has his doubts. He concedes that some heavy alpha "users" express feelings of "being very, very much with it" during high alpha periods but says that most do not get so intense a reward.

Dr. Kamiya's work with practiced Zen meditators indicates that alpha is probably an important part of their art, but not the whole picture. "I do think here again, however, that it will be possible to find the unique neurophysiological signature of meditation by checking out other channels—besides alpha. Once we have the complete physiological pattern that characterizes meditation, there's no reason why we can't train people, with feedback, to mimic it in a relatively short period of time."

One of the leading BFT researchers looking into channels beyond alpha is Dr. Barbara Brown, Chief of Experiential Physiology at the Veterans Administration Hospital in Sepulveda, Calif. A psychopharmacologist and psychophysiologist with the development of five important drugs to her credit, Dr. Brown is one of the strong proponents of BFT. Her laboratory houses what is probably the most sophisticated feedback complex in the country. Apart from alpha, Dr. Brown is working with beta and theta waves and with a number of other physiologic functions.

Her subjects watch the "music" of their minds and bodies flicker across various screens in a dazzling matrix of colors, each coded to a different function. There's feedback for alpha and gastric acidity (the latter picked up by tiny, painless monitors in the stomach), body temperature and beta, eye movements and theta, muscle activity, heart rate and pulse pressure. One literally confronts one's inner self—and learns how to manipulate it. Just as subjects quickly learn to control alpha, so do they become adept at exercising their wills over all of these other functions. It's not difficult to understand why Dr.

Brown's cerebral light shows, starring the subjects themselves, have been attracting volunteers in record numbers. She now has a backlog of more than 500 would-be subjects.

The research in theta and beta waves is already yielding some enticing information. Theta, which Dr. Brown defines as "that rhythmic EEG activity of from four to seven cycles per second," seems to be related, she says, to problem solving, sorting and filing of incoming data and retrieval of information already deposited in the brain's memory bank. Dr. Brown is heartened enough by her findings to declare that "Theta training may very well facilitate awareness, enhance memory and, in general, lead to a sensational increase in the efficiency with which the mind works."

As for beta, which falls into a fast-paced 14 to 28 cycles per second, Dr. Brown has found that heavy smokers generate an unusually large amount of it. And unlike the nonsmoker or light smoker, these individuals exhibit very little alpha. Dr. Brown finds "absolutely irresistible" an experiment in which she will attempt to train some of these highstrung betas to become cool, serene alphas. Will they then stop smoking and settle down to enjoying things at a pace more conducive to longer life? According to Dr. Brown, "It seems entirely possible. Even likely."

In addition to her laboratory work, Dr. Brown is now occupied with the chairmanship of the Bio-Feedback Research Society, which she helped found a little over a year ago. At its first national conference, conducted in California last October, 142 scientists were in attendance. From reports presented at that symposium, Dr. Brown has compiled a list of some of the most significant areas in which BFT may have profound impact. Several of them have already been suggested here. Among others are the following:

Athletics. "Perfection in athletic accomplishments is acquired largely through mental concentration to produce an optimally integrated physical sequence of events," Dr. Brown notes. "The individual can just as easily practice the mental state away from the practice area, using the feedback signals from his brain waves and muscle states to signal moments of optimal preparation.

Appetite Control. "When the compulsion to eat exists," she says, "the physiology and brain waves reflect this 'drive' state. The individual can train himself to recognize such a state by means of signals of his physiologic activity—which are displayed to him. He can then train himself to distinguish between the states and continue to produce a non-compulsive state."

Preventive medicine and psychosomatic ills—"The physiologic activity of each troublesome system can be used to feed back information about its own functioning. These can be heart rate, blood pressure, respiration, skin temperature, gastric acidity, intestinal motility, muscles, etc."

Heart-rate Control. "Here it appears that feedback techniques can be of use in at least two major areas: (1) a wide variety of cardiac irregularities, particularly tacchycardia, bradycardia, extra systoles and auricular flutter; and (2) psychologic anxiety and fear reactions.: Dr. Peter Lang, research professor of psychology at the University of Wisconsin, is one of the researchers who have achieved some success in this area. His subjects learn "to drive their own hearts" with video feedback screens on which are projected lines corresponding to heart rate. The shorter the line, the slower the heart rate, and subjects quickly learn to shorten the lines.

Blood-pressure Control. "This sort of control," says Dr. Brown, "may prove to be a lifesaving procedure, providing the patient with the ability to maintain his blood pressure low enough to prevent development of both the symptoms of high blood pressure (headaches, dizziness) as well as preventing the more serious results of high blood pressure, such as coronary attacks, strokes and kidney damage." Among those most active in this field, building on the animal experiments of Dr. Neal E. Miller of Rockefeller University, are Drs. David Shapiro and Bernard Tursky of Harvard Medical School.

Skin-temperature Control. "A fairly easy physiologic activity that individuals can learn to bring under voluntary control is the temperature of the hand or even a single finger," Dr. Brown observes. "Many processes involve constriction of the blood vessels. With feedback training, this vasoconstriction can be markedly reduced, with the consequent relief from pain and coldness." Scientists getting good results here include Elmer and Alyce Green of the Menninger Foundation in Kansas. Using temperature feedback, several of their subjects have been relieved of chronic headaches of the migraine variety. The Greens also suggest that "starvation and absorption of tumors through blood-flow control" appears possible.

Muscle Control. "Individuals suffering from muscle tension due to anxiety or who suffer muscle fatigue or general fatigue benefit from training to induce muscle relaxation," Dr. Brown explains, noting that Dr. John V. Basmajian of Emory University has trained several of his subjects to "fire" specific, individual muscle cells at will. Firing of the electrical energy within the cell is amplified to provide audio feedback, and some subjects become so skillful that they can actually fire off cells in rhythmic sequences so that it sounds as if they are playing the drums. Among possible applications are control of muscle spasms without drugs, induced relaxation and the manipulation of cellular activity to control prosthetic devices without many of the encumbering mechanisms that are required today.

Education. Here Dr. Brown notes that many have proposed teaming BFT with the upcoming crop of computer-assisted machines. "It is well known," she says, "that the attention span of children is short. An accurate indicator of the length of each span of attention would be extremely useful in maximizing the use of teaching machines. Ideally, the display screen of the teaching machine would be capable of changing color: green, let us say, for periods when the child's attention level is high, constituting a go-ahead signal; and red for periods when attention begins to wander—a stop signal."

All of these things, researchers say, are within our grasp now; some have already been attained. For the future, Dr. Brown foresees the collapse of mental hospitals when "brain-wave analysis reveals an incipient neurosis or psychosis, an individualized program for feedback can be supplied. The potential patient can then visit his neighborhood computer self-treatment center where he inserts the taped treatment program into the computerized feedback system and continues treatment until all signs of the potentially abnormal condition have disappeared." Others have suggested that feedback systems will be devised that will enable women to control their ovulation, providing the ultimate birth control technique. Some even envision—for the more remote future—conscious control over cell death, so that aging can be slowed or even halted.

The Greens of Kansas have suggested that creativity might be enhanced by training in the alpha-theta border region.

"It is interesting to note," they observe, in a scientific paper coauthored with E. Dale Walters, "that the psychological state associated with hypnagogic-like imagery has been reported by many outstanding thinkers as the condition in which their most valuable ideas come to them. To describe this state, they have used such phrases as 'the fringe of consciousness,' the 'off-consciousness,' the 'transliminal mind,' and 'reverie.' It is not difficult to imagine a research program in creativity in which brain-wave feedback is used for voluntary induction of that psychophysiological state, in the alpha-theta border region, which is associated with such descriptive statements." Though theta is normally linked with sleep or deep trance, the Greens have already trained individuals to exert such control over their internal states that some can communicate verbally in the theta condition.

To hurry the day when the common man can reap some of the benefits of BFT, researchers are actively working to create inexpensive portable bio-feedback trainers. Dr. Kamiya says that a number of large companies are developing such machines and predicts that they will be available within the next year at a cost of less than $200 each.

Dr. Brown is developing one of the most exotic pieces of feedback hardware—a device that translates brain and body signals into acceptable musical harmonies. With additional design, she says, the instrument will also be able to translate signals into visual art forms. She envisions mass production of the portable device at reasonable cost. With your own light-and-sound show, she says, you can learn to recognize "your own kind of music" and then detect, in plenty of time to do something about it, when you are "getting out of tune with yourself."

Dr. Kamiya has proposed a similar device, but one that would utilize ordinary television sets for feedback display. And the Greens have already played what they call "the music of the hemispheres" or "biological music"—brain-wave signals filtered through some of their non-portable auditory feedback systems. Dr. Miller in New York envisions feedback systems the size of hearing aids. Such devices may be only five years away, warning patients when their heart rates or blood pressures are beginning to rise, helping others ward off muscle spasms, epileptic seizures and so on.

What sort of controls will be imposed over the manufacture, sale and distribution of these devices remains to be seen. There is a fear among some that everything is moving too fast in this field, that the cultists and the faddists may move in, as they did with LSD, giving the research effort a bad name, inviting uninformed Government control. Indeed, one participant at the national meeting of the Bio-Feedback Research Society, Dr. Jean Houston of the Foundation for Mind Research, observed that before long, everyone will be saying, "Oh, boy, you can program yourself against anxiety, to euphoria, to love, to whatever it is that you ought to. This is what, in cultures, has traditionally been performed by sacramental functions. And there is this emergent sacramentalism with regard to the feedback processes that I am sensing here . . . You are getting into cultic relationships . . . There are emergent shamans in your group."

While some counsel extreme caution, call for Food and Drug Administration control and so on, others point out that it is futile to worry at length about the faddists. One participant at the Bio-Feedback meeting asserted that you can no more stop people from tinkering with feedback than you can stop them from smoking pot or drinking alcohol. Dr. Kamiya notes that feedback systems are relatively easy to construct, and imaginative amateurs are found to come up with models of their own before very long. The best thing that the Society can do, several agreed, is to prepare detailed guidelines for the proper use of feedback devices, pointing out some of the possible dangers inherent in manipulating such things as heart rate and blood pressure.

"This is too important to let isolated cases of abuse stand in the way of research progress," Dr. Brown declares. "We mustn's let hysteria stand in the way, as it did with LSD, which could have become one of the most important research tools ever to come along." Dr. Brown is frankly opposed to FDA interference in biofeedback research. "I don't really think we should have to proceed as we do with a new drug—to determine safety, efficiency—because the effects of feedback are predictable. We've got a tremendous amount of historical data in the Zen and Yoga material. Furthermore, society needs this now. We've got this monstrous limbo area in which people are half sick, the area of psychosomatic distress where they can't get any help, except at great expense and often through long years of therapy. And it is in this very area that feedback can do so much, where tension and anxiety can be alleviated with such ease."

She agrees wholeheartedly with the Greens who, in the paper authored with Dale Walters, conclude that "the most significant thing that may be facilitated through training in the voluntary control of internal states is the establishment of a Tranquility Base, not in outer space but in inner space, on, or within, the lunar being of man."

Excerpts from

Report of the National Advisory Commission on Civil Disorders

3

EDITOR'S NOTE: *The President's "Riot Commission Report" clearly shows to any open-minded truth-seeking reader that the basic cause of persistent mental and physical anguish to black Americans throughout history and yet today, and of the riots which such anguish precipitated is White Racism. This racism, practiced subtly or overtly by most, or possibly all, white Americans and our institutions has pervasive and detrimental effects on the mental and physical health of black Americans—and, yes, on the health of those who practice it! The following selections from this important governmental report intend to point out a few of these health effects.*

Chapter 7, Unemployment, Family Structure and Social Disorganization

The Social Impact of Employment Problems in Disadvantaged Negro Areas

Unemployment and the Family

The high rates of unemployment and underemployment in racial ghettos are evidence, in part, that many men living in these areas are seeking, but cannot obtain, jobs which will support a family. Perhaps equally important, most jobs they can get are at the low end of the occupational scale, and often lack the necessary status to sustain a worker's self-respect, or the respect of his family and friends. These same men are also constantly confronted with the message of discrimination: "You are inferior because of a trait you did not cause and cannot change." This message reinforces feelings of inadequacy arising from repeated failure to obtain and keep decent jobs.

Wives of these men are forced to work and usually produce more money. If the men stay at home without working, their inadequacies constantly confront them and tensions arise between them and their wives and children. Under these pressures, it isn't surprising that many of these men flee their responsibilities as husbands and fathers, leaving home, and drifting from city to city, or adopting the style of "street corner men."

Statistical evidence tends to document this. A close correlation exists between the number of nonwhite married women separated from their husbands each year and the unemployment rate among nonwhite males 20 years old and over. Similarly, from 1948 to 1962, the number of new Aid to Families with Dependent Children cases rose and fell with the nonwhite male unemployment rate. Since 1963, however, the number of new cases—most of them Negro children—has steadily increased even though the unemployment rate among nonwhite males has declined. The impact of marital status on employment among Negroes is shown by the fact that in 1967 the proportion of married men either divorced or separated from their wives was more than twice as high among unemployed nonwhite men as among employed nonwhite men. Moreover, among those participating in the labor force, there was a higher proportion of married men with wives present than with wives absent.

Fatherless Families

The abandonment of the home by many Negro males affects a great many children growing up in the racial ghetto. As previously indicated, most American Negro families are headed by men, just like most other American families. Yet the proportion of families with female heads is much greater among Negroes than among whites at all income levels, and has been rising in recent years.

This disparity between white and nonwhite families is far greater among the lowest income families—those most likely to reside in disadvantaged big-city neighborhoods—than among higher income families. Among families with incomes under $3,000 in 1966, the proportion with female heads was 42 per cent for Negroes but only 23 per cent for whites. In contrast, among families with incomes of $7,000 or more, 8 per cent of Negro families had female heads compared to 4 per cent of whites.

Proportion of Families of Various Types
(In percent)

	Husband-Wife		Female Head	
Date	White	Nonwhite	White	Nonwhite
1950	88.0%	77.7%	8.5%	17.6%
1960	88.7	73.6	8.7	22.4
1966	88.8	72.7	8.9	23.7

The problems of "fatherlessness" are aggravated by the tendency of the poor to have large families. The average poor, urban, nonwhite family contains 4.8 persons, as compared with 3.7 for the average poor, urban, white family. This is one of the primary factors in the poverty status of nonwhite households in large cities.

The proportion of fatherless families appears to be increasing in the poorest Negro neighborhoods. In the Hough section of Cleveland, the proportion of families with female heads rose from 23 to 32 per cent from 1960 to 1965. In the Watts section of Los Angeles it rose from 36 to 39 per cent during the same period.

The handicap imposed on children growing up without fathers, in an atmosphere of poverty and deprivation, is increased because many mothers must work to provide support. The following table illustrates the disparity between the proportion of nonwhite women in the child-rearing ages who are in the labor force and the comparable proportion of white women:

Percentage of Women in the Labor Force

Age Group	Nonwhite	White
20–24	55%	51%
25–34	55	38
35–44	61	45

With the father absent and the mother working, many ghetto children spend the bulk of their time on the streets—the streets of a crime-ridden, violence-prone, and poverty-stricken world. The image of success in this world is not that of the "solid citizen," the responsible husband and father, but rather that of the "hustler" who promotes his own interests by exploiting others. The dope sellers and the numbers runners are the "successful" men because their earnings far outstrip those men who try to climb the economic ladder in honest ways.

Young people in the ghetto are acutely conscious of a system which appears to offer rewards to those who illegally exploit others, and failure to those who struggle under traditional responsibilities. Under these circumstances, many adopt exploitation and the "hustle" as a way of life, disclaiming both work and marriage in favor of casual and temporary liaisons. This pattern reinforces itself from one generation to the next, creating a "culture of poverty" and an ingrained cynicism about society and its institutions.

The "Jungle"

The culture of poverty that results from unemployment and family disorganization generates a system of ruthless, exploitative relationships within the ghetto. Prostitution, dope addiction, casual sexual affairs, and crime create an environmental jungle characterized by personal insecurity and tension. The effects of this development are stark:

- The rate of illegitimate births among nonwhite women has risen sharply in the past two decades. In 1940, 16.8 per cent of all nonwhite births were illegitimate. By 1950 this proportion was 18 per cent; by 1960, 21.6 per cent, by 1966, 26.3 per cent. In the ghettos of many large cities, illegitimacy rates exceed 50 per cent.
- The rate of illegitimacy among nonwhite women is closely related to low income, and high unemployment. In Washington, D.C., for example, an analysis of 1960

census tracts shows that in tracts with unemployment rates of 12 per cent or more among nonwhite men, illegitimacy was over 40 per cent. But in tracts with unemployment rates of 2.9 per cent and below among nonwhite men, reported illegitimacy was under 20 per cent. A similar contrast existed between tracts in which median nonwhite income was under $4,000 (where illegitimacy was 38 per cent) and those in which it was $8,000 and over (where illegitimacy was 12 per cent).

• Narcotics addiction is also heavily concentrated in low-income Negro neighborhoods, particularly in New York City. Of the 59,720 addicts known to the U. S. Bureau of Narcotics at the end of 1966, just over 50 per cent were Negroes. Over 52 per cent of all known addicts lived within New York State, mostly in Harlem and other Negro neighborhoods. These figures undoubtedly greatly understate the actual number of persons using narcotics regularly—especially those under 21.

• Not surprisingly, at every age from 6 through 19, the proportion of children from homes with both parents present who actually attend school is higher than the proportion of children from homes with only one parent or neither present.

• Rates of juvenile delinquency, venereal disease, dependency upon AFDC support, and use of public assistance in general are much higher in disadvantaged Negro areas than in other parts of large cities. Data taken from New York City contrasting predominantly Negro neighborhoods with the city as a whole clearly illustrates this fact.

Social Distress—Major Predominately Negro Neighborhoods in New York City and the City as a Whole

	Juvenile delinquency[1]	Venereal disease[2]	ADC[3]	Public assistance[4]
Brownsville	125.3	609.0	459.0	265.8
East New York	98.6	207.5	148.6	71.8
Bedford-Stuyvesant	115.2	771.3	337.1	197.2
Harlem	110.8	1,603.5	265.7	138.1
South Bronx	84.4	308.3	278.5	165.5
New York City	52.2	269.1	120.7	60.8

[1] Number of offenses per 1,000 persons 7-20 years (1965)
[2] Number of cases per 100,000 persons under 21 years (1964)
[3] Number of children in aid to dependent children cases per 1,000 under 18 years, using 1960 population as base (1965)
[4] Welfare assistance recipients per 1,000 persons, using 1960 population as base (1965)

In conclusion: in 1965, 1.2 million nonwhite children under 16 lived in central city families headed by a woman under 65. The great majority of these children were growing up in poverty conditions that make them better candidates for crime and civil disorder than for jobs providing an entry into American society.

Chapter 8, Conditions of Life in the Racial Ghetto

Health and Sanitation Conditions

The residents of the racial ghetto are significantly less healthy than most other Americans. They suffer from higher mortality rates, higher incidence of major diseases, and lower availability and utilization of medical services. They also experience higher admission rates to mental hospitals.

These conditions result from a number of factors.

Poverty

From the standpoint of health, poverty means deficient diets, lack of medical care, inadequate shelter and clothing and often lack of awareness of potential health needs. As a result, almost 30 per cent of all persons with family incomes less than $2,000 per year suffer from chronic health conditions that adversely affect their employment—as compared with less than 8 percent of the families with incomes of $7,000 or more.

Poor families have the greatest need for financial assistance in meeting medical expenses. Only about 34 per cent of families with incomes of less than $2,000 per year use health insurance benefits, as compared to nearly 90 per cent of those with incomes of $7,000 or more.

These factors are aggravated for Negroes when compared to whites for the simple reason that the proportion of persons in the United States who are poor is 3.5 times as high among Negroes (41 per cent in 1966) as among whites (12 per cent in 1966).

Maternal Mortality. Mortality rates for nonwhite mothers are four times as high as those for white mothers. There has been sharp decline in such rates since 1940, when 774 nonwhite and 320 white mothers died for each 100,000 live births. In 1965, only 84 nonwhite mothers and 21 white mothers died per 100,000 live births —but the gap between nonwhites and whites actually increased.

Infant Mortality

Mortality rates among nonwhite babies are 58 per cent higher than among whites for those under one month old and almost three times as high among those from one month to one year old. This is true in spite of a large drop in infant mortality rates in both groups since 1940.

Number of Infants Who Died Per 1,000 Live Births

	Less Than One Month Old		One Month to One Year Old	
Year	White	Nonwhite	White	Nonwhite
1940	27.2	39.7	16.0	34.1
1950	19.4	27.5	7.4	17.0
1960	17.2	26.9	5.7	16.4
1965	16.1	25.4	5.4	14.9

Life Expectancy

To some extent because of infant mortality rates, life expectancy at birth was 6.9 years longer for whites (71.0 years) than for nonwhites (64.1 years) in 1965. Even in the prime working ages, life expectancy is significantly lower among nonwhites than among whites. In 1965, white persons 25 years old could expect to live an average of 48.6 more years, whereas nonwhites 25 years old could expect to live another 43.3 years, or 11 per cent less. Similar but smaller discrepancies existed at all ages from 25 through 55; some actually increased slightly between 1960 and 1965.

Lower Utilization of Health Services

A fact that also contributes to poorer health conditions in the ghetto is that Negro families with incomes similar to those of whites spend less on medical services and visit medical specialists less often.

Percent of Family Expenditures Spent for Medical Care, 1960-61

Income group	White	Nonwhite	Ratio, white, nonwhite
Under $3,000	9	5	1.8:1
$3,000 to $7,499	7	5	1.4:1
$7,500 and over	6	4	1.5:1

Since the lowest income group contains a much larger proportion of nonwhite families, the overall discrepancy in medical care spending between these two groups is very significant, as shown by the following table:

Health Expenses Per Person Per Year for the Period from July to December 1962

Income by racial group	Total Medical	Hospital	Doctor	Dental	Medicine	Other
Under $2,000 per family per year:						
White	$130	$33	$41	$11	$32	$13
Nonwhite	63	15	23	5	16	5
$10,000 and more per family per year:						
White	179	34	61	37	31	16
Nonwhite	133	34	50	19	23	8

These data indicate that nonwhite families in the lower income group spent less than half as much per person on medical services as white families with similar incomes. This discrepancy sharply declines but is still significant in the higher income group, where total nonwhite medical expenditures per person equal, on the average, 74.3 per cent of white expenditures.

Negroes spend less on medical care for several reasons. Negro households generally are larger, requiring greater nonmedical expenses for each household and leaving less money for meeting medical expenses. Thus, lower expenditures per person would result even if expenditures per household were the same. Negroes also often pay more for other basic necessities such as food and consumer durables, as discussed in the next part of this chapter. In addition, fewer doctors, dentists, and medical facilities are conveniently available to Negroes than to most whites—a result both of geographic concentration of doctors in higher income areas in large cities and of discrimination against Negroes by doctors and hospitals. A survey in Cleveland indicated that there were 0.45 physicians per 1,000 people in poor neighborhoods, compared to 1.13 per 1,000 in nonpoverty areas. The result nationally is fewer visits to physicians and dentists.

Percent of Population Making One or More Visits to Indicated Type of Medical Specialist from July 1963 to June 1964

Type of Medical Specialist	Family Incomes of $2,000 to $3,999		Family Incomes of $7,000 to $9,999	
	White	Nonwhite	White	Nonwhite
Physician	64	56	70	64
Dentist	31	20	52	33

Although widespread use of health insurance has led many hospitals to adopt nondiscriminatory policies, some private hospitals still refuse to admit Negro patients or to accept doctors with Negro patients. And many individual doctors still discriminate against Negro patients. As a result, Negroes are more likely to be treated in hospital clinics than whites and they are less likely to receive personalized service. This conclusion is confirmed by the following data:

Percent of All Visits to Physicians from July 1963 to June 1964, Made in Indicated Ways

Type of Visit to Physician	Family Incomes of $2,000 to $3,000		Family Incomes of $7,000 to $9,999	
	White	Nonwhite	White	Nonwhite
In physician's office	68	56	73	66
Hospital clinic	17	35	7	16
Other (mainly telephone)	15	9	20	18
TOTAL	100	100	100	100

Environmental Factors

Environmental conditions in disadvantaged Negro neighborhoods create further reasons for poor health conditions there. The level of sanitation is strikingly below that which is prevalent in most higher income areas. One simple reason is that residents often lack proper storage facilities for food—adequate refrigerators, freezers, even garbage cans, which are sometimes stolen as fast as landlords can replace them.

In areas where garbage collection and other sanitation services are grossly inadequate—commonly in the poorer parts of our cities—rats proliferate. It is estimated that in 1965, there were over 14,000 cases of ratbite in the United States, mostly in such neighborhoods.

4 No Mañanas for Today's Chicanos

by John Rechy

The Colonia Pancho Villa hangs over the barren hills of Juarez, Mexico, like a worn shroud. Close up, it's a fetid hell of adobe shacks crushed against gaps in the hills. In summer, disease is a presence. Children slide on "haystacks" of garbage. There is no running water. In winter, people freeze to death. Rain erodes their hovels.

In El Paso's south side two-story tenements quiver like giants on tangled stalks. One dark, dank, unlighted outside toilet serves up to six families. Velvety grime from petroleum (some units have no gas) clings stubbornly to walls. Each winter people die from noxious fumes. Water for up to eighteen units is provided by one small sink near the toilets. As many as ten people live in each two-room unit. There are skeleton beds in the unventilated kitchens. Before one unit a small trailer squats like a tombstone; it will carry a family to the fields of California.

Every morning, beginning before dawn, the men and women from the colonias in Juarez will cross the bridge over the waterless Rio Grande into Texas—legally or illegally. They will then join their cousins from El Paso's south side. In front of employment bureaus or

SOURCE. Copyright 1970 by John Rechy. Reprinted by permission of Harold Matson Co., Inc. Published in the March 14, 1970 issue of Saturday Review.

on the streets, they will wait for trucks or cars hunting cheap labor. Some will become strike-breaking scabs. ("I understand," says an El Paso tenement resident. "I would too if my family was starving.") Jobs are scarce; they go to the persons willing to work for least. Such jobs may take them to the lower Rio Grande valley of Texas, where they will subsist—if they do—in wooden shacks, without water, electricity, or sewage system.

These people are descended from the Aztecs, Toltecs, and Mayans. They are the Mexicans—Chicanos—who are heirs to "one of the most ancient cultures, magnificent literatures, and historic universities in the Americas ... (to) learned men whose civilizations compared with the greatest in the world," writes Stan Steiner in *La Raza.*

No people in the New World have an older written history. Before the founding of the University of Mexico in 1553 (nearly a century before the founding of Harvard), school systems among these Indian nations were teaching medicine, art, philosophy, engineering, architecture, and even astrology and the meaning of dreams. Some Olmec writings have been dated as far back as 600 B.C. This heritage was brought to the North American Southwest by the Spanish conquistadors and the Mexican Indians. Thus was born the culture of la raza, a fusion of Spanish and Indian. A rich literature—poetry, history, plays, essays—developed from it.

Steiner's *La Raza* (the phrase is translated as "the race," but is used by Mexicans to indicate pride in their heritage) is a book of panoramic scope and realized intention, an impressionistic history of the Mexican people from their original magnificence through their defeats and on to their burgeoning self-awareness and militancy. It is an intricate, fascinating tapestry, rich, colorful, beautiful. The book is also a relevant and timely chronicle, important because today the noble culture of la raza is all but forgotten in the Southwest, virtually erased from existence.

Luis Valdex, director of El Teatro Campesino, the theater of the field workers of California, says, "There is no textbook of the history of la raza. Yet the history of the Mexican in this country is 400 years old ... Our history has been lost." In the Southwest school books hardly refer to the significant contributions of la raza. Thus the Chicano can rightly claim, in Steiner's words, that he has been "humiliated by the textbooks, tongue-tied by the teachers, de-educated by the schools."

Children in Texas schools have been forced to kneel and ask forgiveness for speaking Spanish. In some, "Spanish monitors" act as spies. Schools, asserts a San Antonio student, "try to brainwash the Chicanos ... try to make us forget our history to be ashamed to being Mexicans ... They succeed in making us feel empty, and angry inside."

In kaleidoscopic chapters that shift from past to present, Steiner traces the outrages against the Mexicans, including the seizing of their territories by land-grabbers—and by the United States in the Mexican-American War, which General Ulysses S. Grant, then a lieutenant in the invading army, called the "most unjust (war) ever waged by a stronger against a weaker nation ... a conspiracy to acquire territory out of which slave states might be formed." The war resulted in the defeat of the Mexicans, who were already weakened by their successful struggle for independence from Spain. The United States Army "committed atrocities to make heaven weep and every American of Christian morals blush for his country ... Murder, robbery and rape of mothers and daughters in the presence of tied-up males of the families" were common, wrote General Winfield Scott, the commander of the United States Army.

That was only a blood-soaked prelude to U.S. savagery against the Mexicans. Steiner chronicles the mass deportations of Mexicans during the frightened 1950s. Contemptuously dubbed "Operation Wetback," a wave of official terror was unleashed by the Border Patrol against Mexican workers entering the U.S. illegally. Yet farmers knowingly employed these destitute, vulnerable "illegals" until the harvest was completed. Then they reported them for deportation—before their wages were paid.

Today hundreds of people are still virtually enslaved on ranches throughout the Southwest. (One Chicano labored for thirty-three years in the fields without pay.) In many other ways Mexicans suffer inhumanity. Once a locked, windowless truck containing more than three dozen workers on their way to the fields was abandoned on a Texas highway. Amid cries and the pounding of bloody fists on steel walls, several of them suffocated to death.

In the area of the Rio Grande valley, which Steiner calls "The Region of the Damned," migrants live under conditions "close to peonage." Ruled despotically by the Texas Ranger mentality, this valley has a history of savagery. The murders of Mexicans may exceed the lynchings of blacks in the South. From a porch—his court—the clownish Judge Roy Bean claimed that there was "no law in his books against killing a Mexican." According to Jovita Gonzales, a respected Texas writer, the Rangers "executed" several hundred Mexicans in the early Twenties without arraignment or trial. There is a brutal saying that "every Texas Ranger has some Mexican blood . . . on his boots."

It is not surprising that a strike by melon pickers against La Casita Farms in that area would be met with violence from the Rangers. Breaking into the home of a "trouble-maker," guns ready, they kicked Magdaleno Dimas, a laborer, and smashed his head with the barrel of a shotgun. A suit brought against the Rangers by the farm workers' union was mysteriously "lost" in the courts.

Poverty—like racism—has haunted the Chicano in America. Pregnant women are so undernourished that in a San Antonio area hospital they are routinely given blood transfusions. In New Mexico's Taos County, malnutrition is comparable with that of war-ravaged peoples. More than half of the New Mexico village families live on incomes below the poverty level of $3,000. Signs in front of their homes often proclaim: "We Are Hungry." A Senate subcommittee on migratory labor heard a woman field worker testify to the constant presence of death, hunger, illness, brutal treatment, and fear of retaliation from employers if they protest.

Yet the myth of the lazy Mexican living happily on welfare persists. A Chicano spokesman points out, "The ranchers and businessmen in the Anglo communities get ten times as much as we do through farm subsidies, oil depletions, crop parities, soil-bank programs." In a single year one district in Texas received $5-million in agricultural payments for 400 farmers; the same district got a measly $224,000 worth of food for 146,000 poor people. "We don't want welfare," says a proud New Mexico farmer. "We want enough of our land to graze a milk cow."

The claim for restoration to Chicanos of their ancestral land constitutes a dramatic struggle in the courts of New Mexico. The claim is based on the Treaty of Guadalupe Hidalgo of 1848, which expressly—and "In the Name of Almighty God"—guarantees, "inviolately," retention of property by owners and their heirs within the annexed territory of New Mexico. Although this treaty is often mentioned in history books, the guarantee of property retention is virtually never quoted nor mentioned.

Destroying archives of land-grant records and using other methods of robbery, speculators, who included two lawyers and perhaps the territorial governor, seized this land. To call attention to the plight of the impoverished New Mexico farmers and to bring the matter of land claims into the courts, Reies Tijerina and a man from the Federal Alliance of Free States made a citizen's arrest of two forest rangers for trespassing in Carson National Forest. In another symbolic act they attempted a raid of the Tierra Amarilla courthouse to arrest the district attorney, whom they accused of persecuting them. Armed troops, tanks, and aircraft were enlisted in the pursuit of Tijerina and his men. Houses were invaded without warrants, and several of Tijerina's supporters were imprisoned and kept under repressive conditions within a corral, also without warrant. Subsequent vindictive charges against Tijerina, now in jail, are inching through the maze of courts.

But others, more militant, are ready to take his place in the barrios of California and the Southwest. Already there are the Brown Berets, born in the streets and dedicated to act in self-defense to protect the rights of Chicanos "by all means necessary." Their motto is "To Serve, Observe, Protect." Their insignia is a holy cross and two crossed rifles. The color of their caps proclaims pride in the color of their skin. Newspapers have described them as a "highly disciplined paramilitary organization." "You think of guns," says a young Chicano leader. "That's not what we mean by self-defense. It's not the vigilante thing, or the Minute-men. Self-defense means protection of your people from the injustices we feel the police subject us to." "Who organized (the Brown Berets)?" asks another. "The police organized them."

In Denver a small seventeen-year-old Chicano boy is shot in the back by a policeman who, arguing self-defense, is acquitted. Another cop, also cleared, claims he tripped and his gun went off, killing a Mexican youth. Other killings take place with frightening regularity under similar circumstances. Writing in a barrio newspaper, a young man claims, "More Chicanos are killed by the cops on the streets of the Southwest than any other minority group in the population." Arbitrary frisking, cruel harassment, racial taunts, savage arrests are daily occurrences in the Chicano barrios from San Antonio to El Paso to Los Angeles.

Precipitated in part by such conditions, a "blowout" occurred in 1968 in East Los Angeles. Calling for reform of abysmal school conditions and demanding the transfer of prejudiced teachers and the revision of the schools' curricula to acknowledge Mexican contributions to the country, 15,000 Chicano students shut down classes throughout their barrio. There followed an invasion by the cops and a blockade of the neighborhood. Thirteen leaders, including a teacher, were jailed and charged with "conspiracy" to disturb the educational process. They were hurriedly tried, convicted, fined, and placed on probation.

"Blowouts, Baby, Blowouts!" proclaimed a young writer in a school newspaper, ominously echoing the blacks' "Burn, baby, burn!" That cry reflects the restiveness and demand for change. "It's time for a new Mexican Revolution," a speaker tells students at UCLA. "We've got to stand up and talk straight to the gabachos (Anglos), saying, 'Hell, no! I won't go!' to your whole lousy system."

To some, that system includes the powerful Catholic Church. "The Church has conspired with those in power," a San Antonio Chicano charges, scoring Archbishop Lucey in particular. "Why? To keep the poor people ignorant. Why? Because in every barrio the Church owns slum property, tenements, rat-holes."

Another "blowout" occurred in a Denver high school where students insisted that a teacher who had made a racial slur be transferred. They were barred from the principal's office by 250 cops. In the ensuing riot men, women, and children were beaten, Maced, and tear-gassed by police. Thirty-six Chicanos were arrested. "Some say it was a riot," reported an eyewitness. "It wasn't. It was more like guerrilla warfare."

Dodollo "Corky" Gonzales, once a prizefighter, now a poet and a presence on the political scene, told the students: "... you have made history. We just talk about revolution, but you act it by facing the shotguns, billies, gas, and Mace. You are the real revolutionaries."

And so they are. In the streets of the barrios of Denver, El Paso, San Antonio, Los Angeles, something beautiful has happened to them. They do not share the crippling ambiguous identity that their parents suffered. Were they Mexicans? Latin-Americans? Spanish-Americans? Indians? Spanish? "Let's end the hangup about identity," says a Chicano in Arizona. "We know who we are."

The revolution is also being waged on another front—the grape fields of California. Peter Matthiessen's *Sal Si Puedes* ("Escape if You Can") documents its own list of horrors surrounding the migrant workers: abysmal living conditions, exposure to dangerous sprays, a 1967 average income of less than $1,500, housing codes specifically excluding laborers' camps (officials of the Farm Bureau Federation in Bakersfield, California, admitted to the Housing Authority that they deliberately created miserable living conditions for the migrants so they would leave immediately after the harvest was completed), violations of child-labor regulations (a skinny boy of ten is described struggling to lift a heavy box of grapes), exclusion from Social Security and Workmen's Compensation, filth and illness, an infant mortality rate 125 per cent higher than the national level.

Protesting such conditions, workers led by Cesar Chavez, himself a field laborer, struck the grape growers of California in 1965. The strike was greeted by violence. Local sheriffs hounded the strikers. Speeding cars dashed against the pickets. One man was permanently crippled; his case crawls through the courts. Nixon, not yet President, declared his intention to eat California grapes at every opportunity.

The strikers had to battle the courts, too. Expediently claiming a labor law unconstitutional, a Los Angeles court granted an injunction that kept the U.S. Immigration Service from enforcing a Justice Department regulation forbidding green-card (legally entered) Mexicans to work in fields where a labor dispute had been certified. Growers quickly hired scabs. As soon as the harvest ended, the courts decided the law was constitutional after all.

"Most good Americans, like 'good Germans,'" Matthiessen says, "have managed to stay unaware of inhumanity in their own country (because) ... misery refutes the American way of life." And he correctly sees the plight of the migrant worker as part of a multifaceted evil, "related to all of America's most serious afflictions: racism, poverty, environmental pollution, and urban crowding and decay—all of these compounded by the waste of war."

Yet the broad scope of Matthiessen's intentions is marred by a staggering insistence on comprehensiveness, and also by his awe of Chavez.

On the first count, his document becomes so tangled in a labyrinth of labor-union details that the drama of the strike itself is sometimes all but lost. Brilliant descriptive flashes, dramatically built confrontations (the excitement of the picket line, with strikers challenging scabs to cross over) indicate what the book might have been.

Matthiessen's admiration for Chavez is boundless. He sees him as the one who, "of all leaders now in sight, best represents the rising generations." That is not so. Mystical, ascetic, dedicated, Chavez is unquestionably a giant figure in the emergency of la raza, much as Martin Luther King is for the blacks. But he is not yet a saint, and Matthiessen seems to attempt his canonization. At the end of his book he remembers Chavez in a San Francisco church. "A man trapped against his will in Heaven ... The hands, the dance cried to the world: Wait! Have Faith! Look, look! Let's go! Good-bye! Hello! I love you!"

The young militant Chicanos are not in the mood for waiting, and their faith in evolutionary social progress is waning—nor do they "love you." Instead they await the fierce warning from a Chicano James Baldwin and search for their own Malcolm X, their own Eldridge Cleaver. They know that a non-violent man like Chavez lives under the constant threat of assassination in a lunatic state.

Despite its honest outrage, Matthiessen's book has too much of the sweet, lovely, idealistic, decent wistfulness of Martin Luther King's "I have a dream." The dream has turned into a nightmare. Steiner knows that, and his book reflects it—and, though unstated, this: that in reconstructing their own violated history, the young Chicanos have also discovered the submerged history of American violence.

"Mañana Is Here!" proclaims a banner appearing recurrently in gatherings of Chicano militants. The ludicrous, false image of the sleepy Mexican waiting for tomorrow is gone. And The Man had better know it, because tomorrow is indeed here.

5 Training the Woman to Know Her Place: The Power of a Nonconscious Ideology

by Sandra L. Bem
and Daryl J. Bem

"In the beginning God created the heaven and the earth ... And God said, let us make man in our image, after our likeness; and let them have dominion over the fish of the sea, and over the fowl of the air, and over the cattle, and over all the earth .... And the rib, which the Lord God had taken from man, made he a woman and brought her unto the man .... And the Lord God said unto the woman, What is this that thou has done? And the woman said, The serpent beguiled me, and I did eat .... Unto the woman He said, I will greatly multiply thy

*Bem, S.L. & Bem, D.J. Case study of a nonconscious ideology: training the woman to know her place. In D.J. Bem, Beliefs, attitudes, and human affairs. Belmont, Calif.: Brooks/Cole, 1970. (Revised: March, 1971)

**Order of authorship determined by the flip of a coin.

sorrow and thy conception; in sorrow thou shalt bring forth children; and thy desire shall be to thy husband, and he shall rule over thee." (Gen. 1, 2, 3)

And lest anyone fail to grasp the moral of this story, Saint Paul provides further clarification:

"For a man .... is the image and glory of God; but the woman is the glory of the man. For the man is not of the woman, but the woman of the man. Neither was the man created for the woman, but the woman for the man." (I Cor. II)

"Let the woman learn in silence with all subjection. But I suffer not a woman to teach, nor to usurp authority over the man, but to be in silence. For Adam was first formed, then Eve. And Adam was not deceived, but the woman, being deceived, was in the transgression. Notwithstanding, she shall be saved in childbearing, if they continue in faith and charity and holiness with sobriety." (I Tim. 2)

And lest it be thought that only Christians have this rich heritage of ideology about women, consider the morning prayer of the Orthodox Jew:

"Blessed art Thou, oh Lord our God, King of the Universe, that I was not born a gentile.

"Blessed art Thou, oh Lord our God, King of the Universe, that I was not born a slave.

"Blessed art Thou, oh Lord our God, King of the Universe, that I was not born a woman."

Or the Koran, the sacred text of Islam:

"Men are superior to women on account of the qualities in which God has given them pre-eminence."

Because they think they sense a decline in feminine "faith, charity, and holiness with sobriety," many people today jump to the conclusion that the ideology expressed in these passages is a relic of the past. Not so. It has simply been obscured by an equalitarian veneer, and the ideology has now become nonconscious. That is, we remain unaware of it because alternative beliefs and attitudes about women go unimagined. We are like the fish who is unaware that his environment is wet. After all, what else could it be? Such is the nature of all nonconscious ideologies. Such is the nature of America's ideology about women. For even those Americans who agree that a black skin should not uniquely qualify its owner for janitorial or domestic service continue to act as if the possession of a uterus uniquely qualifies *its* owner for precisely that.

Consider, for example, the 1968 student rebellion at Columbia University. Students from the radical left took over some administration buildings in the name of equalitarian principles which they accused the university of flouting. Here were the most militant spokesmen one could hope to find in the case of equalitarian ideals. But no sooner had they occupied the buildings than the male militants blandly turned to their sisters-in-arms and assigned them the task of preparing the food, while they—the menfolk—would presumably plan further strategy. The reply these males received was the reply they deserved, and the fact that domestic tasks behind the barricades were desegregated across the sex line that day is an everlasting tribute to the class consciousness of the ladies of the left.

But these conscious coeds are not typical, for the nonconscious assumptions about a woman's "natural" talents (or lack of them) are at least as prevalent among women as they are among men. A psychologist named Philip Goldberg (1968) demonstrated this by asking female college students to rate a number of professional articles from each of six fields. The articles were collated into two equal sets of booklets, and the names of the authors were changed so that the identical article was attributed to a male author (e.g., John T. McKay) in one set of booklets and to a female author (e.g., Joan T. McKay) in the other set. Each student was asked to read the articles in her booklet and to rate them for value, competence, persuasiveness, writing style, and so forth.

As he had anticipated, Goldberg found that the identical article received significantly lower rating when it was attributed to a female author than when it was attributed to a male author. He had predicted this result, for articles from professional fields generally considered the province of men, like law and city planning, but to his surprise, these coeds also downgraded articles from the fields of dietetics and elementary school education when they were attributed to female authors. In other words, these students rated the male authors as better at everything, agreeing with Aristotle that "we should regard the female nature as afflicted with a natural defectiveness." We repeated this experiment informally in our own classrooms and discovered that male students show the same implicit prejudice against female authors that Goldberg's female students showed. Such is the nature of a nonconscious ideology!

It is significant that examples like these can be drawn from the college world, for today's students have challenged the established ways of looking at almost every other issue, and they are quick to reject those practices of our society which conflict explicitly with their major values. But as the above examples suggest, they will find it far more difficult to shed the more subtle aspects of a sex-role ideology which—as we shall now attempt to demonstrate—conflicts just as surely with their existential values as any of the other societal practices to which they have so effectively raised objection. And as we shall see, there is no better way to appreciate the power of a society's nonconscious ideology than to examine it within the framework of values held by that society's avant-garde.

Individuality and Self-Fulfillment

The dominant values of today's students concern personal growth on the one hand, and interpersonal relationships on the other. The first of these emphasizes individuality and self-fulfillment; the second stresses openness, honesty, and equality in all human relationships.

The values of individuality and self-fulfillment imply that each human being, male or female, is to be encouraged to "do his own thing." Men and women are no longer to be stereotyped by society's definitions. If sensitivity, emotionality, and warmth are desirable human characteristics, then they are desirable for men as well as for women. (John Wayne is no longer an idol of the young, but their pop-art satire.) If independence, assertiveness, and serious intellectual commitment are desirable human characteristics, then they are desirable for women as well as for men. The major prescription of this college generation is that each individual should be encouraged to discover and fulfill his own unique potential and identity, unfettered by society's presumptions.

But society's presumptions enter the scene much earlier than most people suspect, for parents begin to raise their children in accord with the popular stereotypes from the very first. Boys are encouraged to be aggressive, competitive, and independent, whereas girls are rewarded for being passive and dependent (Barry, Bacon, & Child, 1957; Sears, Maccoby, & Levin, 1957). In one study, six-month-old infant girls were already being touched and spoken to more by their mothers while they were playing than were infant boys. When they were thirteen months old, these same girls were more reluctant than the boys to leave their mothers; they returned more quickly and more frequently to them; and they remained closer to them throughout the entire play period. When a physical barrier was placed between mother and child, the girls tended to cry and motion for help; the boys made more active attempts to get around the barrier (Goldberg & Lewis, 1969). No one knows to what extent these sex differences at the age of thirteen months can be attributed to the mothers' behavior at the age of six months, but it is hard to believe that the two are unconnected.

As children grow older, more explicit sex-role training is introduced. Boys are encouraged to take more of an interest in mathematics and science. Boys, not girls, are given chemistry sets and microscopes for Christmas. Moreover, all children quickly learn that mommy is proud to be a moron when it comes to mathematics and science, whereas daddy knows all about these things. When a young boy returns from school all excited about biology, he is almost certain to be encouraged to think of becoming a physician. A girl with similar enthusiasm is told that she might want to consider nurse's training later so she can have "an interesting job to fall back upon in case—God forbid—she ever needs to support herself." A very different kind of encouragement. And any girl who doggedly persists in her enthusiasm for science is likely to find her parents horrified by the prospect of a permanent love affair with physics as they would be by the prospect of an interracial marriage.

These socialization practices quickly take their toll. By nursery school age, for example, boys are already asking more questions about how and why things work (Smith, 1933). In first and second grade, when asked to suggest ways of improving various toys, boys do better on the fire truck and girls do better on the nurse's kit, but by the third grade, boys do better regardless of the toy presented (Torrance, 1962). By the ninth grade, 25% of the boys, but only 3% of the girls, are considering careers in science or engineering (Flanagan, unpublished; cited by Kagan, 1964). When they apply for college, boys and girls are about equal on verbal aptitude tests, but boys score significantly higher on mathematical aptitude tests—about 60 points higher on the College Board examinations, for example (Brown, 1965, p. 162). Moreover, girls improve their mathematical performance if problems are reworded so that they deal with cooking and gardening, even though the abstract reasoning required for their solution remains the same (Milton, 1958). Clearly, not just ability, but the motivation and confidence to tackle a mathematical problem have been undermined.

But these effects in mathematics and science are only part of the story. A girl's long training in passivity and dependence appears to exact an even higher toll from her overall motivation to achieve, to search for new and independent ways of doing things, and to welcome the challenge of new and unsolved problems. In one study, for example, elementary school girls were more likely to try solving a puzzle by imitating an adult, whereas the boys were more likely to search for a novel solution not provided by the adult (McDavid, 1959). In another puzzle-solving study, young girls asked for help and approval from adults more frequently than the boys; and, when given the opportunity to return to the puzzles a second time, the girls were more likely to rework those they had already solved, whereas the boys were more likely to try puzzles they had been unable to solve previously (Crandall & Rabson, 1960). A girl's sigh of relief is almost audible when she marries and retires from the outside world of novel and unsolved problems.

This, of course, is the most conspicuous outcome of all: the majority of American women become full-time homemakers. And of those who work, 78% end up in dead-end jobs as clerical workers, service workers, factory workers, and sales clerks. Only 15% of all women workers are classified by the Labor Department as professional or technical workers, and even this figure is misleading. For the poorly paid occupation of non-college teacher absorbs nearly half of these women, and an additional 25% are nurses. Fewer than 5% of all professional women—fewer than 1% of all women workers—fill those positions which, to most Americans, connote "professional": physician, lawyer, engineer, scientist, college professor, journalist, and the like. Such are the consequences of a nonconscious ideology.

But why does this process violate the values of individuality and self-fulfillment. It is *not* because some people may regard the role of homemaker as inferior to other roles. That is not the point. Rather, the point is that our society is managing to consign a large segment of its population to the role of homemaker—either by itself or in conjunction with typing, teaching, nursing, or unskilled labor—just as inexorably as it has in the past consigned the individual with a black skin to the role of janitor or domestic. It is not the equality of the role which is at issue here, but the fact that in spite of their unique identities, the majority of America's women end up in the *same* role.

Even an I.Q. in the genius range does not guarantee that a woman's unique potential will find expression. In a famous study of over 1300 men and women whose I.Q.'s averaged 151 (Terman & Oden, 1959), 86% of the men have achieved prominence in professional and managerial occupations. In contrast, only a minority of the women are even employed. Of those who are, 37% are nurses, librarians, social workers, and non-college teachers. An additional 26% are secretaries, stenographers, bookkeepers, and office workers! Only 11% are in the higher professions of law, medicine, college teaching, engineering, science, economics, and the like. And even at age 44, well after their children have gone to school, 61% of these highly gifted women are full-time homemakers. This homogenization of America's women is the major consequence of our society's sex-role ideology.

Even so, however, several arguments are typically advanced to counter the claim that America's homogenization of its women subverts individuality and self-fulfillment. The three most common arguments invoke, respectively, (1) free will, (2) biology, and (3) complementarity.

1. The free will argument proposes that a 21-year old woman is perfectly free to choose some other role if she cares to do so; no one is standing in her way. But that is hardly the case. Even the woman who has managed to finesse society's attempt to rob her of her career motivations is likely to find herself blocked by society's trump card: the feeling that one cannot have a career and be a successful woman simultaneously. A competent and motivated woman is thus caught in a double-bind which few men have even faced. She must worry not only about failure, but also about success. If she fails in her achieve-

ment needs, she must live with the knowledge that she is not living up to her own—and society's—conception of a feminine woman. Thus, even the woman who is lucky enough to have retained some career motivation is likely to find herself in serious conflict: she has a motive to achieve as well as a motive to avoid success.

This conflict was strikingly revealed in a study which required college women to complete the following story: "After first-term finals, Anne finds herself at the top of her medical-school class" (Horner, 1969). The stories were then examined for unconscious, internal conflict about success and failure. The women in this study all had high intellectual ability and histories of academic success. They were the very women who could have successful careers. And yet, over two thirds of their stories revealed a clearcut inability to cope with the concept of a feminine, yet career-oriented woman.

The most common "fear-of-success" stories showed strong fears of social rejection as a result of success. The women in this group showed anxiety about becoming unpopular, unmarriageable, and lonely:

> Anne starts proclaiming her surprise and joy. Her fellow classmates are so disgusted with her behavior that they jump on her in a body and beat her. She is maimed for life.

> Anne is an acne-faced bookworm .... She studies twelve hours a day, and lives at home to save money. "Well, it certainly paid off. All the Friday and Saturday nights without dates, fun—I'll be the best woman doctor alive." And yet a twinge of sadness comes through —she wonders what she really has ...

> Although Anne is happy with her success, she fears what will happen to her social life. The male med students don't seem to think very highly of a female who has beaten them in their field ... She will be a proud and successful but alas a very lonely doctor.

> Anne is pretty darn proud of herself, but everyone hates and envies her.

> Anne doesn't want to be number one in her class ... She feels she shouldn't rank so high because of social reasons. She drops to ninth and then marries the boy who graduates number one.

In the second "fear-of-success" category were stories in which the women seemed concerned about definitions of womanhood. These stories expressed guilt and despair over success and doubts about their femininity and normality:

> Unfortunately Anne no longer feels so certain that she really wants to be a doctor. She is worried about herself and wonders if perhaps she is not normal ... Anne decides not to continue with her medical work but to take courses that have a deeper personal meaning for her.

> Anne feels guilty ... She will finally have a nervous breakdown and quit medical school and marry a successful young doctor.

A third group of stories could not even face up to the conflict between having a career and being a woman. These stories simply denied the possibility that any woman could be so successful:

> Anne is a code name for a nonexistent person created by a group of med students. They take turns writing for Anne ...

> Anne is really happy she's on top, though Tom is higher than she—though that's as it should be. Anne doesn't mind Tom winning.

> Anne is talking to her counselor. Counselor says she will make a fine nurse.
>
> It was luck that Anne came out on top because she didn't want to go to medical school anyway.

By way of contrast, here is a typical story written not about Anne, but about John:

> John has worked very hard and his long hours of study have paid off ... He is thinking about his girl, Cheri, whom he will marry at the end of med school. He realizes he can give her all the things she desires after he becomes established. He will go on in med school and be successful in the long run.

Nevertheless, there were a few women in the study who welcomed the prospect of success:

> Anne is quite a lady—not only is she on top academically, but she is liked and admired by her fellow students—quite a trick in a man-dominated field. She is brilliant—but she is also a woman. She will continue to be at or near the top. And ... always a lady.

Hopefully, the day is approaching when as many "Anne" stories as "John" stories will have happy endings.

It should be clear that the "free-will" argument conveniently overlooks the fact that the society which has spent twenty long years carefully marking the woman's ballot for her has nothing to lose in that twenty-first year by pretending to let her cast it for the alternative of her choice. Society has controlled not her alternatives, but her motivation to choose any but one of those alternatives. The so-called "freedom-to-choose" is illusory, and it cannot be invoked to justify the society which controls the motivation to choose.

2. The biological argument suggests that there may really be inborn differences between men and women in, say independence or mathematical ability. Or that there may be biological factors beyond the fact that women can become pregnant and nurse children which uniquely dictate that they, but not men, should stay home all day and shun serious outside commitment. Maybe female hormones really are responsible somehow. One difficulty with this argument, of course, is that female hormones would have to be different in the Soviet Union, where one-third of the engineers and 75% of the physicians are women. In America, women constitute less than 1% of the engineers and only 7% of the physicians (Dodge, 1966). Female physiology *is* different, and it may account for some of the psychological differences between the sexes, but America's sex-role ideology still seems primarily responsible for the fact that so few women emerge from childhood with the motivation to seek out any role beyond the one that our society dictates.

But even if there really were biological differences between the sexes along these lines, the biological argument would still be irrelevant. The reason can best be illustrated with an analogy.

Suppose that every black American boy were to be socialized to become a jazz musician on the assumption that he has a "natural" talent in that direction, or suppose that his parents should subtly discourage him from other pursuits because it is considered "inappropriate" for black men to become physicians or physicists. Most liberal Americans, we submit, would disapprove. But suppose that it *could* be demonstrated that black Americans, *on the average*, did possess an inborn better sense of rhythm than white Americans. Would *that* justify ignoring the unique characteristics of a *particular* black youngster from the very beginning and specifically socializing him to become a musician?

We don't think so. Similarly, as long as a woman's socialization does not nurture her uniqueness, but treats her only as a member of a group on the basis of some assumed average characteristic, she will not be prepared to realize her own potential in the way that the value of individuality and self-fulfillment imply she should.

The irony of the biological argument is that it does not take biological differences seriously enough. That is, it fails to recognize the range of biological differences between individuals within the same sex. Thus, recent research has revealed that biological factors help determine many personality traits. Dominance and submissiveness, for example, have been found to have large inheritable components; in other words, biological factors *do* have the potential for partially determining how dominant or submissive an individual, male or female, will turn out to be. But the effects of this biological potential could be detected only in males (Gottesman, 1963). This implies that only the males in our culture are raised with sufficient flexibility, with sufficient latitude given to their biological differences, for their "natural" or biologically determined potential to shine through. Females, on the other hand, are subjected to a socialization which so ignores their unique attributes that even the effects of biology seem to be swamped. In sum, the biological argument for continuing America's homogenization of its women gets hoist with its own petard.

3. Many people recognize that women do end up as full-time homemakers because of their socialization and that these women do exemplify the failure of our society to raise girls as unique individuals. But, they point out, the role of the homemaker is not inferior to the role of the professional man: it is complementary but equal.

This argument is usually bolstered by pointing to the joys and importance of taking care of small children. Indeed, mothers *and* fathers find child-rearing rewarding, and it is certainly important. But this argument becomes insufficient when one considers that the average American woman now lives to age 74 and has her *last* child at about age 26; thus, by the time the woman is 33 or so, her children all have more important things to do with their daytime hours than to spend them entertaining an adult woman who has nothing to do during the second half of her life span. As for the other "joys" of homemaking, many writers (e.g., Friedan, 1963) have persuasively argued that the role of the homemaker has been glamorized far beyond its intrinsic worth. This charge becomes plausible when one considers that the average American homemaker spends the equivalent of a man's working day, 7.1 hours, in preparing meals, cleaning house, laundering, mending, shopping, and doing other household tasks. In other words, 43% of her waking time is spent in activity that would command an hourly wage on the open market well below the federally-set minimum for menial industrial work.

The point is not how little she would earn if she did these things in someone else's home, but that this use of time is virtually the same for homemakers with college degrees and for those with less than a grade school education, for women married to blue-collar workers. Talent, education, ability, interests, motivations: all are irrelevant. In our society, being female uniquely qualifies an individual for domestic work.

It is true, of course, that the American homemaker has, on the average, 5.1 hours of leisure time per day, and it is here, we are told, that each woman can express her unique identity. Thus, politically interested women can join the League of Women Voters; women with humane interests can become part-time Gray Ladies; women who love music can raise money for the symphony. Protestant women play Canasta; Jewish women play Mah-Jongg; brighter women of all denominations and faculty wives play bridge; and so forth.

But politically interested *men* serve in legislatures; *men* with humane interests become physicians or clinical psychologists; *men* who love music play in the symphony; and so forth. In other words, why should a woman's unique identity determine only the periphery of her life rather than its central core?

Again, the important point is not that the role of homemaker is necessarily inferior, but that the woman's unique identity has been rendered irrelevant. Consider the following "predictability test." When a boy is born, it is difficult to predict what he will be doing 25 years later. We cannot say whether he will be an artist, a doctor, or a college professor because he will be permitted to develop and to fulfill his own unique potential, particularly if he is white and middle-class. But if the newborn child is a girl, we can usually predict with confidence how she will be spending her time 25 years later. Her individuality doesn't have to be considered; it is irrelevant.

The socialization of the American male has closed off certain options for him too. Men are discouraged from developing certain desirable traits such as tenderness and sensitivity just as surely as women are discouraged from being assertive and, alas, "too bright." Young boys are encouraged to be incompetent at cooking and child care just as surely as young girls are urged to be incompetent at mathematics and science.

Indeed, one of the errors of the early feminist movement in this country was that it assumed that men had all the goodies and that women could attain self-fulfillment merely by being like men. But that is hardly the utopia implied by the values of individuality and self-fulfillment. Rather, these values would require society to raise its children so flexibly and with sufficient respect for the integrity of individual uniqueness that some men might emerge with the motivation, the ability, and the opportunity to stay home and raise children without bearing the stigma of being peculiar. If homemaking is as glamorous, it would probably still be more fulfilling for some men than the jobs in which they now find themselves.

And if biological differences really do exist between men and women in "nurturance," in their inborn motivations to care for children, then this will show up automatically in the final distribution of men and women across the various roles: relatively fewer men will choose to stay at home. The values of individuality and self-fulfillment do not imply that there must be equality of outcome, an equal number of men and women in each role, but that there should be the widest possible variation in outcome consistent with the range of individual differences among people, regardless of sex. At the very least, these values imply that society should raise its males so that they could freely engage in activities that might pay less than those being pursued by their wives without feeling that they were "living off their wives." One rarely hears it said of a woman that she is "living off her husband."

Thus, it is true that a man's options are limited by our society's sex-role ideology, but as the "predictability test" reveals, it is still the woman in our society whose identity is rendered irrelevant by America's socialization practices. In 1954, the

United States Supreme Court declared that a fraud and hoax lay behind the slogan "separate but equal." It is unlikely that any court will ever do the same for the more subtle motto that successfully keeps the woman in her place: "complementary but equal."

Interpersonal Equality

> Wives, submit yourselves unto your own husbands, as unto the Lord. For the husband is the head of the wife, even as Christ is the head of the church; and he is the savior of the body. Therefore, as the church is subject unto Christ, so let the wives be to their own husbands in everything." (Eph. 5)

As this passage reveals, the ideological rationalization that men and women hold complementary but equal positions is a recent invention of our modern "liberal" society, part of the equalitarian veneer which helps to keep today's version of the ideology nonconscious. Certainly those Americans who value open, honest, and equalitarian relationships generally are quick to reject this traditional view of the male-female relationship; and, an increasing number of young people even plan to enter "utopian" marriages very much like the following hypothetical example:

> "Both my wife and I earned Ph.D. degrees in our respective disciplines. I turned down a superior academic post in Oregon and accepted a slightly less desirable position in New York where my wife could obtain a part-time teaching job and do research at one of the several other colleges in the area. Although I would have preferred to live in a suburb, we purchased a home near my wife's college so that she could have an office at home where she would be when the children returned from school. Because my wife earns a good salary, she can easily afford to pay a maid to do her major household chores. My wife and I share all other tasks around the house equally. For example, she cooks the meals, but I do the laundry for her and help her with many of her other household tasks."

Without questioning the basic happiness of such a marriage or its appropriateness for many couples, we can legitimately ask if such a marriage is, in fact, an instance of interpersonal equality. Have all the hidden assumptions about the woman's "natural" role really been eliminated? Has the traditional ideology really been exercised? There is a very simple test. If the marriage is truly equalitarian, then its description should retain the same flavor and tone even if the roles of the husband and wife were to be reversed.

> "Both my husband and I earned Ph.D. degrees in our respective disciplines. I turned down a superior academic post in Oregon and accepted a slightly less desirable position in New York where my husband could obtain a part-time teaching job and do research at one of the several other colleges in the area. Although I would have preferred to live in a suburb, we purchased a home near my husband's college so that he could have an office at home where he would be when the children returned from school. Because my husband earns a good salary, he can easily afford to pay a maid to do his major household chores. My husband and I share all other tasks around the house equally. For example, he cooks the meals, but I do the laundry for him and help him with many of his other household tasks."

It seems unlikely that many men or women in our society would mistake the marriage *just* described as either equalitarian or desirable, and thus it becomes apparent that the ideology about the woman's "natural" role consciously permeates the entire fabric of such "utopian" marriages. It is true that the wife gains some measure of equality when her career can influence the final place of residence, but why is it the unquestioned assumption that the husband's career solely determines the initial set of alternatives that are to be considered? Why is it the wife who automatically seeks the part-time position? Why is it *her* maid instead of *their* maid. Why *her* laundry? Why *her* household tasks? And so forth throughout the entire relationship.

The important point here is not that such marriages are bad or that their basic assumptions of inequality produce unhappy, frustrated women. Quite the contrary. It is the very happiness of the wives in such marriages that reveals society's smashing success in socializing its women. It is a measure of the distance our society must yet traverse toward the goals of self-fulfillment and interpersonal equality that such marriages are widely characterized as utopian and fully equalitarian. It is a mark of how well the woman has been kept in her place that the husband in such a marriage is often idolized by women, including his wife, for "permitting" her to squeeze a career into the interstices of their marriage as long as his own career is not unduly inconvenienced. Thus is the white man blessed for exercising his power benignly while his "natural" right to that power forever remains unquestioned.

Such is the subtlety of a nonconscious ideology!

A truly equalitarian marriage would permit both partners to pursue careers or outside commitments which carry equal weight when all important decisions are to be made. It is here, of course, that the "problem" of children arises. People often assume that the woman who seeks a role beyond home and family would not care to have children. They assume that if she wants a career or serious outside commitment, then children must be unimportant to her. But of course no one makes this assumption about her husband. No one assumes that a father's interest in his career necessarily precludes a deep and abiding affection for his children or a vital interest in their development. Once again America applies a double standard of judgment. Suppose that a father of small children suddenly lost his wife. No matter how much he loved his children, no one would expect him to sacrifice his career in order to stay home with them on a full-time basis—*even if he had an independent source of income.* No one would charge him with selfishness or lack of parental feeling if he sought professional care for his children during the day. An equalitarian marriage simply abolishes this double standard and extends the same freedom to the mother, while also providing the framework for the father to enter more fully into the pleasures and responsibilities of child rearing. In fact, it is the equalitarian marriage which has the most potential for giving children the love and concern of two parents rather than one. But few women are prepared to make use of this freedom. Even those women who have managed to finesse society's attempt to rob them of their career motivations are likely to find themselves blocked by society's trump card: the feeling that the raising of the children is their unique responsibility and in time of crisis—ultimately theirs alone. Such is the emotional power of a nonconscious ideology.

In addition to providing this potential for equalized child care, a truly equalitarian marriage embraces a more general division of labor which satisfies what might be called "the roommate test." That is, the labor is divided just as it is when two men or two women room together in college or set up a bachelor apartment together. Errands and domestic chores are assigned by preference, agreement, flipping a coin, given to hired help, or—as is sometimes the case—left undone.

It is significant that today's young people, many of whom live this way prior to marriage, find this kind of arrangement within marriage so foreign to their thinking. Consider an analogy. Suppose that a white male college student decided to room or set up a bachelor apartment with a black male friend. Surely the typical white student would not blithely assume that his black roommate was to handle all the domestic chores. Nor would his conscience allow him to do so even in the unlikely event that his roommate would say: "No, that's okay. I like doing housework. I'd be happy to do it." We suspect that the typical white student would still not be comfortable if he took advantage of this offer, if he took advantage of the fact that his roommate had been socialized to be "happy" with such an arrangement. But change this hypothetical black roommate to a female marriage partner, and somehow the student's conscience goes to sleep. At most it is quickly tranquilized by the thought that "she is happiest when she is ironing for her loved one." Such is the power of a nonconscious ideology.

Of course, it may well be that she *is* happiest when she is ironing for her loved one.

Such, indeed, is the power of a nonconscious ideology!

References

Barry, H., III, Bacon, M.K., & Child, I.L. A cross-cultural survey of some sex differences in socialization. *Journal of Abnormal and Social Psychology*, 1957, 55, 327-332.

Brown, R. *Social Psychology.* New York: Free Press, 1965.

Crandall, V.J., & Rabson, A. Children's repetition choices in an intellectual achievement situation following success and failure. *Journal of GEnetic Psychology*, 1960, 97, 161-168.

Dodge, N.D. *Women in the Soviet Economy.* Baltimore: The Johns Hopkins Press, 1966.

Flanagan, J.C. Project talent. Unpublished manuscript.

Friedan, B. *The Feminine Mystique.* New York: Norton, 1963.

Goldberg, P. Are women prejudiced against women? *Transaction,* April 1968, 5, 28-30.

Goldberg, S. & Lewis, M. Play behavior in the year-old infant: early sex differences. *Child Development*, 1969, 40, 21-31.

Gottesman, I.I. Heritability of personality: a demonstration. *Psychological Monographs*, 1963, 77 (Whole no. 572).

Horner, M. Woman's will to fail. *Psychology Today*, November, 1969.

Kagan, J. Acquisition and significance of sex typing and sex role identity. In M.L. Hoffman & L.W. Hoffman (Eds.) *Review of child development research, Vol. 1*, New York: Russell Sage Foundation, 1964. Pp. 137-167.

McDavid, J.W. Imitative behavior in preschool children. *Psychological Monographs*, 1959, 73, (Whole No. 486).

Milton, G.A. Five studies of the relation between sex role identification and achievement in problem solving. Technical Report No. 3, Department of Industrial Administration, Department of Psychology, Yale University, December, 1958.

Sears, R.R., Maccoby, E.E., & Levin, H. *Patterns of Child Rearing.* Evanston, Ill.: Row, Peterson, 1957.

Smith, M.E. The influence of age, sex, and situation on the frequency of form and functions of questions asked by preschool children. *Child Development*, 1933, 3, 201-213.

Terman, L.M., & Oden, M.H. *Genetic Studies of Genius, V. The Gifted Group at Mid-Life: Thirty-five Years' Follow-up of the Superior Child.* Stanford, Ca.: Stanford University Press, 1959.

Torrance, E.P. *Guiding Creative Talent.* Englewood Cliffs, N.Y.: Prentice-Hall, 1962.

The Crime of Punishment

6

by Karl Menninger

Few words in our language arrest our attention as do "crime," "violence," "revenge," and "injustice." We abhor crime: we adore justice; we boast that we live by the rule of law. Violence and vengefulness we repudiate as unworthy of our civilization, and we assume this sentiment to be unanimous among all human beings.

Yet crime continues to be a national disgrace and a world-wide problem. It is threatening, alarming, wasteful, expensive, abundant, and apparently increasing! In actuality it is decreasing in frequence of occurrence, but it is certainly increasing in visibility and the reactions of the public to it.

Our system for controlling crime is ineffective, unjust, expensive. Prisons seem to operate with revolving doors—the same people going in and out and in and out. Who cares?

Our city jails and inhuman reformatories and wretched prisons are jammed. They are known to be unhealthy, dangerous, immoral, indecent, crime-breeding dens of iniquity. Not everyone has smelled them as some of us have. Not many have heard the groans and the curses. Not everyone has seen the hate and despair in a thousand blank, hollow faces. But, in a way, we all know how miserable prisons are. We want them to be that way. And they are. Who cares?

SOURCE. Adapted from the book, *The Crime of Punishment*, Viking Press, 1968. Also published in the September 7 issue of the *Saturday Review.*

Professional and big-time criminals prosper as never before. Gambling syndicates flourish. White-collar crime may even exceed all others, but goes undetected in the majority of cases. We are all being robbed and we know who the robbers are. They live nearby. Who cares?

The public filches millions of dollars worth of food and clothing from stores, towels and sheets from hotels, jewelry and knick-knacks from shops. The public steals, and the same public pays it back in higher prices. Who cares?

Time and again somebody shouts about this state of affairs, just as I am shouting now. The magazines shout. The newspapers shout. The television and radio commentators shout (or at least they "deplore"). Psychologists, sociologists, leading jurists, wardens, and intelligent police chiefs join the chorus. Governors and mayors and Congressmen are sometimes heard. They shout that the situation is bad, bad, bad, and getting worse. Some suggest that we immediately replace obsolete procedures with scientific methods. A few shout contrary sentiments. Do the clear indications derived from scientific discovery for appropriate changes continue to fall on deaf ears? Why is the public so long-suffering, so apathetic and thereby so continuingly self-destructive? How many Presidents (and other citizens) do we have to lose before we do something?

The public behaves as a sick patient does when a dreaded treatment is proposed for his ailment. We all know how the aching tooth may suddenly quiet down in the dentist's office, or the abdominal pain disappear in the surgeon's examining room. Why should a sufferer seek relief and shun it? Is it the fear of unknown complications? Is it distrust of the doctor's ability? All of these, no doubt.

But, as Freud made so incontestably clear, the sufferer is always somewhat deterred by a kind of subversive, internal opposition to the work of cure. He suffers on the one hand from the pains of his affliction and yearns to get well. But he suffers at the same time from traitorous impulses that fight against the accomplishment of any change in himself, even recovery! Like Hamlet, he wonders whether it may be better after all to suffer the familiar pains and aches associated with the old method than to face the complications of a new and strange, even though possibly better way of handling things.

The inescapable conclusion is that society secretly wants crime, needs crime, and gains definite satisfactions from the present mishandling of it! We condemn crime, we punish offenders for it; but we need it. The crime and punishment ritual is a part of our lives. We need crimes to wonder at, to enjoy vicariously, to discuss and speculate about, and to publicly deplore. We need criminals to identify ourselves with, to envy secretly, and to punish stoutly. They do for us the forbidden, illegal things we wish to do and, like scapegoats, of old, they bear the burdens of our displaced guilt and punishment—"the iniquities of us all."

We have to confess that there is something fascinating for us all about violence. That most crime is not violent we know but we forget, because crime is a breaking, a rupturing, a tearing—even when it is quietly done. To all of us crime seems like violence.

The very word "violence" has a disturbing, menacing quality ... In meaning it implies something dreaded, powerful, destructive, or eruptive. It is something we abhor—or do we? Its first effect is to startle, frighten—even to horrify us. But we do not always run away from it. For violence also intrigues us. It is exciting. It is dramatic. Observing it and sometimes even participating in it gives us acute pleasure.

The newspapers constantly supply us with tidbits of violence going on in the world. They exploit its dramatic essence often to the neglect of conservative reporting of more extensive but less violent damage—the flood disaster in Florence, Italy, for example. Such words as crash, explosion, wreck, assault, raid, murder, avalanche, rape, and seizure evoke pictures of eruptive devastation from which we cannot turn away. The headlines often impute violence metaphorically even to peaceful activities. Relations are "ruptured," a tie is "broken," arbitration "collapses," a proposal is "killed."

Meanwhile, on the television and movie screens there constantly appear for our amusement scenes of fighting, slugging, beating, torturing, clubbing, shooting, and the like which surpass in effect anything that the newspapers can describe. Much of this violence is portrayed dishonestly; the scenes are only semirealistic; they are "faked" and romanticized.

Pain cannot be photographed; grimaces indicate but do not convey its intensity. And wounds—unlike violence—are rarely shown. This phony quality of television violence in its mentally unhealthy aspect encourages irrationality by giving the impression to the observer that being beaten, kicked, cut and stomped, while very unpleasant, are not very painful or serious. For after being slugged and beaten the hero rolls over, opens his eyes, hops up, rubs his cheek, grins, and staggers on. The suffering of violence is a part both the TV and movie producers and their audience tend to repress.

Although most of us say we deplore cruelty and destructiveness, we are partially deceiving ourselves. We disown violence, ascribing the love of it to other people. But the facts speak for themselves. We do love violence, all of us, and we all feel secretly guilty for it, which is another clue to public resistance to crime-control reform.

The great sin by which we are all tempted is the wish to hurt others, and this sin must be avoided if we are to live and let live. If our destructive energies can be mastered, directed, and sublimated, we can survive. If we can love, we can live. Our destructive energies, if they cannot be controlled, may destroy our best friends, as in the case of Alexander the Great, or they may destroy supposed "enemies" or innocent strangers. Worst of all—from the standpoint of the individual—they may destroy us.

Over the centuries of man's existence, many devices have been employed in the effort to control these innate suicidal and criminal propensities. The earliest of these undoubtedly depended upon fear—fear of the unknown, fear of magical retribution, fear of social retaliation. These external devices were replaced gradually with the law and all its machinery, religion and its rituals, and the conventions of the social order.

Are there steps that we can take which will reduce the aggressive stabs and self-destructive lurches of our less well-managing fellow men? Are there ways to prevent and control the grosser violations, other than the clumsy traditional maneuvers which we have inherited? These depend basically upon intimidation and slow-motion torture. We call it punishment, and justify it with our "feeling." We know it doesn't work.

Yes, there are better ways. There are steps that could be taken; some are taken. But we move too slowly. Much better use, it seems to me, could be made of the members of my profession and other behavioral scientists than having them deliver courtroom pronunciamentos. The consistent use of a diagnostic clinic would enable trained workers to lay what they can about an offender before the judge who would know best how to implement the recommendation.

This would no doubt lead to a transformation of prisons, if not to their total disappearance in their present form and function. Temporary and permanent detention will perhaps always be necessary for a few, especially the professionals, but this could be more effectively and economically performed with new types of "facility" (that strange, awkward word for institution).

I assume it to be a matter of common and general agreement that our object in all this is to protect the community from a repetition of the offense by the most economical method consonant with our other purposes. Our "other purposes" include the desire to prevent these offenses from occurring, to reclaim offenders for social usefulness, if possible, and to detain them in protective custody, if reclamation is not possible. But how?

The treatment of human failure or dereliction by the infliction of pain is still used and believed in by many non-medical people. "Spare the rod and spoil the child" is still considered wise counsel by many.

Whipping is still used by many secondary schoolmasters in England, I am informed, to stimulate study, attention, and the love of learning. Whipping was long a traditional treatment for the "crime" of disobedience on the part of children, pupils, servants, apprentices, employees. And slaves were treated for centuries by flogging for such offenses as weariness, confusion, stupidity, exhaustion, fear, grief, and even overcheerfulness. It was assumed and stoutly defended that these "treatments" cured conditions for which they were administered.

Meanwhile, scientific medicine was acquiring many new healing methods and devices. Doctors can now transplant organs and limbs; they can remove brain tumors and cure incipient cancers; they can halt pneumonia, meningitis, and other infections; they can correct deformities and repair breaks and tears and scars. But these wonderful achievements are accomplished on willing subjects, people who voluntarily ask for help by even heroic measures. And the reader will be wondering, no doubt, whether doctors can do anything with or for peoples who do not want to be treated at all, in any way! Can doctors cure willful aberrant behavior? Are we to believe that crime is a disease that can be reached by scientific measures? Isn't it merely "natural meanness" that makes all of us do wrong things at times even when we "know better?" Surely there is no medical treatment for the lack of those!

Let me answer this carefully, for much misunderstanding accumulates here. I would say that according to the prevalent understanding of the words, crime is not a disease. Neither is it an illness, although I think it should be! It should be treated, and it could be; but it mostly isn't.

These enigmatic statements are simply explained. Diseases are undesired states of being which have been described and defined by doctors, usually given Greek or Latin appellations, and treated by long-established physical and pharmacological formulae. Illness, on the other hand, is best defined as a state of impaired functioning of such a nature that the public expects the sufferer to repair to the physician for help. The illness may prove to be a disease: more often it is only vague and nameless misery, but something which doctors, not lawyers, teachers, or preachers, are supposed to be able and willing to help.

When the community begins to look upon the expression of aggressive violence as the symptom of an illness or as indicative of illness, it will be because it believes doctors can do something to correct such a condition. At present, some better-informed individuals do believe and expect this. However angry at or sorry for the offender, they want him "treated" in an effective way so that he will cease to be a danger to them. And they know that the traditional punishment, "treatment-punishment," will not effect this.

What will? What effective treatment is there for such violence? It will surely have to begin with motivating or stimulating or arousing in a cornered individual the wish and hope and intention to change his methods of dealing with the realities of life. Can this be done by education, medication, counseling, training? I would answer yes. It can be done successfully in a majority of cases, if undertaken in time.

The present penal system and the existing legal philosophy do not stimulate or even expect such a change to take place in the criminal. Yet change is what medical science always aims for. The prisoner, like the doctor's other patients, should emerge from his treatment experience a different person, differently equipped, differently functioning, and headed in a different direction than when he began the treatment.

It is natural for the public to doubt that this can be accomplished with criminals. But remember that the public used to doubt that change could be effected in the mentally ill. No one a hundred years ago believed mental illness to be curable. Today all people know (or should know) that mental illness is curable in the great majority of instances and that the prospects and rapidity of cure are directly related to the availability and intensity of proper treatment.

The forms and techniques of psychiatric treatment used today number in the hundreds. No one patient requires or receives all forms, but each patient is studied with respect to his particular needs, his basic assets, his interests, and his special difficulties. A therapeutic team may embrace a dozen workers—as in a hospital setting—or it may narrow down to the doctor and the spouse. Clergymen, teachers, relatives, friends, and even fellow patients often participate informally but helpfully in the process of readaptation.

All of the participants in this effort to bring about a favorable change in the patient—i.e., in his vital balance and life program—are imbued with what we may call a therapeutic attitude. This is one indirect antithesis to attitudes of avoidance, ridicule, scorn, or punitiveness. Hostile feelings toward the subject, however justified by his unpleasant and even destructive behavior, are not in the curriculum of therapy or in the therapist. This does not mean that therapists approve of the offensive and obnoxious behavior of the patient; they distinctly disapprove of it. But they recognize it as symptomatic of continued imbalance and disorganization, which is what they are seeking to change. They distinguish between disapproval, penalty, price, and punishment.

Doctors charge fees; they impose certain "penalties" or prices, but they have long since put aside primitive attitudes of retaliation toward offensive patients. A patient may cough in the doctor's face or may vomit on the office rug; a patient may curse or scream or even struggle in the extremity of his pain. But these acts are not "punished." Doctors and nurses have no time or thought for inflicting unnecessary pain even upon patients who may be difficult, disagreeable, provocative, and even dangerous. It is their duty to care for them, to try to make them well, and to prevent them from doing themselves or others harm. This requires love, not hate. This is the deepest meaning of the therapeutic attitude. Every doctor knows this; every worker in a hospital or clinic knows it (or should).

There is another element in the therapeutic attitude. It is the quality of hopefulness. If no one believes that the patient can get well, if no one—not even the doctor—has any hope, there probably won't be any recovery. Hope is just as important as love in the therapeutic attitude.

"But you were talking about the mentally ill," readers may interject, "those poor, confused, bereft, frightened individuals who yearn for help from you doctors and nurses. Do you mean to imply that willfully perverse individuals, our criminals, can be similarly reached and rehabilitated? Do you really believe that effective treatment of the sort you visualize can be applied to people who do not want any help, who are so willfully vicious, so well aware of the wrongs they are doing, so lacking in penitence or even common decency that punishment seems to be the only thing left?"

Do I believe there is effective treatment for offenders, and that they can be changed? Most certainly and definitely I do. Not all cases, to be sure; there are also some physical afflictions which we cannot cure at the moment. Some provision has to be made for incurables—pending new knowledge—and these will include some offenders. But I believe the majority of them would prove to be curable. The willfulness and the viciousness of offenders are part of the thing for which they have to be treated. These must not thwart the therapeutic attitude.

It is simply not true that most of them are "fully aware" of what they are doing, nor is it true that they want no help from anyone, although some of them say so. Prisoners are individuals: some want treatment, some do not. Some don't know what treatment is. Many are utterly despairing and hopeless. Where treatment is made available in institutions, many prisoners seek it even with the full knowledge that doing so will not lessen their sentences. In some prisons, seeking treatment by prisoners is frowned upon by the officials.

Various forms of treatment are even now being tried in some progressive courts and prisons over the country—educational, social, industrial, religious, recreational, and psychological treatments. Socially acceptable behavior, new work-play opportunities, new identity and companion patterns all help toward community reacceptance. Some parole officers and some wardens have been extremely ingenious in developing these modalities of rehabilitation and reconstruction—more than I could list here even if I knew them all. But some are trying. The secret of success in all programs, however, is the replacement of the punitive attitude with a therapeutic attitude.

Offenders with propensities for impulsive and predatory aggression should not be permitted to live among us unrestrained by some kind of social control. But the great majority of offenders, even "criminals," should never become prisoners if we want to "cure" them.

There are now throughout the country many citizens' action groups and programs for the prevention and control of crime and delinquency. With such attitudes of inquiry and concern, the public could acquire information (and incentive) leading to a change of feeling about crime and criminals. It will discover how unjust is much so-called "justice," how baffled and frustrated many judges are by the ossified rigidity of old-fashioned, obsolete laws and state constitutions which effectively prevent the introduction of sensible procedures to replace useless, harmful ones.

The public has a fascination for violence, and clings tenaciously to its yen for vengeance, blind and deaf to the expense, futility, and dangerousness of the resulting penal system. But we are bound to hope that this will yield in time to the persistent, penetrating light of intelligence and accumulating scientific knowledge. The public will grow increasingly ashamed of its cry for retaliation, its persistent demand to punish. This is its crime, our crime against criminals—and, incidentally, our crime against ourselves. For before we can diminish our sufferings from the ill-controlled aggressive assaults of fellow citizens, we must renounce the philosophy of punishment, the obsolete, vengeful penal attitude. In its place we would seek a comprehensive constructive social attitude—therapeutic in some instances, restraining in some instances, but preventive in its total social impact.

In the last analysis this becomes a question of personal morals and values. No matter how glorified or how piously disguised, vengeance as a human motive must be personally repudiated by each and every one of us. This is the message of old religions and new psychiatrics. Unless this message is heard, unless we, the people—the man on the street, the housewife in the home—can give up our delicious satisfactions in opportunities for vengeful retaliation on scapegoats, we cannot expect to preserve our peace, our public safety, or our mental health.

7 A Partial List of Human Potential or Self-Actualization Centers

WEST COAST

Alcoholics Anonymous
(look for local chapters in
the telephone book and in
the classified section of
your newspaper)

Berkeley Center for Human Interaction
1820 Scenic
Berkeley, California 94709

Bridge Mountain Foundation
2011 Alba Road
Ben Lomond, California 95005

The Center
P.O. Box 3014
Stanford, California 94305

Center for Human Communication
Family Therapy Institute, Group Ctr.
120 Oak Meadow Drive
Los Gatos, California 95030

Esalen Institute
Big Sur, California 93920

Esalen Institute
P.O. Box 31389
San Francisco, California 94131

Explorations Institute
P.O. Box 1254
Berkeley, California 94701

Gestalt Institute of San Francisco, Inc.
1719 Union Street
San Francisco, California 94123

Institute For Group & Family Studies
347 Alma
Palo Alto, California 94301

Interracial House
2062 85 Avenue
Oakland, California

Kairos
The Ranch
P.O. Box 350
Rancho Santa Fe, California 92067

The National Center For The Exploration
Of Human Potential
8080 El Paseo Grande
La Jolla, California 92037

Northwest Family Therapy Institute
P.O. Box 94278
Tacoma, Washington 98494

Recovery Inc.
The Association of Nervous and
Former Mental Patients
(local chapters in the telephone book)
National Headquarters
116 S. Michigan Avenue
Chicao, Illinois 60603

Seminars in Group Process
8475 S.W. Bohmann Parkway
Portland, Oregon 97223

Society For Comparative Philosophy, Inc.
P.O. Box 857
Sausalito, California 94965

Star Weather Ranch Institute
P.O. Box 923
Hailey, Idaho 83333

Tahoe Institute
P.O. Box DD
South Lake Tahoe, California 95705

Topanga Center For Human Development
P.O. Box 480
Reseda, California 91335

CENTRAL STATES

Amare: The Institute of Human
Relatedness
Box 108
Bowling Green, Ohio 43402

Cambridge House
1900 N. Cambridge Avenue
Milwaukee, Wisconsin 53202

Center For Creative Interchange
602 Center Street
Des Moines, Iowa 50309

Communications Center I
1001 Union Blvd.
St. Louis, Missouri 63113

Espirtu
1214 Miramar
Houston, Texas 77005

Evergreen Institute
3831 W. Wagon Trail Drive
Littleton, Colorado 80120

Gestalt Institute of Cleveland, Inc.
12921 Euclid Avenue
Cleveland, Ohio 44112

Kopavi, Inc.
4841 11th Avenue South
Minneapolis, Minnesota 55417

The Laos House
700 West 19th
Austin, Texas 78701

Midwest Personal Growth Center
200 South Hanley Road
Clayton, Missouri 63105

Oasis: Midwest Center For
Human Potential
Stone-Brandel Center
1439 South Michigan Avenue
Chicago, Illinois 60605

Shadybrook House
RR 1
Mentor, Ohio 44060

EAST COAST

Associates For Human Resources
387 Sudbury Road
Concord, Massachusetts 01742

Aureon Institute
71 Park Avenue
New York, New York 10016

Center For The Whole Person
1633 Race Street
Philadelphia, Pennsylvania 19103

The Center of Man
Micanopy, Florida 32667

EAST COAST

The Family Relations Institute
3509 Farm Hill Drive
Falls Church, Virginia 22044

Human Dimensions Institute
at Rosary Hill College
4380 Main Street
Buffalo, New York 14226

Institute for Experimental Education
P.O. Box 446
Lexington, Massachusetts 02173

Institute For Rational Living
Pennsylvania Branch
300 South 19th Street
Philadelphia, Pennsylvania 19103

Plainfield Consultation Center
831 Madison Avenue
Plainfield, New Jersey 07060

CANADA AND MEXICO

Cold Mountain Institute
P.O. Box 4362
Edmonton 60, Alberta

Shalal
750 West Broadway
Vancouver, B.C.

Bibliography and Suggested Readings

BIBLIOGRAPHY

Advisory Commission on the Status of Women: *California Women*, State of California Printing Office, Sacramento, California, 1971.

Cohn, Edgar S., ed.: *Our Brother's Keeper: The Indian in White America*, New Community Press Book distributed by the World Publishing Company, New York, 1969.

Gustaitis, Rasa: *Turning On;* The MacMillan Company, New York, 1969.

"Report of the National Advisory Commission on Civil Disorders," Washington, D.C., U.S. Government Printing Office, 1969.

Rogers, Carl: "The Concept of the Fully Functioning Person;" Center for Studies of the Person, La Jolla, California (unpublished paper).

SUGGESTED READINGS

"Conscious Control of Brain Waves," *Psychology Today*, 1968, pp. 58-59.

Lederman, Janet: *Anger and the Rocking Chair*, McGraw-Hill Book Company, 1969.

Rogers, Carl: "The Person of Tomorrow," Commencement Address at Sonoma State College, 1969.

Rogers, Carl: "Toward a Modern Approach to Values: The Valuing Process in the Mature Person, "*Person to Person: The Problem of Being Human*, Real Peoples Press, 1967.

Szasy, Thomas: "The Crime of Committment," *Psychology Today*, March, 1969.

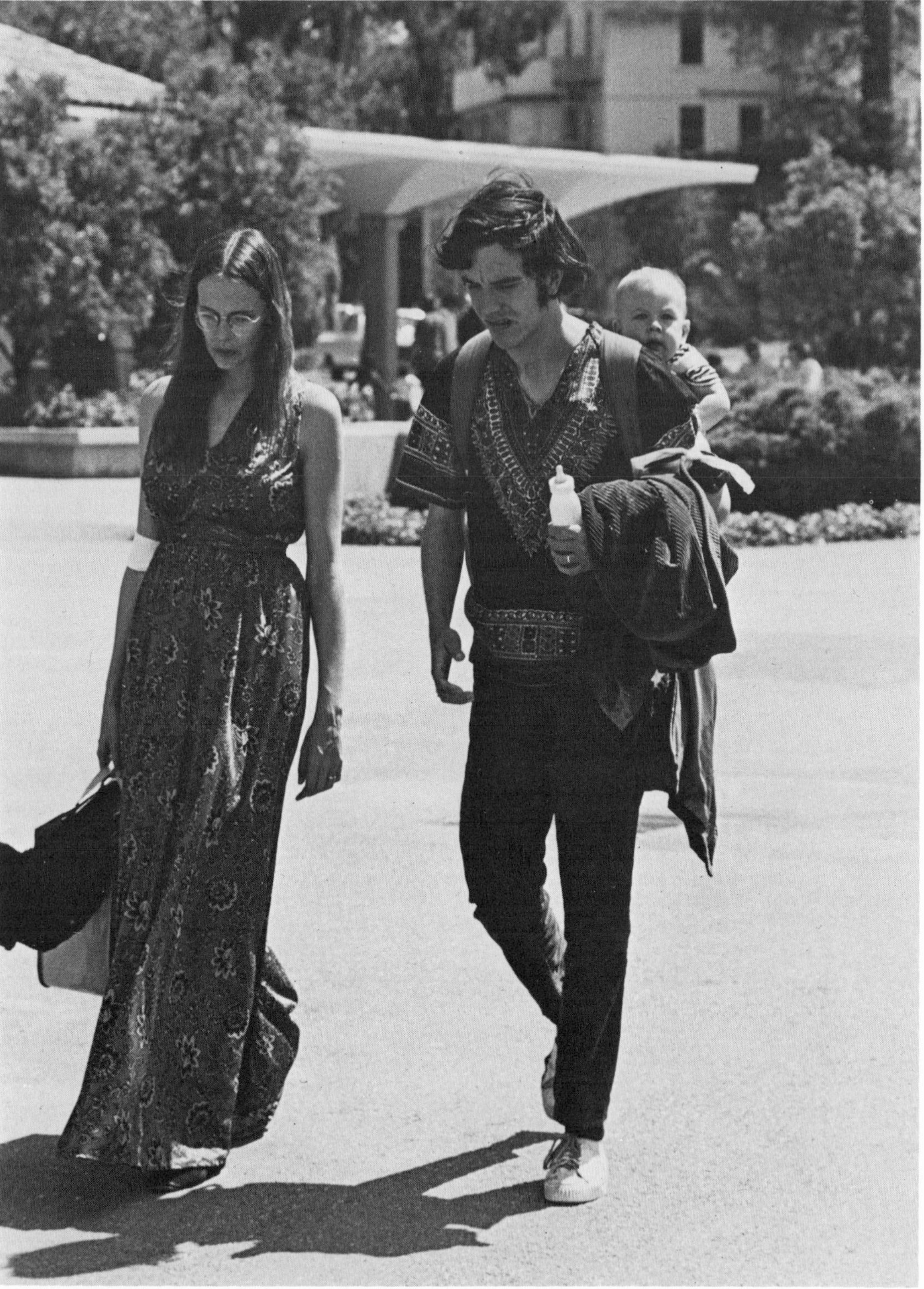

UNIT 2

Human Sexuality

There is no part of human life that is more troublesome than the area of human sexuality. This consists of "in bed" sex, as well as every area of life that is touched by the fact of your biological sex. Human sexuality includes a variety of physiological problems, a whole area of contrived behavioral standards, and attempts to "fit" your sex role designation.

A few of the physiological problems women must face are learning about and caring for menstrual periods, protecting themselves against unwanted pregnancy, menopausal problems, and various disease problems peculiar to females. Men must also be aware of their physiological problems such as: nocturnal emissions, protecting themselves against fathering an unwanted child, and certain diseases (infection of the prostate gland) peculiar to males.

The behavioral problems will vary with the society, the time in history, and the sex of the individual. These include such diverse problems as relating to other people from your sex role in finding and holding a job, acceptable "dating" and other "relating" problems, and whether to accept or how to manage the "marriage partner" or "parent" role.

Ideas concerning all the attitude and behavioral aspects of sexuality are now openly in a period of study and transition. Women are reviewing and questioning the relation between the "female role" they have been accepting and their true human potential (Unit I) and men should be considering the "male role" that has caused them so many emotional and physical health problems. Sociologists and other interested individuals are concerned about the nature of what is generally considered to be *the* American family style (the Nuclear Family), what purpose it serves, some ideas about its shortcomings and possible remedies. Others are looking at styles of marriage. Even more basic are the speculations and evidence concerning the assumed biological drive to become a "mother." This unit includes papers pertaining to all these topics.

There are many problems having to do with the "in bed" part of sexuality. Most of these are behavioral, and a few are physiological.

For those outside of marriage we try to repress the fact that all normal healthy humans have a sex drive that must be satisfied by one of three ways: (1) masturbation (2) sublimation, or (3) intercourse. When it does slip into the conscious level we demand that *other* unmarried people sublimate the drive. Sublimation is the channeling of a drive into another direction, preferably physical, creative, or religious activity. This is impossible for all but very few, if any, to attain. For those of us who masturbate (92% of all men and 62% of all women according to Kinsey) a great variety of horror stories have been concocted. Such fables as: it leads to mental retardation, insanity, impotence or frigidity in later life, hair on the palm of the hand or loss of the organ are the most common ones. Psychiatrist Murry Banks proclaims the nonsense and harmfulness of such tales and states that the only physical effect of masturbation is a strong arm.

The remaining outlet is intercourse, and there is no part of life about which more myths occur or against which there are more sanctions. All states with the exception of Illinois specify illegal methods and positions even for husbands and wives! The new Illinois penal code specifies only that the people involved in any sex act be "consenting adults." In other states there are no legal outlets in intercourse for unmarried people, in spite of our vast population of premarital, divorced, and widowed.

The Kinsey Report and our own personal observations, however, show that people *are finding* outlets, and we know that in spite of the frequency of premarital and extra marital intercourse the laws are seldom implemented.

On the wedding night some of us expect the virgin bride to miraculously become a proficient lover (the "male role" specifications usually prize experience, with the more notches on the steering post the better). Even after years of marriage many couples still worry about the acceptableness of certain positions or practices; whereas in actuality anthropologists have found that essentially any imaginable position or practice has been considered normal at some time in some society. The Kinsey Report shows that essentially all have been practiced in secret by varying numbers of people in our society.

With about 18 million illegitimate people alive in the United States today (one in twelve born across the nation) and the social stigma linked with illegitimacy, roughly a million abortions each year, only 26% of all married couples having no more than the number of children they wanted, and the myriad problems of too many people in the country, obviously conception and contraception are important problems. This unit discusses these problems.

One of the greatest problems today in American society has to do with homosexuality. With such a multitude of contrived specifications for each "sex role" and so many difficulties in trying to fit into them, a great many people have psychological problems over homosexuality. People who *aren't* overtly homosexual, or who have on occasion had a homosexual experience are afraid they may be homosexual. People who *are* overtly homosexual either wish they weren't or wish they could live their lives without the stigma and oppression that exists. A more enlightened view than is usually found in the mass media is given in this unit (from TIME).

The Homosexual: Newly Visible, Newly Understood

1

An exclusive formal ball will mark Halloween in San Francisco this week. In couturier gowns and elaborately confected masquerades, the couples will whisk around the floor until 2 a.m., while judges award prizes for the best costumes and the participants elect an "Empress." By then the swirling belles will sound more and more deep-voiced, and in the early morning hours dark stubble will sprout irrepressibly through their Pan-Cake Make-Up. The celebrators are all homosexuals, and each year since 1962 the crowd at the annual "Beaux Arts Ball" has grown larger. Halloween is traditionally boys' night out, and similar events will take place in Los Angeles, New York, Houston, and St. Louis.

Though they still seem fairly bizarre to most Americans, homosexuals have never been so visible, vocal or closely scrutinized by research. They throw public parties, frequent exclusively "gay" bars (70 in San Francisco alone), and figure sympathetically as the subjects of books, plays and films. Encouraged by the national climate of openness about sex of all kinds and the spirit of protest, male and female inverts have been organizing to claim civil rights for themselves as an aggrieved minority.

Political Pressure

Their new militancy makes other citizens edgy, and it can be shrill. Hurling rocks and bottles and wielding a parking meter that had been wrenched out of the sidewalk, homosexuals rioted last summer in New York's Greenwich Village after police closed one of the city's 50 all-gay bars and clubs on an alleged liquor-law violation. Pressure from militant self-styled "homophiles" has forced political candidates' views about homosexuality into recent election campaigns in New York, San Francisco and Los Angeles. Homosexuals have picketed businesses, the White House and the Pentagon, demanding an end to job discrimination and the right to serve in the Army without a dishonorable discharge if their background is discovered.

Some 50 homophile organizations have announced their existence in cities across the country and on at least eight campuses. Best known are the Mattachine societies (named for 16th century Spanish masked court jesters), and the Daughters of Bilitis (after French poet Pierra Louys' The Songs of Bilitis, a 19th century series of lyrics glorifying lesbian love). W. Dorr Legg, educational director at Los Angeles' 17-year-old ONE, Inc., claims, "I won't be happy until all churches give homosexual dances and parents are sitting in the balcony saying 'Don't John and Henry look cute dancing together?' " Radical groups such as the Gay Liberation Front chant "Gay power" and "Gay is good" and turgidly call for "the Revolution of Free and Frequent Polysexuality."

Last week's report to the National Institute of Mental Health (TIME, Oct. 24) urged legislation of private homosexual acts between adults who agree to them.* It was the latest sign that the militants are finding grudging tolerance and some support in the "straight" community. The Federal Appeals Court in Washington, D.C., for example, has responded to a recent case by declaring that a governmental agency could not dismiss an employee without first proving that his homosexuality would palpably interfere with the efficiency of the agency's operations. The New York TIMES, which for years shied from the word homosexual, in June permitted a homosexual writing under his own name, Freelance Critic Donn Teal, to contribute an article on "gay" themes in theater. In large cities, homosexuals have reached tacit agreements with police that give them the de facto right to their own social life.

Homosexual organizations across the country run discussion groups and record hops. A San Francisco group known as S.I.R. (Society for Individual Rights) organizes ice-skating parties, chess clubs and bowling leagues. Nor is it necessary for a homosexual to join a homophile organization to enjoy a full social life: homosexuals often are the parlor darlings of wealthy ladies ("fag hags"). Marriage in these circles can involve a homosexual and a busy career woman who cooly take the vows for companionship—so that they can pool their incomes and tax benefits for a glittering round of entertaining.

Seduction and Sodomy

Homosexuals with growing frequency have sought the anonymity and comparative permissiveness of big cities. It is this concentration of homosexuals in urban neighborhoods rather than any real growth in their relative numbers that has increased their visibility and made possible their as-

*Three dissenting members of the study group shied away from making policy recommendations, claiming that the issues were moral and not scientific in nature.

sertiveness. According to the Kinsey reports, still the basic source for statistics on the subject, 10% of American men have long periods of more or less exclusive homosexuality; only 4% (2% of women) are exclusively homosexual all their lives. These may be inflated figures, but most experts think that the proportion of homosexuals in the U.S. adult population has not changed drastically since Kinsey did his survey, giving the country currently about 2,600,000 men and 1,400,000 women who are exclusively homosexual. Despite popular belief, these numbers are not substantially increased by seduction: most experts now believe that an individual's sex drives are firmly fixed in childhood.

Inevitably, the homosexual life has attracted eager entrepreneurs. A firm in Great Neck, N.Y., runs a computer-dating service for homosexuals; San Francisco's Adonis bookstore has some 360 different magazines on display that carry everything from lascivious photos of nude men to reports on the homophile movement and lovelorn advice by "Madame Soto-Voce." Police and homosexuals agree that operating a gay bar is still an occupation that often appeals to Mafiosi. In New York City, sleazy movie houses along Broadway now match their traditional offerings of cheesecake with "beefcake."

Off-Broadway producers have found that homosexuals will flock to plays about themselves. Yet most dramas about deviates are written for heterosexual audiences. The New York stage currently offers John Osborns's *A Patriot for Me*, Mart Crowley's *The Boys in the Band* and John Herbert's *Fortune and Men's Eyes*, a 1967 drama about prison life. Revived last week in a new production, it has been rewritten so that a scene of forcible sodomy that used to take place out of the audience's sight is now grimly visible (though simulated). In movies, too, homosexuality is the vogue: *Staircase*, starring Rex Harrison and Richard Burton, *Midnight Cowboy* and Fellini's forthcoming *Satyricon.* On the lesbian side there are *The Fox*, *Therese and Isabelle*, and *The Killing of Sister George.*

The quality of these works ranges from excellent to nauseating. But it is a fact that treatment of the theme has changed. "Homosexuality used to be a sensational gimmick," says Playwright Crowley. "The big revelation in the third act was that the guy was homosexual, and then he had to go offstage and blow his brains out. It was associated with sin, and there had to be retribution." These days a movie or play can end, as *Staircase* does, with a homosexual couple still together, or, as *Boys in the Band* winds up, with two squabbling male lovers trying desperately to save their relationship. Beyond that, the homosexual is a special kind of anti-hero; his emergence on center stage reflects the same sympathy for outsiders that has transformed oddballs and criminals from enemies into heroic rebels against society in such films as *Bonnie and Clyde* and *Alice's Restaurant.*

Is there a homosexual conspiracy afoot to dominate the arts and other fields? Sometimes it seems that way. The presence of talented homosexuals in the field of classical music, among composers, performers, conductors and management, has sometimes led to charges by disappointed outsiders that the music world is a closed circle. The same applies to the theater, the art world, painting, dance, fashion, hairdressing and interior design, where a kind of "homintern" exists: a gay boss will often use his influence to help gay friends. The process is not unlike the ethnic favoritism that prevails in some companies and in big-city political machines; with a special sulky twist, it can be vicious to outsiders. Yet homosexual influence has probably been exaggerated. The homosexual cannot go too far in foisting off on others his own preferences: the public that buys the tickets or the clothes is overwhelmingly heterosexual. Genuine talent is in such demand that entrepreneurs who pass it by on the grounds of sex preference alone may well suffer a flop or other damage to their own reputations.

The Dark Side of Love

Discrimination aside, what about the more indirect propagation of homosexual points of view? Homosexual taste can fall into a particular kind of self-indulgence as the homosexual revenges himself on a hostile world by writing grotesque exaggerations of straight customs, concentrates on superficial stylistic furbelows or develops a "campy" fetish for old movies. Somerset Maugham once said of the homosexual artist that "with his keen insight and quick sensibility, he can pierce the depths, but in his innate frivolity he fetches up from them not a priceless jewel but a tinsel ornament."

In many cases, including Maugham's own, that is an exaggeration. Indeed the talented homosexual's role as an outsider, far from disqualifying him from commenting on life, may often sharpen his insight and esthetic sensibility. From Sappho to Colette to Oscar Wilde and James Baldwin, homosexual authors have memorably celebrated love—and not always in homosexual terms. For example, W.H. Auden's *Lullaby* —"Lay your sleeping head, my love/Human on my faithless arm"—must rank as one of the 20th century's most exquisite love lyrics.

In recent years, writes Critic Benjamin DeMott, "the most intense accounts of domestic life and problems, as well as the few unembarrassedly passionate love poems, have been work of writers who are not heterosexual . . . Tennessee Williams, Edward Albee, Allen Ginsberg, Jean Genet and Auden. They have a steady consciousness of a dark side of love that is neither homo- nor heterosexual but simply human." New York *Times* Drama Critic Clive Barnes muses, "Creativity might be a sort of psychic disturbance itself, mightn't it? Artists are not particularly happy people anyway."

Despite the homosexual's position in the arts, it is easy to overestimate the acceptance he has achieved elsewhere. Most straight Americans still regard the invert with a mixture of revulsion and apprehension, to which some authorities have given the special diagnostic name of homosexual panic. A Louis Harris poll released last week reported that 63% of the nation consider homosexuals "harmful to American life," and even the most tolerant parents nervously watch their children for real or imagined signs of homosexuality, breathing sighs of relief when their boy or girl finally begins dating the opposite sex.

Such homophobia is based on understandable instincts among straight people, but it also involves innumerable misconceptions and oversimplifications. The worst of these may well be that all homosexuals are alike. In fact, recent research has uncovered a large variation among homosexual types. With some overlap, they include:

The Blatant Homosexual. Chaucer's Pardoner in *The Canterbury Tales* had a voice "small as a goat's. He had no beard nor ever would have, his face was as smooth as if lately shaven; I trow he were a mare or a gelding." This is the eunuch-like caricature of femininity that most people associate with homosexuality. In the 1960s he may be the catty hairdresser or the lisping, limp-wristed interior decorator. His lesbian counterpart is the "butch,"

Nice, looking Men

the girl who is aggressively masculine to the point of trying to look like a man. Blatants also include "leather boys," who advertise their sadomasochism by wearing leather jackets and chains, and certain transvestites, or "Tvs." (Other transvestites are not homosexuals at all and, while they enjoy dressing in female clothing, may also have women as sex partners.) Actually, such stereotype "queers" are a distinct minority. Paul Gebhard, director of Alfred Kinsey's Institute for Sex Research, estimates that only around 10% of all homosexuals are immediately recognizable. Blatants often draw sneers from other homosexuals, and in fact many of them are only going through a phase. Having recently "come out"—admitted their condition and joined the homosexual world—they feel insecure in their new roles and try to re-create their personalities from scratch. Behaving the way they think gay people are supposed to behave, they too temporarily fall victim to the myth.

The Secret Lifer. The other 90% of the nation's committed inverts are hidden from all but their friends, lovers, and occasionally, psychiatrists. Their wrists are rigid, their "s's" well formed; they prefer subdued clothes and closecropped hair, and these days may dress more conservatively than flamboyant straights. Many wear wedding rings and have wives, children and employers who never know. They range across all classes, all races, all occupations. To lead their double lives these full or part-time homosexuals must "pass" as straight, and most are extremely skilled at camouflage. They can cynically tell—or at least smile at—jokes about "queers;" they fake enjoyment when their boss throws a stag party with nude movies.

The Desperate. Members of this group are likely to haunt public toilets ("tearooms") or Turkish baths. They may be pathologically drawn to sex but emotionally unable to face the slightest strains of sustaining a serious human relationship, or they may be married men who hope to conceal their need by making their contacts as anonymous as possible

The Adjusted. By contrast, they lead relatively conventional lives. They have a regular circle of friends and hold jobs, much like Los Angeles Businessman "Charles Eliott" or Manhattan Secretary "Rachel Porter" described on the last page. Their social lives generally begin at the gay bars or in rounds of private parties. Often they try to settle down with a regular lover, and although these liaisons are generally short-lived among men, some develop into so-called "gay marriages," like the 14-year union between Poets Allen Ginsberg and Peter Orlovsky.

The Bisexual. Many married homosexuals are merely engaging in "alibi sex," faking enjoyment of intercourse with their wives. Some researchers, however, have found a number of men and women who have a definite preference for their own sex but engage in occasional activity with the opposite sex and enjoy it. The description of Julius Caesar's protean sex life probably contained a core of fact: "He was every man's wife and every woman's husband." (Caesar's wife was a different case.)

The Situational Experimental. He is a man who engages in homosexual acts without any deep homosexual motivation. The two Kinsey reports found that almost 40% of white American males and 13% of females have some overt sexual experience to orgasm with a person of their own sex between adolescence and old age. Yet a careful analysis of the figures shows that most of these experiences are only temporary deviations. In prisons and occasionally in the armed forces,* for example, where no women are available. Thus the men frequently turn to homosexual contacts, some in order to reassert their masculinity and recapture a feeling of dominance.

The homosexual subculture, a semipublic world, is, without question, shallow and unstable. Researchers now think that these qualities, while inherent in many homosexuals, are also induced and inflamed by social pressures. The notion that homosexuals cause crime is a homophobic myth: studies of sex offenders show that homosexuals are no more likely to molest young children than are heterosexuals. Homosexuals are more likely to be victims of crime: Sociologists John Gagnon, of the State University of New York at Stony Brook, and William Simon, of the Illinois Institute of Juvenile Research, in a recent survey of homosexuals found that only 10% of them had ever been arrested; by contrast, 10% had been blackmailed and over 25% had been robbed, frequently after being attacked and beaten.

Insecurity and promiscuity go hand in hand. One man told U.C.L.A. Researcher Evelyn Hooker that he had had relations with 1,500 different partners during a 15-year span. Since homosexual couples cannot comfortably meet in mixed company, the gay bars become impersonal "meat racks"—not unlike "swinger" bars for heterosexual singles—whose common denominator is little more than sex. Keeping a gay marriage together require unusual determination, since the partners have no legal contract to stay together for worse or better; there are no children to focus the couple's concern.

The strain of the covert life shows clearly in brittle homosexual humor, which swings between a defensive mockery of the outside world and a self-hating scorn for the gay one. Recent research projects at the Indiana Sex Research Institute and elsewhere have sought out homosexuals who are not troubled enough to come to psychiatrists and social workers and have found them no worse adjusted than many heterosexuals. Nonetheless, when 300 New York homosexuals were polled several years ago, only 2% said that they would want a son of theirs to be a homosexual. Homophile activists contend that there would be more happy homosexuals if society were more compassionate; still, for the time being at least, there is a savage ring of truth to the now famous line from *The Boys in the Band*: "Show me a happy homosexual, and I'll show you a gay corpse."

How and Why?

What leads to homosexuality? No one knows for sure, and many of the explanations seem overly simple and unnecessarily doctrinaire. Sociologist Gagnon says: "We may eventually conclude that there are as many causes for homosexuality as there are for mental retardation—and as many kinds of it." The only thing most experts agree on is that homosexuality is not a result of any kinky gene or hormone predispositions—at least none that can be detected by present techniques. Male and female homosexuals do not constitute a "third sex"; biologically, they are full men and women.

The reason that the invert's sex behavior is not dictated by his anatomy is related to a remarkable finding of sex researchers:

*As Winston Churchill said of the traditions of the Royal Navy just before World War I: "What are they? Rum, sodomy and the lash."

no one becomes fully male or female automatically. The diverse psychological components of masculinity and femininity—"gender role identity"—are learned. Gender is like language, says John Hopkins University Medical Psychologist John Money: ',Genetics ordains only that language can develop, not whether it will be Nahuatl, Arabic or English."

This does not mean that homosexuality is latent in all mature humans, as has been widely believed from a misreading of Freud. In American culture, sex roles are most powerfully determined in the home, and at such a young age (generally in the first few years of life) that the psychological identity of most homosexuals—like that of most heterosexuals—is set before they know it. In the case of homosexuality, parents with emotional problems can be a powerful cause, leaving their child without a solid identification with the parent of the same sex and with deeply divided feelings for the parent of the opposite sex. In an exhaustive study of homosexuals in therapy, a group of researchers headed by Psychoanalyst Irving Bieber observed that a large number of homosexuals came from families where the father was either hostile, aloof or ineffectual and where the mother was close-binding and inappropriately intimate (CBI in scientific jargon). Bieber's wife, Psychologist Toby Bieber, has found many of the same patterns in the parents of lesbians, although in reverse.

Yet scientists have begun to realize that the homosexual hang-up is not exclusively homemade. For one thing, social pressures can unbalance parents' child-raising practices. Marvin Opler, an anthropologist trained in psychoanalysis who teaches at the State University of New York at Buffalo, says that Western culture generally, and the U.S. in particular, puts such a high premium on male competition and dominance that men easily become afraid that they are not measuring up, and take out their frustrations by being hostile to their sons.

The accepted notion that boys and girls should ignore each other until puberty and then concentrate heavily on dating can also distort parental attitudes. If a mother catches a little boy playing doctor with a little girl under the porch and tells him he has been bad, says Gebhard, she may be subtly telling him that sex with girls is bad: "Anything that discourages heterosexuality encourages homosexuality." If an uptight parent or teacher catches an impressionable adolescent boy in sexual experiments with other boys and leaps to the conclusion that he is a homosexual, the scoldings he gets may make him freeze up with girls in another way. He may start to think that if everyone considers him a homosexual, he must be one. Many schools compound the problem by enshrining the supermale and overemphasizing sports. The inevitable peer group yelling "Sissy!" at the drop of a fly ball can also start the long and complicated process by which a boy can come to think of himself as "different."

So potent is the power of suggestion, says Psychologist Evelyn Hooker, that one male need never have been sexually aroused by another to begin thinking of himself as gay. The unathletic, small, physically attractive youth is particularly prone to being singled out for "sissyhood," and authorities agree that it is this social selection rather than anything genetic that makes homosexuality somewhat more common among so-called "pretty boys."

Most experts agree that a child will not become a homosexual unless he undergoes many emotionally disturbing experiences during the course of several years. A boy who likes dolls or engages in occasional homosexual experiment is not necessarily "queer": such activities are often a normal part of growing up. On the other hand, a child who becomes preoccupied with such interests or is constantly ill at ease with the opposite sex obviously needs some form of psychiatric counseling. While only about one-third of confirmed adult inverts can be helped to change, therapists agree that a much larger number of "pre-homosexual" children can be treated successfully.

Changing Sexual Roles

A more elusive question is whether or to what extent homosexuality and acceptance of it may be symptoms of social decline. For varying reasons, homosexual relations have been condoned and at times even encouraged among certain males in many primitive societies that anthropologists have studied. However, few scholars have been able to determine that homosexuality had any effect on the functioning of those cultures. At their fullest flowering, the Persian, Greek, Roman and Moslem civilizations permitted a measure of homosexuality; as they decayed, it became more prevalent. Sexual deviance of every variety was common during the Nazis' virulent and corrupt rule of Germany.

Homosexuality was also common in Elizabethan England's atmosphere of wholesale permissiveness. Yet the era not only produced one of the most robust literary and intellectual outpourings the world has ever known but also laid the groundwork for Britain's later imperial primacy—during which time homosexuality became increasingly stigmatized.

In the U.S. today, homosexuality has scarcely reached the proportions of a symptom of widespread decadence (though visitors sometimes wonder as they observe the lounging male whores on New York's Third Avenue or encounter male couples embracing effusively in public parks). Still, the acceptance or rejection of homosexuality does raise questions about the moral values of the society: its hedonism, its concern with individual "identity." The current conceptions of what causes homosexuality also pose a fundamental challenge to traditional ideas about the proper role to be played by all men and women. In recent years, Americans have learned that a man need not be a Met pitcher or suburban Don Juan to be masculine: the most virile male might well be a choreographer or a far-out artist. Similarly, as more and more women become dissatisfied with their traditional roles, Americans may better understand that a female can hold a highly competitive job—or drive a truck—without being forced to sacrifice her sexuality or the satisfactions of child rearing. A nation that softens the long and rigid separation of roles for men and women is also less likely to condemn the homosexual and confine him to a netherworld existence.

Morality and Tolerance

The case for greater tolerance of homosexuals is simple. Undue discrimination wastes talents that might be working for society. Police harassment, which still lingers in many cities and more small towns, despite a growing live-and-let-live attitude, wastes manpower and creates unnecessary suffering. The laws against homosexual acts also suggest that the nation cares more about enforcing private morality than it does about preventing violent crime. To be sure, it is likely that a more permissive atmosphere might convince many people, particularly adolescents, that a homosexual urge need not be resisted since the condition would, after all, be "respectable." On the other hand, greater tolerance might mitigate extreme fear of not being able to live up to exaggerated standards of heterosexual performance—and might thus reduce the number of committed homosexuals.

A violently argued issue these days is whether the confirmed homosexual is mentally ill. Psychoanalysts insist that homosexuality is a form of sickness; most homosexuals and many experts counter that the medical concept only removes the already fading stigma of sin, and replaces it with the charge—even more pejorative nowadays—that homosexuality is pathological. The answers will importantly influence society's underlying attitude. While homosexuality is a serious and sometimes crippling maladjustment, research has made clear that it is no longer necessary or morally justifiable to treat all inverts as outcasts. The challenge to American society is simultaneously to devise civilized ways of discouraging the condition and to alleviate the anguish of those who cannot be helped, or do not wish to be.

A Discussion: Are Homosexuals Sick?

One of the crucial issues in the public discussion about homosexuality is whether or not the condition is a mental illness. To try to find out, TIME asked eight experts on homosexuality—including two admitted homosexuals—to discuss the subject at a symposium in New York City. The participants: Robin Fox British-born anthropologist at Rutgers University; John Gagnon, sociologist at the State University of New York; Lionel Tiger, a Canadian sociologist also at Rutgers; Wardell Pomeroy, a psychologist who co-authored the Kinsey reports on men and on women and who is now a psychotherapist; Dr. Charles Socarides, a psychoanalyst who has seen scores of homosexuals in therapy and is associate clinical professor of psychiatry at Albert Einstein College of Medicine in The Bronx; the Rev. Robert Weeks, an Episcopal priest who has arranged for the meetings of a homosexual discussion group to take place at his Manhattan church; Dick Leitsch a homosexual who is executive director of the Mattachine Society of New York; and Franklin Kameny, an astronomer and homosexual who is founder-president of the Mattachine Society of Washington.

Kameny: All the homosexuals whom you have explored in depth were patients or others in clinical circumstances. So how do you know that all the ones who wouldn't come near you are sick and suffer from severe anxieties?

Socarides: We do hear, from people who are in treatment, about their friends in homosexual life and some of these also come to us. They see around them a complete disaster to their lives. They see that the most meaningful human relationship is denied them—the male-female relationship.

Tiger: There is a lack of a tragic sense here. All people have problems. I have all kinds of anxieties: everybody I know has anxieties. Some of them are severe; some of them are not severe. Often they are severe at different stages of the life cycle and for different reasons. To pick on homosexuals in this particular way, as on Communists or Moslems in another, is to shortchange their option for their own personal destiny.

Socarides: By God, they should live in the homosexual world if they want to! No one is arguing that point; no one is trying to say that a homosexual should be forced to seek help. Everybody is now saying that the homosexual needs compassion and understanding, the way the neurotic does or anybody else suffering from any illness. That is true. I agree with that.

Weeks: I think that historically the church has had a very hypocritical view of homosexuality. Instead of accepting the totality of sexuality, the church is still a little uncomfortable with the total sexual response; it still insists that people conform to a certain type of sexual behavior.

Fox: I was talking to a very pretty American girl recently who said that her first reaction to European males was one of considerable shock because the kind of touching behavior between males, was something that she would have been horrified to see in the men she had grown up with. This strikes me as a very American attitude, because of its rigidity, because of its absolute exclusiveness, because of its treatment of this as something horrible and beyond the pale.

Gagnon: There is no explanation for this attitude unless you want to take Ken Tynan's explanation, which is that people think that people ought to be alike, and anyone who didn't get wife, have spear and carry shield was bad juju, and you threw him out of the crowd.

Leitsch: It has always struck me that one of the primary reasons for the American attitude toward homosexuality is that we are so close to our agrarian background. When America was first settled, we had a hell of a big country to fill up, and we had to fill it up in a hurry. We have never been big enough to be decadent before.

Fox: Yes, America has to learn to be decadent gracefully, I think.

Weeks: I just finished counseling a person who was addicted to the men's room in Grand Central Station. He knows he is going to get busted by the cops; yet he has to go there every day. I think I did succeed in getting him to cease going to the Grand Central men's room, perhaps in favor of gay bars. This is a tremendous therapeutic gain for this particular man. But he is sick; he does need help. However, I don't think Dr. Socarides is talking about people like another acquaintance of mine, a man who has been "married" to another homosexual for fifteen years. Both of them are very happy and very much in love. They asked me to bless their marriage, and I am going to do it.

Pomeroy: I think they are beautiful. I don't think they are sick at all.

Socarides: In medicine we are taught that sickness is the failure of function. For example, a gall bladder is pathological precisely when it ceases to function or its functioning is impaired. A human being is sick when he fails to function in his appropriate gender identity, which is appropriate to his anatomy. A homosexual who has no other choice is sick in his particular way. Is the man who goes to the "tearooms" any more or less sick than the two men in this "married" relationship? No. I think they are all the same. However, I think that perhaps the element of masochism or self-punitive behavior is greater in the man who will go openly, publicly, and endanger himself in this particular way.

Fox: You seem to say that the anxieties provoke a homosexual into seeking a partner of the same sex. Isn't it possible that he prefers such a partner, and that this provokes anxieties?

Socarides: If his actions are a matter of preference, then he would not be considered a true obligatory homosexual.

Gagnon: I am troubled here by the sense of intellectual and historical narrowness.

We should not get hung up on the 20th century nuclear family as the natural order of man, living in the suburbs and having three kids, or on the kind of Viennese-Jewish comparison that Freud really created. All of a sudden, I find a new penisology—that somehow the shape of the penis and of the vagina dictate the shape of human character. I have a minimum definition of mental health. You don't end up in a psychiatrist's office or in the hands of the police, you stay out of jail, you keep a job, you pay your taxes, and you don't worry people too much. That is called mental health. Nobody ever gets out of it alive. There is no way to succeed.

Socarides: Freud's test was a person's ability to have a healthy sexual relationship with a person of the opposite sex and to enjoy his work.

Fox: A psychoanalyst says that we are destined to heterosexual union, and anything that deviates from this must by definition be sick. This is nonsense even in animal terms. Animal communities can tolerate quite a lot of homosexual relationships. The beautiful paradigm of this is geese. Two male geese can form a bond that is exactly like the bond between males and females. They function as a male-female pair; and geese, as far as I can see, are a very successful species.

So far as the two "married" individuals are concerned, they are engaged in what to them is a meaningful and satisfying relationship. What I would define as a sick person in sexual terms would be someone who could not go through the full sequence of sexual activity, from seeing and admiring to following, speaking, touching, and genital contact. A rapist, a person who makes obscene telephone calls—these seem to me sick people, and I don't think it matters a damn whether the other person is of the same sex or not.

Socarides: The homosexuals who come to our office tell us: "We are alone, we are despairing, we cannot join the homosexual society—this would be giving up. We like what they are doing, but we will not join them in terms of calling ourselve normal. We are giving up our heritage, our very lives. We know how we suffer. Only you will know how we suffer, because we will tell only you how we suffer." As a physician, I am bothered by this, because I deal with the suffering of human beings.

Pomeroy: I am not speaking facetiously, but I think it would be best to say that all homosexuals are sick, that all heterosexuals are sick, that the population is sick. Let us get rid of this term and look at people as people. I have heard psychiatrists perfectly soberly say that 95% of all the population in the U.S. is mentally ill.

Gagnon: The issue is that the society can afford it and the homosexuals cannot. The society can afford 4% of its population to be homosexuals and treat them as it wishes, as it does the 10% who are black. The homosexual pays a terrible price for the way the society runs itself. This is central to the daily life of the homosexual. Can he get a job? Can he do this? Can he do that? If we took the law off the books tomorrow, the homosexual would still pay a very high price.

Kameny: One of the major problems we have to face is the consequences of these attitudes, which are poisonous to the individual's self-esteem and self-confidence. The individual is brainwashed into a sense of his own inferiority, just as other minorities are. When we are told "You are sick," and "You are mentally ill," that finishes the destruction.

Pomeroy: If I were to base my judgment of homosexuals, both male and female, on the people who come to me in my practice, I think I would agree that they are sick, that they are upset in many, many different ways. But I had 20 years of research experience prior to this, in which I found literally hundreds of people who would never go to a therapist. They don't want help. They are happy homosexuals.

Socarides: I guess some of you feel that obligatory homosexuality is not an illness, that homosexuality should be proposed as a normal form of sexuality to all individuals. I think that this would be a disaster. A little boy might go next door to the Y and an older man might say to him, "Look, this is normal, my son. Just join me in this." If you sell this bill of goods to the nation, you are doing irreparable harm, and there will be a tremendous backlash against the homosexual.

Fox: I went through the English school system, which everybody knows is a homosexual system in the very fullest sense. Speaking as an obligatory heterosexual on behalf of myself and the other 90%, we went through it, we enjoyed it, we came out the other end, and we are fine. Some people have strayed about somewhere in the middle. This notion, therefore, that if you catch somebody and tell him that homosexuality is normal and practice it with him, he is necessarily going to get stuck in it, is absolutely nonsense. And I cite my three daughters as evidence.

Socarides: The only place to get the material that will tell us the truth about what the homosexual suffers is in-depth analysis. Sociologists, anthropologists, even psychologists do not tell us what is going on in the basic psyche of the homosexual. I believe we should change the laws. I believe that homosexuals have been persecuted. The homosexual must be seen as a full-fledged citizen in a free society and must be given all the rights and prerogatives that all other citizens enjoy, neither more nor less. I think, however, that we must do one other thing. It must be declared that homosexuality is a form of emotional illness, which can be treated, that these people can be helped.

Kameny: With that, you will surely destroy us.

Four Lives in the Gay World

The personal experiences related below are those of a male homosexual, a lesbian and a girl who calls herself bisexual, and a former homosexual who has undergone extensive psychotherapy. In otherwise candid interviews with TIME correspondents, all four requested that they be identified by pseudonyms.

Charles Eliott, 40, owns a successful business in Los Angeles. In the den of his $60,000 house he has a bronze profile of Abe Lincoln on the wall and a copy of *Playboy* on the coffee table. Wearing faded chinos and a button-down Oxford shirt, he looks far more subdued than the average Hollywood male; he might be the happily married coach of a college basketball team—and a thoroughgoing heterosexual. In fact, his male lover for the past three months has been a 21-year-old college student. He says: "I live in a completely gay world. My lawyer is gay, my doctor is gay, my dentist is gay, my banker is gay. The only person who is not gay is my housekeeper, and sometimes I wonder how he puts up with us."

Eliott has never been to an analyst; introspection is not his forte. Why did he become homosexual? "Well, my mother was an alcoholic; my brother and I ate alone every night. I was the person who always went to the circus with the chauffeur. But I wouldn't say I was exactly sad as a child; I was rather outward-going."

He went to prep school at Hotchkiss, and on to Yale. There he discovered his homosexual tendencies.

Eliott returned home to Chicago to run the family business; to maintain his status in the community, he married. It lasted five months. After the divorce he married again, this time for two years; "She began to notice that I didn't enjoy sex, and that finally broke it up. I don't think she knows even today that I am a homosexual."

It took ten years to make Eliott give up his double life in Chicago for the uninhibited world of Los Angeles. He avoids the gay bars, instead throws catered parties around his pool. "I suppose most of my neighbors know," he says. "When you have 100 men over to your house for cocktails, people are going to suspect something. Now that I no longer try to cope with the straight world, I feel much happier."

"If Katie were a man, I would marry her and be faithful to her the rest of my life." So vows Rachel Porter, 21, who is slightly plump, wears her blonde hair in a pert pixy cut, and works as a secretary in a Manhattan publishing firm. Rachel has been seeing Katie Burns, a tall, strikingly handsome private secretary in a large corporation, for three years now, and sharing an apartment with her for three months. Yet Rachel's feelings are mixed. "I don't really say to this day that I am a lesbian," she says. "I'm bisexual. My interests are definitely guys, and eventually I'd like to have a child or two, probably out of wedlock." Katie, by contrast, in the past three years has given up dates with men.

Rachel grew up in the large family of a plumber who was too poor to send her to college. "I probably wouldn't know that a good relationship was possible if it wasn't for my mother and father. I was pretty much of a loner, and to this day I do horrible things like going to the movies alone. I never had a crush on a girl; I had an affair with a boy behind my parents' back when I was 18."

Rachel met Katie shortly after that affair ended. "Gradually there was definitely a growing feeling," she recalls. "When I realized it, I was very upset. I didn't want to be gay. When I first went to a psychologist, I thought, "Gee, I'm such a creep!" I thought that being in love with a girl made me a boy. He told me that I most certainly was not a boy. I couldn't erase the fact that I loved another woman, but I began thinking that as long as I was a woman too, things couldn't be all that bad."

Rachel and Katie have both told their parents about their relationship. "Our mothers both said, 'You're my daughter and I love you anyway,' " says Rachel. They refuse to live an exclusively gay life and engage in tennis, horseback riding and softball games with a circle of many straight friends (who also know the nature of their relationship). Muses Rachel: "Do I see myself living with Katie the rest of my life? Off and on, yes. I will probably date, because it's nice to get involved with other people, but that's difficult to work out. I certainly don't think our relationship ought to be exclusive. All I know is that life ought to be loving."

What was it like to be gay? "There were peaks and valleys of despair," says Tom Kramer, 28, a tall New York City public relations man who was a practicing homosexual until 2-1/2 years ago. "Throughout high school and college, I would try to put it out of my mind. I had sissified gestures, and when I was with people I would concentrate on not using them. I would constantly think they were talking about my homosexuality behind my back. In my homosexual contacts, I'd try to be surreptitious, not telling my name or what kind of work I did. When I read about somebody being a pervert, it was like a slap in the face—my God, that's what I am!"

Two years after college, and weighed down with feelings of hopelessness, Tom heard that therapy was possible for homosexuals and went into treatment with an analyst. His prognosis was good: unlike many homosexuals, he desperately wanted to change. Twice a week for two years he discussed his past: the disciplinarian father who said Tom should have got straight A's when he got only A-minuses; the mother who made Tom her favorite. Gradually, Tom says, "I learned that my homosexuality was a way of handling anxiety. Some men drink. My way was homosexuality.

The process went slowly. Strengthened by insights gained in treatment, at one point Tom finally brought himself to kiss a girl good night—and became so terrified that he "cruised" on the way home for a homosexual partner. Two and a half years ago, however, he had his last male assignation, and several months later he "met a wonderful girl. We dated steadily. We had an affair. It was the first time I had had actual intercourse, and it was the happiest moment of my life." Six months ago, he and the girl were married.

Tom is still in analysis, attempting to cope with problems stemming from the same fears that led to his homosexuality. But he is self-confident about sex. "Women arouse me now," he says. "It's a total reversal." He has discussed his therapy with homosexual friends and urged them to attempt the same thing—so far without success. Ironically, though he is no longer attracted to them sexually, Tom says: "I like men better now than I did before. I'm no longer afraid of them."

Motherhood: Who Needs It?

2

by Betty Rollin

Motherhood is in trouble, and it ought to be. A rude question is long overdue: Who needs it? The answer used to be (1) society and (2) women. But now, with the impending horrors of overpopulation, society desperately doesn't need it. And women don't need it either. Thanks to The Motherhood Myth—the idea that having babies is something that all normal women instinctively want and need and will enjoy doing—they just think they do.

The notion that the maternal wish and the activity of mothering are instinctive or biologically predestined is baloney. Try asking most sociologists, psychologists, psychoanalysts, biologists—many of whom are mothers—about motherhood being instinctive; it's like asking department-store presidents if their Santa Clauses are real. "Motherhood—instinctive?" shouts distinguished sociologist/author Dr. Jessie Bernard. "Biological destiny? Forget biology! If it were biology, people would die from not doing it."

"Women don't need to be mothers any more than they need spaghetti," says Dr. Richard Rabkin, a New York psychiatrist. "But if you're in a world where everyone is eating spaghetti, thinking they need it and want it, you will think so too. Romance has really contaminated science. So-called instincts have to do with stimulation. They are not things that well up inside of you."

SOURCE: Reprinted from the September 22, 1970 issue of LOOK, Volume 34, No. 19.

"When a woman says with feeling that she craved her baby from within, she is putting into biological language what is psychological," says University of Michigan psychoanalyst and motherhood-researcher Dr. Frederick Wyatt. "There are no instincts," says Dr. William Goode, president-elect of the American Sociological Association. "There are reflexes, like eye-blinking, and drives, like sex. There is no innate drive for children. Otherwise, the enormous cultural pressures that there are to reproduce wouldn't exist. There are no cultural pressures to sell you on getting your hand out of the fire."

There are, to be sure, biologists and others who go on about biological destiny, that is, the innate or instinctive goal of motherhood. (At the turn of the century, even good old capitalism was explained by a theorist as "the instinct of acquisitiveness.") And many psychoanalysts still hold the Freudian view that women feel so rotten about not having a penis that they are necessarily propelled into the child-wish to replace the missing organ. Psychoanalysts also make much of the psychological need to repeat what one's parents of the same sex has done. Since every woman has a mother, it is considered normal to wish to imitate one's mother.

There is, surely, a wish to pass on love if one has received it, but to insist women must pass it on in the same way is like insisting that every man whose father is a gardener has to be a gardener. One dissenting psychoanalyst says, simply, "There is a wish to comply with one's biology, yes, but we needn't and sometimes shouldn't," (Interestingly, the woman who has been the greatest contributor to child therapy and who has probably given more to children than anyone alive is Dr. Anna Freud, Freud's magnificent daughter, who is not a mother.)

Anyway, what an expert cast of hundreds is telling us is, simply, that biological possibility and desire are not the same as biological need. Women have childbearing equipment. To choose not to use the equipment is no more blocking what is instinctive than it is for a man who, muscles or no, chooses not to be a weight lifter.

So much for the wish. What about the "instinctive" activity of mothering. One animal study shows that when a young member of a species is put in a cage, say, with an older member of the same species, the latter will act in a protective, "maternal" way. But that goes for both males and females who have been "mothered" themselves. And studies indicate that a human baby will also respond to whoever is around playing mother—even if it's father. Margaret Mead and many others frequently point out that mothering can be a fine occupation, if you want it, for either sex. Another experiment with monkeys who were brought up without mothers found them lacking in maternal behavior toward their own offspring. A similar study showed that monkeys brought up without other monkeys of the opposite sex had no interest in mating—all of which suggests that both mothering and mating behavior are learned, not instinctual. And, to turn the cart (or the baby carriage) around, baby ducks who lovingly follow their mothers seemed, in the mother's absence, to just as lovingly follow wooden ducks or even vacuum cleaners.

If motherhood isn't instinctive, when and why, then, was The Motherhood Myth born? Until recently, the entire question of maternal motivation was academic. Sex, like it or not, meant babies. Not that there haven't always been a lot of interesting contraceptive tries. But until the creation of the diaphragm in the 1880's, the birth of babies was largely unavoidable. And, generally speaking, nobody really seemed to mind. For one thing, people tend to be sort of good sports about what seems to be inevitable.

For another, in the past, the population needed beefing up. Mortality rates were high, and agricultural cultures, particularly, have always needed children to help out. So because it "just happened" and because it was needed, motherhood was assumed to be innate.

Originally, it was the word of God that got the ball rolling with "Be fruitful and multiply," a practical suggestion, since the only people around then were Adam and Eve. But in no time, super-moralists like St. Augustine changed the tone of the message: "Intercourse, even with one's legitimate wife is unlawful and wicked where the conception of the offspring is prevented," he, we assume, thundered. And the Roman Catholic position was thus cemented. So then and now, procreation took on a curious value among people who viewed (and view) the pleasures of sex as sinful. One could partake in the sinful pleasure, but feel vindicated by the ensuing birth. Motherhood cleaned up sex. Also, it cleaned up women, who have always been considered somewhat evil, because of Eve's transgression (". . . but the woman was deceived and became a transgressor. Yet woman will be saved through bearing children . . .", I Timothy, 2:14-15) and somewhat dirty because of menstruation.

And so, based on need, inevitability and pragmatic fantasy—the Myth worked, from society's point of view—the Myth grew like corn in Kansas. And society reinforced it with both laws and propaganda—laws that made woman a chattel, denied her education and personal mobility, and madonna propaganda that said she was beautiful and wonderful doing it and it was all beautiful and wonderful to do. (One rarely sees a madonna washing dishes.)

In fact, the Myth persisted—breaking some kind of record for long-lasting fallacies—until something like yesterday. For as truth about the Myth trickled in—as women's rights increased, as women gradually got the message that it was certainly possible for them to do most things that men did, that they live longer, that their brains were not tinier—then, finally, when the really big news rolled in, that they could choose whether or not to be mothers—what happened? The Motherhood Myth soared higher than ever. As Betty Friedan made oh-so-clear in The Feminine Mystique, the '40's and '50's produced a group of ladies who not only had babies as if they were going out of style (maybe they were) but, as never before, they turned motherhood into a cult. First, they wallowed in the aesthetics of it all—natural childbirth and nursing became maternal musts. Like heavy-bellied ostriches, they grounded their heads in the sands of motherhood, only coming up for air to say how utterly happy and fulfilled they were. But, as Mrs. Friedan says only too plainly, they weren't. The Myth galloped on, moreover, long after making babies had turned from practical asset to liability for both individual parents and society. With the average cost of a middle-class child figured conservatively at $30,000 (not including college), any parent knows that the only people who benefit economically from children are manufacturers of consumer goods. Hence all those gooey motherhood commercials. And the Myth gathered momentum long after sheer numbers, while not yet extinguishing us, have made us intensely uncomfortable. Almost all of our societal problems, from minor discomforts like traffic to major ones like hunger, the population people keep reminding us, have to do with there being too many people. And who suffers most? The kids who have been so mindlessly brought into the world, that's who. They are the ones who have to cope with all of the difficult and dehumanizing conditions brought on by overpopulation. They are the ones who have to cope with psychological nausea of feeling unneeded by society. That's not the only reason for drugs, but, surely, it's a leading contender.

Unfortunately, the population curbers are tripped up by a romantic, stubborn, ideological hurdle. How can birth-control programs really be effective as long as the concept of glorious motherhood remains unchanged? (Even poor old Planned Parenthood has to euphemize—why not Planned Unparenthood?) Particularly among the poor, motherhood is one of the few inherently positive institutions that are accessible. As Berkeley demographer Judith Blake points out, "Poverty-oriented birth control programs do not make sense as a welfare measure . . . as long as existing pronatalist policies . . . encourage mating, pregnancy and the care, support, and rearing of children." Or, she might have added, as long as the less-than idyllic childrearing part of motherhood remains "in small print."

Sure, motherhood gets dumped on sometimes: Philip Wylie's Momism got going in the '40's and Philip Roth's *Portnoy's Complaint* did its best to turn rancid the chicken-soup concept of Jewish motherhood. But these are viewed as the sour cries of a black humorist here, a malcontent there. Everyone shudders, laughs, but it's like the mouse and the elephant joke. Still, the Myth persists. Last April, a Brooklyn woman was indicted on charges of manslaughter and negligent homocide—11 children died in a fire in a building she owned and criminally neglected—"But, sputtered her lawyer, "my client, Mrs. Breslow, is a mother, a grandmother and great-grandmother!"

Most remarkably, the Motherhood Myth persists in the face of the most overwhelming maternal unhappiness and incompetence. If reproduction were merely superfluous and expensive, if the experience were as rich and rewarding as the cliche would have us believe, if it were a predominantly joyous trip for everyone riding—mother, father, child—then the going everybody should-have-two-children plan would suffice. Certainly there are a lot of joyous mothers, and their children and (sometimes, not necessarily) their husbands reflect their joy. But a lot of evidence suggests that for more women than anyone wants to admit, motherhood can be miserable. ("If it weren't," says one psychiatrist wryly, "the world wouldn't be in the mess it's in.")

There is a remarkable statistical finding from a recent study of Dr. Bernard's, comparing the mental illness and unhappiness of married mothers and single women. The latter group, it turned out, was both markedly less sick and overtly more happy. Of course, it's not easy to measure slippery attitudes like happiness. "Many women have achieved a kind of reconciliation —a conformity," says Dr. Bernard, "that they interpret as happiness. Since feminine happiness is supposed to lie in devoting one's life to one's husband and children, they do that; so ipso facto, they assume they are happy. And for many women, untrained for independence and 'processed' for motherhood, they find their state far preferable to the alternatives, which don't really exist." Also, unhappy mothers are often loath to admit it. For one thing, if in society's view not to be a mother is to be a freak, not to be a blissful mother is to be a witch. Besides, unlike a disappointing marriage, disappointing motherhood cannot be terminated by divorce. Of course, none of that stops such a woman from expressing her dissatisfaction in a variety of ways. Again, it is not only she who suffers but her husband and children as well. Enter the harridan housewife, the carping shrew. The realities of motherhood can turn women into terrible people. And, judging from the 50,000 cases of child abuse in the U.S. each year, some are worse than terrible.

In some cases, the unpleasing realities of motherhood begin even before the beginning. In *Her Infinite Variety*, Morton Hunt describes young married women pregnant for the first time as "very likely to be frightened and depressed, masking these feelings in order not to be considered contemptible. The arrival of pregnancy interrupts a pleasant dream of motherhood and awakens them to the realization that they have too little money, or not enough space, or unresolved marital problems . . ."

The following are random quotes from interviews with some mothers in Ann Arbor, Michigan, who described themselves as reasonably happy. They all had positive things to say about their children, although when asked about the best moment of their day, they all confessed it was when the children were in bed. Here is the rest:

"Suddenly I had to devote myself to the child totally. I was under the illusion that the baby was going to fit into my life, and I found that I had to switch my life and my schedule to fit him. You think, 'I'm in love, I'll get married, and we'll have a baby.' First there's two, then three, it's simple and romantic. You don't even think about the work" . . . "You never get away from the responsibility. Even when you leave the children with a sitter, you are not out from under the pressure of the responsibility . . ." "I hate ironing their pants and doing their underwear, and they never put their clothes in the laundry basket . . . As they get older, they make less demands on your time because they're in school, but the demands are greater in forming their values . . . Best moment of the day is when all the children are in bed . . . The worst time of day is 4 p.m., when you have to get dinner started, the kids are tired, hungry and crabby—everybody wants to talk to you about their day . . . your day is only half over."

"Once a mother, the responsibility and concern for my children became so encompassing . . . It took a great deal of will to keep up other parts of my personality . . . To me, motherhood gets harder as they get older because you have less control . . . In an abstract sense, I'd have several . . . In the non-abstract, I would not have any" . . . "I had anticipated that the baby would sleep and eat, sleep and eat. Instead, the experience was overwhelming. I really had not thought particularly about what motherhood would mean in a realistic sense. I want to do other things, like to become involved in things that are worthwhile—I don't mean women's clubs—but I don't have the physical energy to go out in the evenings. I feel like I'm missing something . . . the experience of being somewhere with people and having them talking about something—something that's going on in the world."

Every grown-up person expects to pay a price for his pleasures, but seldom is the price as vast as the one endured "however happily" by most mothers. We have mentioned the literal cost factor. But what does that mean? For middle-class American women; it means a life-style with severe and usually unimagined limitations; i.e., life in the suburbs, because who can afford three bedrooms in the city? And what do suburbs mean? For women, suburbs mean other women and children and leftover peanut-butter sandwiches and car pools and seldom-seen husbands. Even the Feminine Mystiqueniks—the housewives who finally admitted that their lives behind brooms (OK, electric brooms) were driving them crazy—were loath to trace their predicament to their children. But it is simply a fact that a childless married woman has no child-work and little housework. She can live in a city, or, if she still chooses the suburbs or the country, she can leave on the commuter train with her husband if she wants to. Even the most ardent job-seeking mother will find little in the way of great opportunities in Scarsdale. Besides, by the time she wakes up, she usually lacks both the preparation for the outside world and the self-confidence to get it. You will say there are plenty of city-dwelling working mothers. But most of those women do additional-funds-for-the-family kind of work, not the interesting career kind that takes plugging during "childbearing years."

Nor is it a bed of petunias for the mother who does make it professionally. Says writer/critic Marya Mannes: "If the creative woman has children, she must pay for this indulgence with a long burden of guilt, for her life will be split three ways between them and her husband and her work . . . No woman with any heart can compose a paragraph when her child is in trouble . . . The creative woman has no wife to protect her from intrusion. A man at his desk in a room with closed door is a man at work. A woman at a desk in any room is available."

Speaking of jobs, do remember that mothering, salary or not, is a job. Even those who can afford nurses to handle the nitty-gritty still need to put out emotionally. "Well-cared-for" neurotic rich kids are not exactly unknown in our society. One of the more absurd aspects of the Myth is the underlying assumption that, since most women are biologically equipped to bear children, they are psychologically, mentally, emotionally and technically equipped (or interested) to rear them. Never mind happiness. To assume that such an exacting, consuming and important task is something almost all women are equipped to do is far more dangerous and ridiculous than assuming that everyone with vocal chords should seek a career in the opera.

A major expectation of the Myth is that children make a not-so-hot marriage hotter, or a hot marriage, hotter still. Yet almost every available study indicates that childless marriages are far happier. One of the biggest, of 850 couples, was conducted by Dr. Harold Feldman of Cornell University, who states his finding in no uncertain terms: "Those couples with children had a significantly lower level of marital satisfaction than did those without children." Some of the reasons are obvious. Even the most adorable children make for additional demands, complications and hardships in the lives of even the most loving parents. If a woman feels disappointed and trapped in her mother role, it is bound to affect her marriage in any number of ways: she may take out her frustrations directly on her husband, or she may count on him too heavily for what she feels she is missing in her daily life.

". . . You begin to grow away from your husband," says one of the Michigan ladies. "He's working on his career and you're working on your family. But you both must gear your lives to the children. You do things the children enjoy, more than things you might enjoy." More subtle and possibly more serious is what motherhood may do to a woman's sexuality. Often when the stork flies in, sexuality flies out. Both in the emotional minds of some women and in the minds of their husbands, when a woman becomes a mother, she stops being a woman. It's not only that motherhood may destroy her physical attractiveness, but its madonna concept may destroy her feelings of sexuality.

And what of the payoff? Usually, even the most self-sacrificing maternal self-sacrificers expect a little something back. Gratified parents are not unknown to the Western world, but there are probably at least just as many who feel, to put it crudely, shortchanged. The experiment mentioned earlier—where the baby ducks followed vacuum cleaners instead of their mothers—indicates that what passes for love from baby to mother is merely a rudimentary kind of object attachment. Without necessarily feeling like a Hoover, a lot of women become disheartened because babies and children are not only not interesting to talk to (not everyone thrills at the wonders of da-da-ma-ma talk) but they are generally not empathetic, considerate people. Even the nicest children are not capable of empathy, surely a major ingredient of love, until they are much older. Sometimes they're never capable of it. Dr. Wyatt says that often, in later years particularly, when most of the "returns" are in, it is the "good mother" who suffers most of all. It is then she must face a reality: The child—the appendage with her genes—is not an appendage, but a separate person. What's more, he or she may be a separate person who doesn't even like her—or whom she doesn't really like.

So if the music is lousy, how come everyone's dancing? Because the mother hood minuet is taught free from birth, and whether or not she has rhythm or likes the music, every woman is expected to do it. Indeed, she wants to do it. Little girls start learning what to want—and what to be—when they are still in their cribs. Dr. Miriam Keiffer, a young social psychologist at Bensalem, The Experimental College of Fordham University, points to studies showing that "at six months of age, mothers are already treating their baby girls and boys quite differently. For instance, mothers have been found to touch, comfort, and talk to their females more. If these differences can be found at such an early stage, it's not surprising that the end product is as different as it is. What is surprising is that men and women are, in so many ways, similar." Some people point to the way little girls play with dolls as proof of their "innate motherliness." But remember, little girls are given dolls. When Margaret Mead presented some dolls to New Guinea children, it was the boys, not the girls, who wanted to play with them, which they did by crooning lullabies and rocking them in the most maternal fashion.

By the time they reach adolescence, most girls, unconsciously or not, have learned enough about role definition to qualify for a master's degree. In general, the lesson has been that no matter what kind of career thoughts one may entertain, one must, first and foremost, be a wife and mother. A girl's mother is usually her first teacher. As Dr. Goode says, "A woman is not only taught by society to have a child; she is taught to have a child who will have a child." A woman who has hung her life on The Motherhood Myth will almost always reinforce her young married daughter's early training by pushing for grandchildren. Prospective grandmothers are not the only ones. Husbands, too, can be effective sellers. After all, they have The Fatherhood Myth to cope with. A married man is supposed to have children. Often, particularly among Latins, children are a sign of potency. They help him assure the world—and himself—that he is the big man he is supposed to be. Plus, children give him both immortality (whatever that means) and possibly the chance to become "more" in his lifetime through the accomplishments of his children, particularly his son. (Sometimes it's important, however, for the son to do better, but not too much better.)

Friends, too, can be counted on as myth-pushers. Naturally one wants to do what one's friends do. One study, by the way, found an absolute correlation between a woman's fertility and that of her three closest friends. The negative sell comes into play here, too. We have seen what the concept of non-mother means (cold, selfish, unwomanly, abnormal). In practice, particularly in the suburbs, it can mean, simply, exclusion—both from child-centered activities (that is, most activities) and child-centered conversations (that is, most conversations). It can also mean being the butt of a lot of unfunny jokes. ("Whaddya waiting for? An immaculate conception? Ha, ha.") Worst of all, it can mean being an object of pity.

In case she's escaped all of those pressures (that is, if she was brought up in a cave), a young married woman often wants a baby just so that she'll (1) have something to do (motherhood is better than clerk/typist, which is often the only type of job she can get, since little more has been expected of her and, besides, her boss also expects her to leave and be a mother); (2) have something to hug and possess, to be needed by and have power over; and (3) have something to be—e.g., a baby's mother. Motherhood affords an instant identity. First, through wifehood, you are somebody's wife; then you are somebody's mother. Both give not only identity and activity, but status and stardom of a kind. During pregnancy, a woman can look forward to the kind of attention and pampering she may not ever have gotten or may never otherwise get. Some women consider birth the biggest accomplishment of their lives, which may be interpreted as saying not much for the rest of their lives. As Dr. Goode says, "It's like the gambler who may know the roulette wheel is crooked, but it's the only game in town." Also, with motherhood, the feeling of accomplishment is immediate. It is really much faster and easier to make a baby than paint a painting, or write a book, or get to the point of accomplishment in a job. It is also easier in a way to shift focus from self-development to child-development—particularly since, for women, self-development is considered selfish. Even unwed mothers may achieve a feeling of this kind. (As we have seen, little thought is given to the aftermath.) And, again, since so many women are underdeveloped as people, they feel that, besides children, they have little else to give—to themselves, their husbands, to their world.

You may ask why then, when the realities do start pouring in, does a woman want to have a second, third, even fourth child? OK, (1) Just because reality is pouring in doesn't mean she wants to face it. A new baby can help bring back some of the old illusions. Says psychoanalyst Dr. Natalie Shainess, "She may view each successive child as a knight in armor that will rescue her from being a 'bad/unhappy mother' ". (2) Next on the horror list of having no children, is having one. It suffices to say that only children are not only OK, they even have a high rate of exceptionality. (3) Both parents usually want at least one child of each sex. The husband, for reasons discussed earlier, probably wants a son. (4) The more children one has, the more of an excuse one has not to develop in any other way.

What's the point? A world without children? Of course not. Nothing could be worse or more unlikely. No matter what anyone says in LOOK or anywhere else, motherhood isn't about to go out like a blown bulb, and who says it should? Only the Myth must go out, and now it seems to be dimming.

The younger-generation females who have been reared on the Myth have not rejected it totally, but at least they recognize it can be more loving to children not to have them. And at least they speak of adopting children instead of bearing them. Moreover, since the new non-breeders are "less hungup" on ownership, they seem to recognize that if you dig loving children, you don't necessarily have to own one. The end of The Motherhood Myth might make available more loving women (and men) for those children who already exist.

When motherhood is no longer culturally compulsory, there will, certainly, be less of it. Women are now beginning to think and do more about development of self, of their individual resources. Far from being selfish, such development is probably our only hope. That means more alternatives for women. And more alternatives mean more selective, better, happier motherhood—and children and husbandhood (or manhood) and peoplehood. It is not a question of whether or not children are sweet and marvelous to have and rear; the question is, even if that's so, whether or not one wants to pay the price for it. It doesn't make sense any more to pretend that women need babies, when what they really need is themselves. If God were still speaking to us in a voice we could hear, even He would probably say, "Be fruitful. Don't multiply."

3 The New Marriage: Marriage as a Framework for Developing Personal Potential

by Herbert A. Otto

Introduction

It is currently the assumption of many leading behavioral scientists (Abraham Maslow, Margaret Mead, Gardner Murphy, Carl Rogers, and Gordon Allport) that the average healthy human being is functioning at a fraction of his capacity. We often hear that the productive person of today is functioning at 10 per cent of his ability. Margaret Mead quotes a 6 per cent figure, and my own estimate is closer to 5 per cent.[1,2,3]

If we accept this hypothesis, the actualizing of our potential can become the most exciting adventure of our lifetime. Conversely, if we

SOURCE: This Chapter is a revision of an address delivered at the 1969 Convention of the California Personnel and Guidance Association, Anaheim, California.

do not use our energies in a continuous process of self-realization and personal growth, the very same energies are directed into destructive channels. If we do not employ these energies positively to actualize our potential, the energies are "short-circuited" and become destructive to the organism as a whole. In the not-too-distant future, we will discover that there is nothing more destructive to the human personality than the damming, blocking, and shutting off of the processes associated with ongoing personality growth and the actualizing of personal potential.

The lack of commitment to self-realization, together with the lack of framework and opportunity for self-realization, are responsible for much of what is labeled as pathological or asocial behavior, "acting out," etc. Actually, this type of symptomatology must be understood as a symbolic form of communication and is really a cry for help. It is a type of flailing about and seeking of change to the best of the person's ability at that time and moment in his life space. The very anger and hostility that such behavior arouses in us is a very clear indication that the individual is still fighting, that he is still attempting to actualize and has not given up his efforts. I am far more concerned about the vast segments of our population who have, in a sense, given up on life. These people live in quiet desperation, believing themselves trapped, yet fearing to leave the comfort of their entrapment. Most tragically, they do not know that they have a potential to actualize, and therefore, they have little reason to hope.

We must begin to reach this segment of our society which feels relatively hopeless, is committed to the status quo, is dulled by routine, and permeated by boredom. We must reach them with our human potentiality concepts and with opportunities to actualize their potential. It is especially important to reach out to this segment of our society because they form a reservoir of hate and destructiveness which may well set off an epidemic of hate. Yet this reservoir of hatred does offer a dynamic opportunity for social change and regeneration, for by channeling this energy toward the development of individual abilities and talents and the actualizing of personal potential, leadership is thereby created which can then be applied to the regeneration of our social institutions and structures.

Our societal structures and institutions have a great influence on what we call "personality" and the dimensions of our human functioning. The actualizing of our human potential is closely bound to the regeneration of our human institutions. As always, we must begin with ourselves and the institutions with which we are most intimately concerned and connected. Those of us who are married can begin with an assessment of the institution we call marriage.

If two partners envision their marriage as a framework for actualizing personal potential, the following key question becomes pertinent: "Are both partners satisfied with their rate of personal growth while engaged in this ongoing relationship we call marriage?" All too often, marriage results in a dull, stultifying routine, deadly to the growth processes of both marital partners. Many times, boredom and satiation with each other is made tolerable

[1]Herbert A. Otto, ed., Explorations in Human Potentialities (Springfield, Ill., Charles C. Thomas, 1966).
[2]Herbert A, Otto, Guide to Developing Your Potential (New York, Charles Scribner's Sons, 1967).
[3]Herbert A. Otto, ed., Human Potentialities: The Challenge and The Promise (St. Louis, Warren H. Green, 1968).

largely by the devotion and responsibilities attendant to the upbringing of the children. The three ingredients of such a marriage, which are the children, habit, and fear of social stigma, form an unhealthy glue, when it is the only glue which keeps a marriage together. There are more such marriages than we would care to admit. This is the tremendous clinical substratum of "indifferent" or "tolerable" marriages. This type of marriage unfortunately never reaches the counselor, but contributes to massive unhappiness, discontent, and finally the utter capitulation of a life endured, but not lived joyously.

Conversely, marriage can be envisioned as a framework for actualizing personal potential. The concepts, approaches, and methods which have been the outgrowth of research in the area of Human Potentialities can revitalize marriage as an institution. In a large number of instances, where marriage ends in a divorce, one or both partners, consciously or unconsciously, recognize that the nature of the relationship has become progressively inimical to their personality growth and actually impedes, or is destructive to, the actualizing of personal potential. In contrast, the New Marriage offers an ongoing adventure of self-discovery, personal growth, unfoldment, and fulfillment. Growth by its very nature is not smooth or easy, for growth involves change and the emergence of the new. But growth and the actualizing of personal potential is also a joyous and deeply satisfying process which can bring to marriage a new quality of zest for living, of joie de vivre, and of excitement.

The New Marriage: Some Dimensions and Characteristics

There are a number of dimensions and characteristics which, in the aggregate, form a unique Gestalt and distinguish the New Marriage from contemporary marriage patterns.

1. There is clear acknowledgement by both partners concerning the personal relevance of the Human Potentialities hypothesis: that the healthy individual is functioning at a fraction of his potential.

This hypothesis is not yet widely known and is still restricted to a relatively small percentage of the population, mostly to the group with a college education. And, to most of those who are acquainted with the Human Potentialities hypothesis, it remains an idle fact, to be filed away in the storehouse of knowledge. There is no awareness that this datum is personally relevant and should be, or is, leading to personal involvement and action designed to develop potential.

2. Love and understanding become dynamic elements in the actualization of the marital partners' personal potential.

Love and understanding become strong supportive forces which encourage and sustain the marital partners in their commitment to self-unfoldment and personal growth. Both partners are aware that there are methods and approaches available, designed to deepen understanding and strengthen the love relationship. They utilize these techniques to bring their love to fuller flowering, to deepen and expand the affectional flow, and to expand the quality of their understanding. Utilizing their love and understanding, both partners foster and support each other's efforts to become more self-actualizing human beings. They help each other to help themselves. To use contemporary language, in the New Marriage, the two persons are devoted to turning each other on and this turns them on.

3. Both partners in the New Marriage are interested in, and participate in, ongo-

ing growth groups, or groups designed to help them to actualize personal potential.

There is recognition that "we grew into what we are through relationships with people; we grow into what we can be through relationships with people." Husband and wife seek those group experiences which they feel will help them to grow as persons. They are involved in both ongoing group experiences, as well as in individual experiences designed to actualize their personal potential. If possible, they will verbally share these experiential encounters with their marital partner. Currently there are over eighty Growth Centers in the United States, similar to Esalen Institute and Kairos Institute, both in California. (See Appendix for a list of growth centers.) This recent development is often referred to as the Human Potentialities Movement. Growth Centers offer ongoing group experiences, weekend marathons, and seminars led by professionals (psychologists, psychiatrists, counselors, social workers, etc.), all of which are designed to help participants actualize more of their possibilities. The Humanistic psychologists have played a strong role in the genesis of this movement. A very large range of exciting new methods and approaches are available, and new ones are constantly developed. The movement represents the growing edge in the exploration of man's inner universe and the realization of his powers.

4. There is clear recognition by both partners that personality and the actualizing of human potential have much to do with the social institutions and structures within which man functions. The need for institutional regeneration is acknowledged by both partners as being personally relevant, leading to involvement in social action.

The husband and wife of the New Marriage recognize that social concern and social responsibility must lead to their involvement as change agents in the local institutions of which they are a member or in which they participate. They know that by the exercise of social responsibility through action, they develop their leadership potential and that this has an effect on the development of other latent abilities and capacities. They realize that to achieve the regeneration of our society we must examine our institutions in the light of the following question: "To what extent does the function of the institution foster the realization of human potential?"

5. There is clear awareness by husband and wife that their interpersonal or relationship environment as well as their physical environment directly affects the actualization of individual potential.

The husband and wife together examine their acquaintanceship and friendship circle with the aim of seeking closer relationships with those people who stimulate them, encourage them, and enhance either partner's creativity. They seek to deepen and extend friendship relations and to seek out new people who, by the nature of their being, provide growth experiences. Husband and wife keep their home environment dynamic, both supporting and reflecting their own growth and change. Both partners recognize that the pollution of the air that we breathe, the water we drink and swim in, and the plundering and spoiling of our natural resources and wilderness areas is for the profit of the few and to the detriment of the many. They become involved in action to help shape a physical environment favorable to man's development.

6. The New Marriage is Here-and-Now oriented and not bound to the past.

More important than the past history of the marriage is what the partners wish to do in the Here-and-Now to accomplish change and growth. Emphasis is on employment of the will and on the utilization of growth processes. A marriage is not its past, but what both partners envision it can be, and what they are willing to invest to make it so.

7. Partners in the New Marraige conceive of their union as an evolving, developing, flexible institution.

Both partners together decide what is right for them, and in a very real sense, they determine the dimensions, structures, and function of their marriage. This is an ongoing process, with changes determined both by individual growth needs and by helping to unfold and actualize each other. There is recognition that the New Marriage is a flexible framework which may lead to other structures of togetherness. There is ongoing commitment to experimental living, to seeking of new experiences, to providing for new inputs. Most importantly, emphasis is placed on the development of a life-affirmative, positive attitude. Joy and pleasure are placed in the service of unfolding the individual's potential. There is a strong focus on joy as an important component of living and on joy as a creative experience. There is an emphasis on the cultivation of ecstasy and on the joyous celebration of life.

8. Husband and wife have an interest in exploring the spiritual dimensions of the New Marriage.

Both partners explore in depth the relationship of their value and belief structure vis-a-vis their marriage. They examine the relationship of values and beliefs to their functioning inside and outside of the marriage—they live as they believe. They explore and develop spiritual dimensions in their sexual relationship. They discover how their involvement in religious organizations can regenerate these structures. They seek to deepen their understanding of God, the Godhead, or the Universe.

9. In the New Marriage, there is planned action and commitment to achieve realization of marriage potential.

The concept of "marriage potential" means that in every marriage there is a potential for greater happiness, for increased productivity, creativity, enjoyment, communication, for more love, understanding, and warmth. Since it is often difficult for two people to actualize more of their marriage potential by themselves, participants in the New Marriage will seek out group experiences designed to deepen their relationship and functioning as a couple. Such experiences are now being offered at many of the Growth Centers.

If we conceive of the New Marriage as an exciting union which has as its main purpose the involvement of both partners in the adventure of actualizing each other's potential, then this purpose becomes a dynamic bond which fosters closeness while at the same time it meets the privacy needs of the partners. Implicit in the concept of the New Marriage is a deep respect for each other as a unique person with many individual capacities, talents, powers, and abilities which can be developed and brought to full flowering.

Also implicit is the concept that two parents who, in love and understanding, are dedicated to help each other actualize individual potential, are thereby doing more for the family than the heads of a child-centered marriage, where the efforts of the parents are subordinated to the needs of the children. The family devoted to the actualizing of the personal potential of its members provides necessary structure, as well as the freedom of group experiences, for growth as a family and individual growth experiences away from the family. These experiences are consciously designed and worked out by the family as a group, with primary emphasis on the needs and the wishes of the individuals involved. The actualization of a member's potential is first and foremost his own concern, but it is also the concern of the other family members who encourage, help, and assist. The primary emphasis, however, is on the individual's efforts to help himself. From this emphasis emerges a new freedom within the structure, and this marks the emergence of The New Family.

Much of what happens (or what doesn't happen) in a contemporary marriage is determined by the implicit assumptions underlying the union. Some of these change during a marriage, others do not. To a considerable extent, these underlying assumptions define the course of the marriage and provide a framework which shapes the nature of the relationship. Some of these assumptions are verbalized at some time during the marriage while others are rarely, if ever, put into words. Among these assumptions are:

1. Marriage furnishes a means for the giving and taking of love, understanding, and for sexual fulfillment.
2. Sexual relations should take place only (or largely) between the two partners.
3. Marriage offers a measure of security, comfort, and stability, so that both partners soon learn to know what they can expect. Boundaries are set by husband and wife and it is their expectation that these will be respected.
4. Marriage involves a set of responsibilities and duties. It also involves certain roles—"what a husband is and should be" and "what a wife is and should be."
5. Marriage is for the raising and rearing of children and "having a family."
6. Marriage is a means of "weathering life's storms and ups-and-downs."
7. Marriage means companionship, someone to talk to.
8. Marriage is an insurance against a lonely old age.

In a similar manner, the implicit and explicit assumptions underlying the New Marriage will determine its course. For this reason, a New Marriage must begin with an exploration of these assumptions by both marital partners. As husband and wife enter into this process, openness and self-disclosure lead to increased personal authenticity and the emergence of a deeper understanding and vital togetherness. The concept of the New Marriage can offer new opportunities, open new doors, and add new creativity, excitement, and joy to married living.

4 Marriage as a Human-Actualizing Contract

by Virginia Satir

When I was asked to write this paper, the idea excited me. I have many thoughts about this subject. As I sit down now to write, I am overwhelmed at the enormity of their implications. My power of imagination fails me in visualizing how all these changes could be accomplished, given this world as it is today, with its vast numbers of people and the prevailing low image of a human being; this world, where love and trust are rarities and suspicion and hate are expected.

Person-person, male-female, and adult-child relations, as they exist today, seem pretty inhuman and many times even anti-human. The current legal and social structure frequently acts to aid and abet these inhuman contacts. Given the state of human relations today, it is not hard to understand current human behavior in marriage, the family, and other human transactions.

The effect of these inhuman and anti-human relations seems abundantly obvious in the widespread presence of mistrust and fear between human beings. If relationships are experienced as mistrust and fear, how can love and trust come about? Statistics on alcoholism, drug addiction, suicide, murder, mental illness, and crimes against

SOURCE: *The Family in Search of a Future*, edited by Herbert Otto, Appleton Century Crofts, New York, 1970, pp. 57-66.

persons or property are more specific indications of inhuman and anti-human treatment. Continuing wars between nations, racial strife, and poverty are global evidence of these same practices.

While these statistics do not include every person in our population, enough are included to make it more than just a random or accidental occurrence. This raises the basic question: *Is this how man really is inherently or is this the result of how he has been taught?* I would have to stop this paper right now if I believed that man's present behavior is the result of what he is, inherently. I believe man's behavior reflects what he has learned and I take hope in the fact that anything that has been learned can be unlearned and new learning can be introduced.

This, of course, raises another basic question: *What are these new learnings?* To talk about a change in the marriage relationship without talking about making changes in the human beings who make the marriage is, in my opinion, putting the cart before the horse. I would like to present some ideas which might go a long way toward moving us all a notch forward in our whole human existence and consequently in the marriage relationship.

What Would Happen If:

1. *Children were conceived only by mature adults?* If these parents felt prepared and knew, beyond few questions of doubt, that they had the skills to be wise, patient, and joyful teachers of human beings, of creative, loving, curious, real persons? Further, if this conception were an active mutual choice representing a welcome addition, instead of a potential deprivation or a substitute for a marital disappointment?

2. *Parenting were seen as probably the most crucial, challenging, and interesting job for each adult engaged in it?*

a. The business and the working world would manage in such a way that young fathers would not be asked to be gone from Monday to Friday. Men are essential; their non-presence hands child-rearing almost exclusively over to women. This skews the kind of parenting a child gets, which is reflected in his image of himself and others. An integrated person needs to have an intimate, real familiarity with both sexes. For many children, fathers are ghosts, benign or malevolent. If they are males, this leaves them with a hazy and incomplete model for themselves. If they are females, their relations and expectations of men evolve more from fantasy than reality. It seems to me that knowledge about, and familiarity with, the other sex in the growing-up years is a large factor in satisfaction in married life. Furthermore, male absence overdraws on the woman's resources, paving the way for all kinds of destructive results for herself, her children, and her husband. However we slice it, we come into the world with life equipment, but it remains for our experiences to teach the uses of it. After all, the husbands and fathers, the wives and mothers of today are the boys and girls of yesterday.

b. Women who are mothers and men who are fathers could have auxiliary help without stigma in their parenting. Parenting for the first five years is a twenty-four-hour-a-day job. This gets pretty confining if there is no relief. Auxiliary help might go a long way toward breaking the possession aspect of parenthood and move it more toward the real responsibility of developing the child's humanity.

c. There would be family financial allowances to people who needed them, not on the basis of being poor and just making survival possible, but because it was needed to facilitate optimum growth.

d. Preparation for parenting would be seen as something to be actively learned instead of assuming that the experience of conception and birth automatically provided all the know-how one needed. Nobody calling himself an engineer would even be considered for an engineering job if all the preparation he had consisted of his wish to be one, and the knowledge he gained by watching his engineer father.

3. *The idea of developing human beings was considered so important and vital that each neighborhood had within walking distance a Family Growth Center which was a center for learning about being human, from birth to death.* These might well replace public welfare offices, among other institutions. In my opinion, this process, learning how to be human, will never end; I believe the human potential is infinite. We have barely scratched the surface.

4. *The literal context surrounding the birth event included full awareness for the woman giving birth, the active witnessing of the birth process by the father of the child, and the rooming-in of all three for at least the first two weeks.* Everyone would get a chance to be in on the getting-acquainted process that necessarily takes place. In a first birth, the female would meet her husband in his father role for the first time; the male would meet his wife in her mother role for the first time; each would meet a slightly new person. Many men and women feel like strangers to each other when they meet as fathers and mothers despite the fact that they have previously been husbands and wives.

The subsequent celebration following the birth could celebrate not only a birth of a new human being, but a birth of new roles for the adults as well. (The way some celebrations have gone would suggest immaculate conception.) Men often feel like useless appendates at this time. No wonder there are fears of replacement on their part. I wonder whether it would be as possible for men who are fathers to leave their families as readily as they now do if they were part of the literal birth proceedings, openly hailed and honored as being and having been essential, as are women. I wonder too, if this were done, whether the birth of a baby would create as much estrangement between husband and wives as it often does.

5. *Child-rearing practices were changed.*

a. The emphasis in child rearing would be on helping the child find out, crystal-clearly, how he looked and sounded, how to tune in on how he felt and thought, how to find out how he experienced others and affected them, instead of only the admonishment to be good and find out how to please others.

b. From the moment of birth he would be treated as a person with the capacity to hear, to see, to feel, to sense, and to think, different from the adult only in body development and, initially, in putting his sensory and thought experiences into words.

c. He would have a predictable place in time and space.

d. He would have real and openly welcomed opportunities to feel his power and his uniqueness, his sexuality and his competence as soon as his resources permitted it.

e. He would be surrounded by people who openly and clearly enjoyed each other and him, who were straight and real with one another and with him, thus giving him a model for his own delight in interacting with people. Thus, the joy in relationships might overcome the grimly responsible outlook "becoming an adult" often has for a child.

f. "Yes" and "no" would be clear, reliable, appropriate, and implemented.

g. Realness would be valued over approval when there had to be a choice.

h. At every point in time, regardless of age or label, he would always be treated as a whole person and never regarded as too young to be a person.

i. Every child's feelings would be regarded with dignity and respect, listened to and understood; those around him would do the same with each other. There would be a basic difference between his awareness and expression of his feelings and thoughts, and the action he took in relation to them.

j. Every child's actions would be considered separately from his expressions, instead of linking expressions of feeling with an automatic specific act. He would be taught that actions had to be subject to time, place, situation, other persons, and purpose, rather than being given a stereotyped "should" that applies universally.

k. Difference from others would be seen clearly as an opportunity for learning, holding an important key to interest in living and real contact with others, instead of being seen primarily as something to be tolerated, or destroyed, or avoided.

l. Every child would have continuing experience that human life is to be revered, his and that of all others.

m. Every child would openly receive continuing knowledge of how he and all his parts work—his body, his mind, and his senses. He would receive encouragement for expressing, clarifying, and experimenting with his thoughts, his feelings, his words, his actions, and his body, in all its parts.

n. He would look forward to each new step in growth as an opportunity for discovery, encompassing pain, pleasure, knowledge, and adventure. Each phase of growth has special learnings that could be particularly planned for; evidence showing that a new growth step had been achieved would be openly and obviously validated, like celebrating with a party the onset of menstruation for girls and maybe a change of voice party for boys at the time of puberty. Further examples would be: parties for the first step, first tooth, first day at school, first over-night visit with non-familial members, first date, first sexual intercourse, and the first obvious and costly mistake. Mistakes are an inevitable part of risk-taking, which is an essential part of growth, and needs to be so understood.

o. He could see males and females as different, yet interesting and essential to each other, free to be separate instead of being implicit enemies or feeding on each other.

p. He could get training in male-female relations, could prepare openly for mating and parenting in turn, which would be explained as desirable, and demonstrated as such.

q. He would be openly let in on the experiences of adults in parenting, maritalling, and selfing.

6. *He could freely experience in an openly welcoming way the emergence of the sexual self.* This would require lifting the cover of secrecy on the genitals and all that it entails.

7. *The goal of being human was being real, loving, intimate, authentic, and alive as well as competent, productive, and responsible.*

We have never had people reared anything like this on a large enough scale to know how this would affect marriage, the family, and, in general, people-to-people relationships. We have never realized what impetus to a really better world and a socially more evolved people might be created for tackling the "insurmountable" problems of suicide, murder, alcoholism, illegitimacy, irresponsibility, incompetence, war, racial and national conflicts. I think this is worth trying.

In our society, marriage is the social and legal context in which new humans originate and are expected to grow into fully developed human beings. The very life of our society depends upon what happens as a result of marriage. Looking at the institution of marriage as it exists today raises real questions about its effectiveness.

The marriage contract in the Western Christian world has no provision for periodic review or socially acceptable means of termination. I would offer that this contrast, as it stands, is potentially inhuman and anti-human, and works against the development of love, trust, and connectedness with other human beings. It is made with the apparent assumption that the conditions present at its inception will continue without change for eternity. This asks people to be wiser than they can possibly be. It is made at a time in the lives of the respective parties when they have the least preparation in fact with which to make this contract.

The contract exacts an explicit agreement that other intimate relationships with the same and the other sex shall cease and each partner shall be the sole resource of total comfort and gratification for the other. Implicitly, the current marriage contract abolishes individual autonomy and makes togetherness mandatory. Independent wishes and acts, or contradictory opinions are seen as threats to marriage.

If marriage partners hold on to their integrity and their individuality, their independent wishes and acts, or contradictory opinions, they may retain their integrity but lose the relationship. So, to preserve the marriage, one has to lose one's integrity if to manifest the integrity loses the marriage.

Almost any recent study of the sexual practices of married people reports that many marital partners do not live completely monogamously. Marital partners report from few to many extra-marital sexual relationships, which are largely secret. Frequently-married persons practice a consecutive spousing which is a sort of polygamy done in parts. Mate-swapping, which is polygamy in the open, is becoming more frequent. The myth is monogamy; the fact is frequently polygamy. Evidently, the expectation that each mate should completely suffice the other is failing, and may, by its failure, demonstrate the unreality of this expectation.

Maybe with these facts we have to consider the possibility that human beings are not naturally monogamous.

Maybe monogamy is the most efficient and economic way to organize heterosexual relationships to permit child raising. If so, could monogamy as well as being efficient and economic also be creative, enjoyable, and growth-producing? Maybe this hinges on making possible individual autonomy as well as togetherness. Right now it looks all too often as though monogamy is experienced, after a relatively short time, as grim, lifeless, boring, depressing, disillusioning—a potential context for murder, suicide, mental human decay. Perhaps persons who had rearing of the kind I described would make marriage an exciting and alive experience, and then maybe monogamy could become the rich and fulfilling experience the poets describe.

The marriage contract with its implicit social expectation of chastity is based on the assumption that the expectation of an experience is the same as the actual experience. Chastity all too often disguises ignorance, naivete, and inhibition. These attitudes in too many cases contaminate the marital relationship rather than enhance it.

At this point, I can only fantasy how the sexual relationship in marriage would be changed if the marital partners had been brought up with openness, frankness, love, acceptance, and knowledge of their whole body and that of the other sex.

The current Western marriage contract has been derived from a chattel economic base, which stresses possessing. This frequently gets translated into duty and becomes emotional and sometimes literal blackmail. The quality of joy is lost in the game of scoreboard. "Who loses, who wins, and who is on top?" The result is the grimness I referred to earlier.

Obviously, only mature people can make workable contracts with some hope of achievement, not because they can predict the events, but because they have a workable, growth-producing, coping process to meet whatever comes along. Few people have had open access to the information and experience that could prepare them for being persons, let alone marriage partners.

From the time of puberty the underlying message is be careful of the other sex—the other sex is dangerous. The symbol of this is genital contact, namely intercourse. Many marriages are made by persons who secretly fear that the other sex is dangerous. Out of this is supposed to come intimacy, tenderness, and joining of efforts. How do potential enemies easily translate their relationship into one of intimacy and tenderness?

Maybe there needs to be something like an apprentice period which is socially approved, that precedes an actual marriage, in which potential partners have a chance to explore deeply and experiment with their relationship. This is not exactly a new idea.

In a period of living together, which was socially approved and considered desirable, each could experience the other and find out whether his fantasy matched the reality. Was it really possible through daily living to have a process enabling each to enhance the growth of the other while at the same time enhancing his own? What is it like to have to undertake joint ventures and being with each other every day? It would seem that in this socially approved context, the changes of greater and continuing realness and authenticity would be increased, and the relationship would deepen since it started on a reality base.

Right now such important learning is denied in an effort to preserve the fiction of chastity. It seems to me that this puts undue weight on something that is peripheral to the big goal—healthy, intimate, human relationships.

We have to have a socially accepted and desirable way to terminate a marriage when it appears that it no longer works. What if it could happen just by mutual consent and the only problem was how to plan for the continuing parenting of the children? I doubt that, between people who were authentic and real, this would be either so destructive or so frequent. Human beings with the best intentions and integrity make errors. There needs to be an honorable way to treat this most important error.

If we could truly see that the act of sexual intercourse has much to do with enriching self-esteem in the partners, and that it can represent the highest and most satisfying form of male-female contact, we would be more discriminating. Further, we could openly teach ways to make this possible. To accomplish this we must lift the cover of secrecy and ignorance. At the present time sexual contact is frequently seen as degrading, a form of war, merchandise, lust, a means of scalp-hunting, or as a scoreboard. In these circumstances, when conception results, the child is potentially doomed to the "psychiatric couch," to prison, to poverty, to premature death, or maybe worse yet, to conformity or boredom. How can one degrade or be destructive toward that which he considers openly, truly beautiful and part of his joy in existence?

If we were all to see the sexual act as the renewal value of the other and the increase of self-esteem in the self, if the decision to procreate was a voluntary, mutually-shared one entered into *after* the intimate, satisfying, renewing experience had been achieved by a male and female pair, what magnitude of revolution might we stimulate in a new model for person-to-person relations?

Anyone who has studied family process at all can see with one eye how (1) the sexual relationship is symbolic of the heterosexual interrelationship and this carries the significance of the person-to-person relationship, and (2) that the fate of the child hangs on this interrelationship.

Intercourse is a fact, not a symbol. Conception, pregnancy, and birth are also facts, not symbols. The child is a result of these facts, but his maturing is guided by the feelings that surround these facts.

I am implying three changes:

1. That the cover of secrecy be removed from the sexual part of the human being. With this cover off, ignorance can be removed.

2. That there be as much attention, care, and implementation, openly, creatively, and confidently given to the care, maintenance, and use of the genitals as there is, for instance, to the teeth.

3. That a couple have a means to know when they have achieved intimacy in their relationship, which is based on their experience with, and awareness of, each other as real persons whom they value, enjoy, and feel connected with.

If we were taught from childhood on that our most important goal as human beings is to be real and in continuing touch with ourselves, this in turn would ensure a real connection with others. Were we taught that creativity, authenticity, health, aliveness, lovingness, and productivity were desirable goals, we would have a much greater sense of when this was achieved, and would also find it much easier to do so.

With the expectation of the age of marriage being around twenty and life expectancy being around seventy, close to fifty years of a person's life can be expected to be lived under the aegis of a marriage contract. If the contract does not permit an alive, dynamic experience with growth possible for both, the result is outrage, submission, destructiveness, withdrawal, premature death, or destructive termination. Maybe this type of marriage contract is impossible. If it is, then perhaps what we need to do is to find a way to conceive and bring up children that does not depend on a permanent relationship between the parents. The act of conception and birth could be entirely separated from the process of raising children. We could have child manufacturers and child raisers. We have much of this now except that it is socially stigmatizing. We work awfully hard to make adoption unsuccessful. "He is not my real child," or "She is not my real mother." Actually most of us know that the significance of the blood tie is mostly in our heads.

Maybe the most important thing is that new humans get born and then they are raised. Who does either or both may not be as important as that it is done and how it is done. Maybe if such a "division of labor" were effected, the energies of all the adults of the world would be more available for work and joy and less tied up with what they "should" be.

Procreation—coming about as it does, with little evidence that it will change much in the near future—guarantees that there will always be males and females around, and that they will be attracted to one another, in or out of marriage. Maybe this could be openly acknowledged and we could find ways to use it for our mutual benefit.

As for me, I think a relationship of trust, worth, and love between people is the highest and most satisfying way of experiencing one's humanity. I think this is where real spirituality takes place. Without it, humans become shrivelled, destructive, and desolate.

Right now, our current forms of human interaction, our fears, our suspicions, and our past are working against us. We have all the resources for the needed change, but we do not yet know how to use them. Our survival as a society may well depend upon finding these uses.

5 Thou Shalt Not Something or Other

by Arthur Hoppe

SCENE: The summit of Mt. Sinai.

TIME: The present. Moses, holding two stone tablets in his hand, enters nervously.

Moses: Sorry to bother you again, Sir, but I'm afraid we need another revision in the original copy.

The Lord (with a sigh): Another? What now?

Moses: Well, Sir, it's where You say here, "Thou shall not kill."

The Lord: That seems perfectly clear and concise.

Moses: But it's causing an awful haggle among Your theologians, Sir. The Catholics feel it applies to spermatozoa and ova; the Conservatives only after the union of the two; the Moderates would reserve it for 20-week-old embryos and up; and the Liberals feel it takes effect precisely at the moment of birth.

The Lord (puzzled): But why would anyone want to kill an unborn child?

Moses: Primarily, Sir, on the chance it might emerge deformed.

The Lord: In that case, why don't they wait to see whether it does before they kill it?

Moses: Oh, all theologians oppose killing children after they're born. Except, of course, at a distance of more than 500 yards.

The Lord: Why 500 yards?

Moses: In wartime, Sir, it is a terrible thing to kill a child with a rifle bullet and an atrocity to do so with a bayonet. But all recognized theologians agree that it is permissible, if regrettable, to blow them up with high explosives or incinerate them, with jellied gasoline, as long as it is dropped from an airplane or fired from an artillery piece—particularly, the Christians feel, if you do so to save them from Godless Communism.

The Lord: I suppose it does do that.

Moses: Of course, once a male child reaches the age of 18 he may be killed in virtually any fashion on the battlefield except with poison gas. The use of poison gas in war, all the theologians agree, is the greatest atrocity.

The Lord: Then where do they use it?

Moses: Only in State-operated gas chambers. It is used there, with the approval of theologians, because it is the most humane way to kill people.

The Lord: But if it's the most humane . . . . Never mind. Is that all?

Moses: I almost overlooked germ warfare. It is also unconscionable to save people from Godless Communism by inflicting them with any fatal sickness—except radiation sickness which causes a lingering and painful death.

The Lord (shaking his head): Moses, I don't know what to do.

Moses (briskly): Well, first off, Sir, I'd suggest setting aside a five-mile stretch of the Pasadena Freeway.

The Lord: Whatever for?

Moses: You certainly aren't going to get the necessary revisions on one of these stone tablets, Sir. Now, I've got a rough draft here of an effective compromise that should mollify all factions. It begins: "Thou shall not kill any person between the ages of minus four months (see Appendix) and 18 years (asterisk) at a distance of less than 500 yards (see Footnote 7a, Chapter Three), with any of the following. . . ."

The Lord (in measured tones): Never mind, Moses. I have a better idea. Gabriel! Gabriel, come here. And bring your trumpet.

6 Be Responsible for Your Own Sexuality

by L. Allure Jefcoat

1. Reason for Concern

At least one-third and possibly over 50 per cent of all children conceived in the United States were not planned and were not totally wanted! This is the startling conclusion to which I have come after reviewing the statistics, reading the results of many studies, counseling and talking with women who have had abortions or given birth to children they did not plan and at least initially did not want!

I further believe that if there were a means of evaluating the number of *planned* conceptions which would not have occurred had the people involved not been conditioned by the society by (1) lack of education that would free them to understand and realize their own potential and their own real needs, (2) by the prevalence of the myths claiming an innate desire and need to have children, and (3) by a confused but very strong training in sex role definition (see "The Motherhood Myth") one could count an additional large percentage of conceptions that were, *without the brainwashing*, certainly unwanted.

In brief, some of the data which have led me to these conclusions are:

A quarter of a million girls under age 18 bore children in 1970.

At least half of all brides ages 20 and under are pregnant at the wedding.

Across the nation one in 10 births is "illegitimate"; and, while philosophies and life styles are changing so that some of these were planned and wanted, most were not.

In 1970, about 50,000 women in California received legal, therapeutic abortions; and, according to the State Health Department, an estimated 20,000 to 60,000 underwent *illegal* abortions.

During 1970 in at least one county in California one out of seven known conceptions ended in legal therapeutic abortion.

In the 1965 National Fertility Study only 26 per cent of the married women reported that they had given birth to only the number of children they wanted.

The psychological, financial and other problems caused to the parents in an unwanted pregnancy usually have life-long reverberations. If the parents are unmarried, in American society where social stigma is so tremendous in general, in spite of its frequency, women particularly suffer emotional disturbances which affect all areas of their lives. Even for the married, the burden of a child one cannot afford financially or emotionally, either because it came at the wrong time or after all the children that couple could raise in a healthy way had been born, is tremendous.

Looking at the situation from a national or international point of view, the strain on every system—health services, educational, economic, governmental, etc.—from population pressures should be in the conscious awareness of every American by now. Note the following:

— Problems of pollution of the air, water and food as a result of trying to provide for the needs and wants of too many people.
— The political tension that is created trying to obtain raw materials from other nations to replace the rapidly depleting stocks of the United States.
— The exorbitant financial commitment to this end and for related political protection.
— The increasing need and demand for health, education and welfare for an exploding population, with a greatly insufficient amount of financing we are willing or able to spend on these needs.
— The increase in physiological and psychological disease directly associated with population pressures and the "stress syndrome."

For anyone who will allow himself to become aware of these problems it becomes obvious that there are *already* too many people!

2. What is Needed?

Education

Why, then, at the personal level do we fail to protect ourselves from conceiving children we cannot support either emotionally or financially? At the national level must we continue increasing our numbers in the face of great social turmoil associated with our inability or failure to provide for the needs of a huge population? Must we either follow India's footsteps or resort to legislated governmental control on the number of children we may have as some have proposed? Or will we take responsibility for this aspect of our sexuality?

I personally do not want governmental control on family size! That is, I do not want governmental control *unless*, after a massive educational program on every mass medium concerning the health and ecological dangers due to over population, we individuals *still* have not taken the responsibility to regulate our births. SUCH A TOTAL EDUCATION HAS NEVER BEEN ATTEMPTED—even now, with air, water, solid waste and other pollution constantly in the news how often is the primary cause of the pollution—TOO MANY PEOPLE—ever mentioned? How many "ecology minded" legislators ever propose bills for educating or providing clinics and contraceptives for this basic need, or even *mention* it? I have faith and a great deal of evidence that education really does work, and I'd like to see it tried in the nation as a whole.

Social Services—Information, Clinics and Contraceptives

There should be an adequate number of well publicized free and inexpensive clinics conveniently placed in every county of every state. These clinics should provide information, materials and professional medical services for every individual who wants contraception, sterilization, or abortion for those for whom contraception fails.

At the present time these services are few, usually too expensive, and information about the ones that do exist is effectively non-existant or at least spotty. I believe that with education about the need for control and the ways and services to control the numbers of children, personal sexual responsibility will be the result!

The effectiveness of a good family planning service is exemplified by the following story: In 1964 a Tulane University team under the direction of Dr. Joseph Beasley began a research program involving 368 men and 540 women between the ages of fifteen and forty five who had been married or had children. They were researching Dr. Beasley's contention that overproduction of children traps people in a life of poverty from which they cannot escape. They also researched the usual claim that poor people *want* large families.

During the interviewing they discovered an alarming amount of sexual ignorance, with one third of the people not even knowing that conception was the result of the union of an egg and a sperm. Though one third of the population was Roman Catholic they found an overwhelming desire for family planning help, with 95% of the people believing that there should be free family planning service for the poor.

In 1965 the first family planning clinic opened in Lincoln Parish, a county of 35,000. The goal was to reach all poor women of child bearing age within two years. At the end of eighteen months, even before their goal was accomplished, the births among the poor of that county had dropped 32% as compared with 5% in adjacent counties. Illegitimate births had dropped to 40% while they had risen 2% in adjacent counties. (Westoff and Westoff)

More general indications that education about, and availability of the means to limit family size *does* lead to greater personal responsibility comes from several sources.

The 1965 National Fertility Study showed a positive correlation between the use of the most effective contraceptive, "the pill," and education, with 37% of the college graduates using them as compared with 12% of non-high school graduates in the same age brackets.

Since this time the number of pill users has doubled, and the difference between usage by those with varying amounts of formal education has decreased, but again the increased usage by those with less than high school education can be attributed to education—informal education by the mass media and by word of mouth.

I am certain that these differences could also disappear if the mass media were used for education about other aspects of this important area of our lives. It is my belief that most women are consciously aware to some level or have feelings that, if they could integrate the feelings with their total needs, tell them when they have had enough children. It is too often a whim, a *momentary* response to some unconscious motivation to conceive, that becomes a *destiny* for a woman. In an individual case perhaps it is an attempt to compensate for a character inadequacy by adding a socially accepted role, "Mother;" or an excuse to keep from developing one's character; or a short-sighted attempt to trap the other into a marriage, which has little chance of success under the circumstances; or a frantic attempt to cement a cracking marriage; or any number of other attempts to fit the "role" she has been set up for by her life programming.

There is a need for in-depth education on the psychological, economic and ecological consequences of each child, a need to integrate the total picture of the effects of these "extra" children on our lives. There is a need for acceptable and readily available means of limiting our families. With this help and information I feel certain that we as individuals will voluntarily take the responsibility of limiting our families.

Essentially everyone who is able to conceive uses or plans to use contraception. The methods used vary from the 100% sterilization and the almost 100% effective pill to the almost 100% failure douche. The consistency of use likewise varies. Both method used and consistency are dependent primarily upon education and secondarily upon religion, race, age, economic status, and number of children already born. Although harder to tabulate than some of the other factors, the emotional health of the woman is also an important factor, with the less stable person having a substantially greater likelihood of misuse or failure to use contraception. The 1965 National Fertility Study found that 97% of married couples used or planned to use some method of contraceptive, but it also showed that only 26% of the couples were completely successful in having the number of children wanted at the time wanted.

This study showed that for married couples where the wife was under 45 years of age, 57% of white couples and 49% of black couples were using contraception at that time. Of the remaining couples 28% of white couples and 30% of black couples were unable to conceive due to sterilizing surgery, hormonal, anatomy or disease problems; 8% of each group was pregnant; 1% white couples and 3% black couples had just delivered; and 3% white couples and 7% black couples were "just not using anything." Of the people using contraception 28% of the white couples and 25% of the black couples used the very effective "pill." Second choice of white couples was the reasonably effective condom (used by 24%) and for 21% of black couples the ineffective douche. Third in frequency for 12% of white couples was the poorly effective rhythm method and for 19% of black couples the condom. Another racial difference, which is primarily a function of education, is the number of children born, as already cited: more children are born to poorly educated black couples than to white couples of the same educational level, but fewer children are born to black couples with college level education than to white couples, of the same educational level.

Income, which is usually a function of education and/or race, is also a determinant. In this study 14% of poor women used no method of contraception while 11% used the douche, which is ineffective, leaving 25% totally unprotected. It was noted earlier that the douche was the second most prevalent method for black couples, who are considerably more likely to be poor. In general, families with lower incomes have more children than families with higher incomes. Non-white couples with lower incomes have more children than white couples in the same income bracket, but non-white couples in higher income brackets have fewer children than white couples in the same income bracket.

There are some religious differences, too, which are greatly influenced by education. In 1965, 75% of Catholic grade school graduates believed in using some form of contraception, as compared with 96% of Catholic High School and college graduates. Among Catholics attending mass at least weekly in 1955, 22% were using contraceptives other than rhythm, and by 1965 this figure had increased to 44%. Contraceptive sterilization is nearly as high for Catholics as for non-Catholics, as reviewed later in this paper.

3. Personal Responsibility

Methods of Contraception

Never in history has there been such widespread reporting, both responsible and irresponsible, in the mass media or by word of mouth about a medication; never have there been so many people taking potent drugs voluntarily for anything but the control of contagious disease, as for "the pill."

In spite of widely publicized alarming reports about side effects of "the pill" over four million American women were consuming 2,660 tons of these contraceptive tablets in 1965; and by 1969 this amount had doubled. In 1969 there were 20 preparations of oral contraceptives of two basic kinds being distributed in the United States.

Most of the preparations act primarily to prevent ovulation by inhibiting the production by the pituitary gland of ovary-stimulating hormones. With inhibition of FSH (follicle stimulating hormone) and LH (leutenizing hormone) of the pituitary the follicle cells of the ovary are not stimulated to mature and release an egg cell; without an egg cell there can be no pregnancy.

Of the two basic kinds of pills the *combination pill* is by far the most widely used, and is more effective with fewer side effects.

Each pill of the cycle is the same, containing a balanced amount of both synthetic estrogen and progestin. Instructions for consumption will vary with the preparation, but a new cycle of pills is usually started 5 to 7 days after the last menstrual cycle and one pill is taken every day for 20 or 21 days. A menstrual period usually begins 1 to 5 days after the last pill is taken, and a new cycle begins. With combination pills, a person may safely "forget" to take one or possibly two pills, take the missed pills as soon as discovered, and continue on with the cycle. If more than two are missed, a person should continue on with the cycle, but use an additional method such as condoms or foam for the rest of the cycle.

The theoretic effectiveness of the combination pill is 0.2%, so that two women per 1000 are expected to be pregnant by the end of the year using the pill. Considering the theoretic failures and human failure in consistent usage, about seven women per 1000 actually become pregnant.

The other basic type of pill is the *Sequential Pill.* There are two kinds of pills in a cycle which must be taken in the right order. For the first 16 days a pill of synthetic estrogen alone is taken daily, followed by the daily consumption of a pill made of both estrogen and progestin for five or six days. If even one pill is missed during a cycle an additional method of contraception should be used along with the remainder of pills of that cycle. The theoretic effectiveness of the sequential pills is 0.7 and the use-effectiveness is 1.4, so that 14 women per 1000 become pregnant yearly using the sequential pills.

Of all the annoying and harmful side effects at various times attributed to oral contraceptives, there is only one dangerous effect with any substantial evidence for it, that of *thromboembolism*, or blood clots. Blood clots occur among both men and women, and the occurrence in women increases with pregnancy or the use of the pill. The 1969 Federal Drug Administration Report on the Oral Contraceptives showed a mortality rate for thromboembolic disease (blood clot disease) has been increasing in the United States for both males and females between the ages of 15-64. Although more men get the disease the increase is slightly greater for females, and the increase was accelerated within the period 1962-1966 as compared with the pre-pill period 1956-1961. These facts are consistent with the hypothesis that the pill is responsible for some thromboembolic mortality, and an FDA study group calculated the numbers of thromboembolic deaths due to oral contraception to be about 3 per 100,000 women per year.

There is no medication, including the common aspirin, without its risk to sensitive people in the population. Both the risks and the benefits of any medication must be weighed. One gynecologist commented that if "the pill" were prescribed for rheumatism rather than for a sex-related problem the public would never hear a word about the harmful effects! With an average rate of 24 per 100,000 women dying due to all complications of pregnancy and childbirth, including blood clots, the risk of the pill appears not so great. Westoff and Westoff have tried to put the risks into perspective this way: (1) Considering the numbers of couples using each of the various contraceptive methods, (2) the failure rate of the contraceptive methods and the consequent number of pregnancies, (3) the mortality rate per pregnancy due to abortion, problems of pregnancy, childbirth and its aftermath, and (4) the calculated number of deaths due to "the pill," they calculated that 324 deaths per year would occur to the 8.5 million women on the pill due to blood clots and pregnancy caused by pill failure and 1,179 deaths to the same number of women using other contraceptive means. Thus, they calculate the risk of dying is about 3-1/2 times greater without the pill!

This is small consolation for the person who happens to be sensitive to drugs in the pill, however. The FDA now requires a warning on each pill package and the American Medical Association has made an 800 word statement which is used on a brochure to be given to women receiving prescriptions for pills to inform her and to alert her of signs of danger. The FDA and the drug companies have committed themselves to the development of contraceptives that are safer and easier to use; and we, the public, must continue to pressure for this. At the present time many such preparations are being tested.

Another contraceptive method of great promise is the *Intra-Uterine Device* or *IUD*. At the time of the 1965 U.S. Fertility Study the IUD was used by only 1% of the couples using contraception. It is estimated that about 5% were using the IUD by 1969, and the number is increasing. This small plastic device, coming in a variety of shapes, is inserted into the uterus by a doctor. There is no further responsibility by the women except to check occasionally during the first months to see if it has been expelled. This check is performed by the woman feeling for a plastic string attached to the IUD and left hanging through the cervix. Most women tolerate the IUD very well, though some experience cramps, spotting between periods and excessively long periods to an extent where some women choose to have them removed. The FDA reports a pregnancy rate of 2.7-2.8 per 100 women per year. A new IUD, the Dalkon shield, made of a soft shield-shaped piece of plastic, reportedly is well tolerated by even women who have borne no children and is nearly as effective a contraceptive as the pill. Advantages to this method for women who can wear them is that it is carefree and not subject to human forgetfulness, and it adds no additional chemicals to the system.

All other methods of contraception are considerably less effective and generally inconvenient. The next two, ranked in order of effectiveness after the pill and the IUD, are the *diaphragm* and the *condom* with an FDA pregnancy rating of 17.9 per 100.

The *diaphragm* is a soft circular rubber shield which is used with a vaginal jelly to form a barrier over the cervix to prevent the entrance of sperms into the uterus. The size needed by an individual is determined by a doctor, and a larger size is ordinarily needed after each birth. Before "the pill" this was the method of contraception most commonly used by educated women. Its use has declined so that many drug stores no longer stock them, but must order them upon request. They are inconvenient to use in that they must be inserted before intercourse and should not be removed for at least eight hours after. A copious amount of vaginal jelly is applied around the rim and a "blob" in the middle, the diaphragm is inserted into the vagina and applied over the cervix against the upper back wall of the vagina. The jelly forms a tight seal blocking entrance of sperm into the uterus and contains a spermicidal chemical.

The *condom* or "rubber" is a sheath made to fit over the erect penis where it acts as a mechanical barrier to the sperm's entrance into the uterus. This is the most effective contraceptive for which no doctor is involved. They can be purchased in a drug store in a variety of types, including some with reservoir ends and some very thin "skins" which don't cut down on sensation as the thicker types do. The failure rate, given by the FDA as 17.9, could be cut to approach the theoretical rate of 2.6 per 100 if four commonly ignored rules were observed: (1) put it on before *any* genital contact. Secretions from the Cowper's gland during the pre-ejaculatory excitement phase often wash out living sperms that were stranded along the tract in a previous ejaculation. (2) be certain to leave room at the end to contain the semen. If it is the reservoir end type this has already been allowed for. Otherwise don't pull it all the way on, or semen will flow up the sides and over the top into the vagina. (3) withdraw before the penis becomes so flacid it no longer fits tightly. Semen can spill over the top. (4) hold the top while withdrawing the penis, as the erection probably has subsided and the condom may slip off.

Vaginal foam can be purchased at a drugstore without a prescription. Used alone, however, its FDA effectiveness rating is 28.3 pregnancies per 100 women per year! These foams are applied in the vagina over the cervix where they act as a not-so-effective mechanical barrier and spermicide. They have the further disadvantage of being cumbersome, having to be applied just before intercourse after which the woman must remain lying down until after intercourse; otherwise the foam barrier will drain away from the cervix.

If a woman either cannot use the pill or an IUD, or she has not taken steps to protect herself with one of these contraceptives, she can have almost their effectiveness by her use of foam and her partner's simultaneous use of a condom.

The same *vaginal jelly* that is used with the diaphragm and a similar product, *vaginal cream*, can be used separately in the same way as vaginal foam. Each is inserted with an applicator. Neither holds its position as well as foam and the FDA gives them a failure rating of 36.8.

The *rhythm method* relies upon abstinance from intercourse during the part of the ovulatory cycle when it is believed a sperm may encounter an egg in the fallopian tube. Sperm cells generally remain alive four days after ejaculation and an egg cell up to two days after ovulation. A woman using this method must refrain from intercourse for at least four days before and two days after her *ovulation* period. To help determine her ovulation period a woman under a doctor's direction takes her temperature each morning before arising for 8-12 months. A slight rise in temperature indicates ovulation. Many women ovulate too irregularly for a pattern to be established; and, even the most regular woman may ovulate off schedule if an emotional upset or viral infection upsets her system. One study involving 1342 women who became pregnant when having intercourse only one time during their entire menstrual cycle showed that some women will get pregnant from intercourse at all times during a cycle. Some women even got pregnant from a single act of intercourse that took place during the menstrual cycle. The greatest number of women in the study got pregnant from intercourse on day 6, and the fewest pregnancies occurred from intercourse the last few days before the menstrual period. The FDA gives no rating on the rhythm method, but Planned Parenthood gives it a rating of 10-40 pregnancies per 100 women per year; and, one doctor speaking for Planned Parenthood says, "There is only one word to call a woman who uses the rhythm method, and that word is 'mother'!" It is obvious that there is need to revise the current rationale for usage of this method.

It must now be apparent that only the pills and the IUDs (particularly the new Dalkon Shield) or the simultaneous use of foam and a condom approach 100% effectiveness. It is difficult to understand the use of a contraceptive less effective than the condom by any responsible person who wants to avoid a pregnanct.

Sterilization as Contraception

Sterilization is the only 100% effective method of contraception. For those who are certain they don't want any children or have all the children they want it is a safe reliable method which needs no further concern.

The 1965 National Fertility Study found that among married white couples with wife aged 20-54, 8% had undergone a sterilizing operation for contraception. In the west the per cent is twice as high with 16% having such an operation. At least one population pocket, a suburban area near San Francisco, had a total sterilization rate of 31% for married white couples, with 23% being for contraceptive purposes, as reported by Dr. Nancy Phillips in *Demography*, May, 1971. The tubal ligation rate of 7% was not greatly increased over the west rate (6%) or the total United States rate (5%). The greatest difference was in 16% vasectomies compared with 10% for the west and 3% for the total United States.

This study was made of the married white women in the Walnut Creek Kaiser Foundation service area. This service area covers 100,000 people in the eleven surrounding communities, who have an education level and median income level above the national average. Forty per cent of the wives surveyed have attended college and 12% have graduated from college. The

1967 median family income was above \$10,000 with less than 2% below \$5,000.

Twenty-five per cent of this population is Catholic. When both partners are Catholic 15% of the couples have either a vasectomy or a tubal ligation for contraceptive purposes. Where only the wife is Catholic 21% of the couples have a sterilizing operation, with 6.6% being tubal ligation and 14.4% being vasectomy. When only the husband is Catholic 18% of couples have sterilization, with 11% being vasectomy. Of the Catholic group over 50% attended church at least monthly and 45% attended weekly.

A vasectomy is a simple operation which can be performed in a doctor's office within a few minutes, requires only a local anesthesia, and costs from \$15 to over \$200, depending upon the doctor, and by law is now covered by most medical plans.

California Senate Bill No. 834, signed by Governor Reagan September 15, 1970 as an amendment to the Insurance Code, states that if a medical plan pays for all or part of a "sterilizing operation or procedure" then it cannot place limitations upon reasons for the operation for either male or female, nor can they vary the fee. Previous to this, arbitrary rules were generally made; for example, the couple must have four children, or a pregnancy must be a danger to the woman's health. Such restrictions can no longer be applied.

This law will have explosive effects on the case loads of hospitals in most areas. Hospital boards must make decisions on how to deal with this new law. A possible way to handle it is to establish special vasectomy clinics operating on a regular schedule. A changing staff would alleviate the boredom for individual doctors and would minimize interference with their scheduling of other necessary operations.

Contrary to the belief still held by some adult men, a vasectomy per se in no way interferes with sex drive or activity. Semen is still released, the only difference being that it carries no sperm cells. The operation consists of cutting and tying the vas deferens, or sperm tubes, just above the testis to prevent passage of sperms. Passage of the male sex hormone, testosterone, is still accomplished by direct release into the blood stream by way of thousands of capillaries. Testosterone does *not* use the vas deferens for its conveyance. Indeed the only way to stop the passage of testosterone through the entire body is to remove the testicles, by castration, which is entirely different from sterilization!

Until very recently, tubal ligation, the sterilizing operation for women, was a much more serious operation than vasectomy, and still is in most cases. An incision is made through the abdominal wall, the fallopian tubes cut and tied. Several days hospitalization is required for this method. A new operation called laproscopic sterilization is completed in a few minutes, does not require overnight hospitalization, and does not leave a noticable scar. The operation is performed with a slender complex instrument through a small cut just under the navel. The fallopian tubes are sealed electrically and cut. The incision requires a "band-aid" type dressing and no stitches. The operation requires the instruments and specialized training and therefore is not yet available to all.

Sterilization, though reversible in some cases, should not be used until the people involved are reasonably sure they have had all the children they want to produce. It has up to now been used primarily by couples for whom some other method has failed and who have already borne more children than they wanted.

Abortion

We have reviewed the fact that with use of even the most effective method of contraception (besides sterilization), the pill with a theoretic effectiveness of .2% and a use-effectiveness of .7%, there are a small percentage but a large number of pregnancies.

.7% failure for 8.5 million pill-using women is 59,500 unwanted pregnancies per year. Considering that some of these women use the less effective sequential pill the number is still higher. Considering the number of women using the less effective contraceptives (283 pregnancies per 1000 women using foam and 179 pregnancies per 1000 women using condoms compared to 7 per 1000 using combination pills), and the women who fail to use any contraceptive, there are a very large number of women wanting abortions.

Abortion is considerably more common than the general public is aware, and has been throughout history. The 1957 Arden House Conference on Abortion reported that the number of illegal abortions performed yearly in the United States might be as low as 200,000 or as high as 1,200,000. In 1970 the illegal abortion figure was fixed at 1,000,000 or 300 abortions for every 1,000 births, nearly a 1 to 3 ratio. At least 80% of those were performed by medical doctors.

The legal abortion figure for the United States has ranged from 8000 per year in the mid-sixties to 20,000 by 1969 to 200,000 in 1970. In California alone 50,000 received legal therapeutic abortions in 1970 and there were an estimated 20,000 to 60,000 illegal abortions. In my county, Contra Costa County, one out of seven pregnancies was terminated in legal therapeutic abortion in that year.

This tremendous increase in legal abortions is due to the complex social changes and new value systems that are occurring across the country and in the resulting liberalized abortion laws.

In California abortion has been a legal method of terminating an unwanted pregnancy for the following reasons: in case of rape or incest she must go through special legal procedures; in case of pregnancy to an unmarried girl under age 15 the right to legal abortion is automatic; or when continuing the pregnancy would gravely impair the mental or physical health of the mother. In the case of a woman over age 21 the consent of the husband is not required. The state Supreme Court ruled in 1971 that parents of a minor girl do not legally have to give consent or be informed of the abortion. The California State Court of Appeals recently ruled unconstitutional the requirement that every abortion receive advance approval by a committee of physicians. Judge Richard Sims and Norman Elkington concurred in the 2-1 decision in an appeal from a criminal abortion case in Alameda County. The decision said "We are impelled to consider that a woman has a Constitutional right to terminate her pregnancy, subject only to reasonably imposed state restrictions designed to safeguard the health of the woman and to protect the advanced fetus." We can expect continuing legal and attitudinal changes concerning abortion in the near future.

In California the average abortion costs between $600 and $700, although costs are covered by the Kaiser Medical Plan and by some medical insurance policies. Furthermore, it is possible for a woman to have an abortion completely or partially paid for by Medi-Cal if she is unmarried and not living with the father or if she is married and her husband is unemployed. Another inexpensive route for obtaining an abortion is to go through social services at a county hospital. If there is a local chapter of Planned Parenthood nearby, their marriage counselors will advise a woman who is pregnant against her wishes of all the alternatives available to her and help her achieve her choice. If abortion is her choice Planned Parenthood counselors will provide her with a list of psychiatrists who interpret the "mental health" part of the 1967 Therapeutic Abortion Act such that they consider the mental health of any woman who has an unwanted pregnancy to be impaired, or will inform her of the newest legislation on abortion. They also will provide her with a list of doctors who will do the abortion and help her with numerous other details.

The 1967 law required that no less than two licensed medical doctors shall approve the abortion and no fewer than three after the 13th week. Abortion done up to the 12th week is considerably safer for the mother than bearing the child. Fewer than 6 per 100,000 die due to abortion; 24 per 100,000 deaths occur due to all the complications of childbirth.

The two usual methods used up to 12 weeks are *D and C* and the *vacuum method.* With D and C (dilation and curretage) the woman is anesthetized, her cervix dilated or stretched, and the contents scraped off the uterine wall. A woman ordinarily remains one or two nights in the hospital. The newer vacuum or suction method *may* be done with local anesthesia on an out-patient basis. Some hospitals have the policy of keeping the patient overnight. A vacuum sucks out the contents of the uterus with little loss of blood. Abortions performed after the 12th week of pregnancy become increasingly more dangerous, and relatively few are performed after this time.

The state of New York, which passed a new abortion bill in 1970 that stipulates that abortions are available on demand to any woman up to 24 weeks of pregnancy without required residency, naturally received many requests from out-of-state women who were well into their pregnancies. During the first two months of the new law 31% of the women were between 12 and 24 weeks into the pregnancy. The mortality rate during the first year in New York was above the national average at eight deaths per 100,000 women receiving abortions. The percentage of late abortions declined rapidly as more women had their abortion needs cared for at an earlier stage. Statistics from countries allowing abortions on demand show the safety of early abortion by trained medical personnel, with Hungary and Czechoslovakia having such a law and a death rate of 2.8 per 100,000 abortions.

Saline injection or "salting out" is one method used in late abortions. A saline solution is injected into the amniotic fluids surrounding the fetus. After a period of time death to the fetus occurs, and labor contractions expel the fetus. An operation much like a Caesarean can also be performed and the fetus removed. It is highly preferable to arrange for an abortion very early in the pregnancy.

A Kaiser gynecologist told a college audience that the local Kaiser facility has 15-20% as many abortions as live births. He stated that he will perform an abortion for any woman who requests one, though he highly resents their carelessness and irresponsibility for not using contraception and thus taking the time he could use for other important and unavoidable health problems. It is true that most, but not all, unwanted pregnancies are due to failure to face an important part of one's sexuality—outright ignorance or carelessness in protecting oneself.

A number of surveys of college students have shown that less than half of college students who are having intercourse are using any method of contraception! This appears contradictory to results of the 1965 National Fertility study and to several other studies which show that effective contraceptive use is higher among *married people of college level* than among *married people of less than college level.* The difference appears to be the marital state. What kinds of unconscious motivations to get pregnant are at work in unmarried college students? Or, why the failure to know oneself and take responsibility for oneself as a mature sexual being?

There certainly needs to be more study of this sensitive area of unconscious motivation to get pregnant; and more open discussion must take place on research findings. We must not place total responsibility on "the professionals," however. We must retain primary responsibility for ourselves, in this important area no less than in other areas of our lives, if we are to be self-actualized fully functioning people. Both are needed: (1) more responsibility by governmental and private health sectors to aid us in understanding the total picture and providing medical services, and (2) more individual responsibility for understanding our own needs and for putting the information, materials and services already available to use! Most important—Be Responsible for Your Own Sexuality.

Following is a brief review of contraceptive methods presently available and their effectiveness ratings:

Methods of Birth Control

CONTRACEPTIVE	RATING*	TYPE OF CONTROL	PROCEDURE	APPROXIMATE COST	DOCTOR INVOLVED?
Sterilization	0	Mechanical Barrier	Vas deferens severed in male; fallopian tubes tied or uterus removed in female. Does not affect sex drive.	Vasectomy *can* be inexpensive. Operation on female more extensive and expensive. Most California medical plans are required by law to cover this operation.	Yes!
Combination pill	.7 (7 per 1000 per year).	Chemical (prevents ovulation)	Combination pill of estrogen and progestin taken from day 5 of menstrual cycle to day 25.	About $1.50 a month or more.	Doctor prescribes. Cost of follow-up visits.
Sequential pill	1.4 (14 per 1000 per year)	Chemical (prevents ovulation	Estrogen pill taken from day 5 through 19 of menstrual cycle, then combination pill taken day 20-25.	$1.50 a month or more.	Doctor prescribes. Cost of follow-up
Intrauterine Device (I.U.D.)	1.5 (The new Dalkan Shield is almost as effective as the pill)	Believed to cause egg to reach uterus at wrong time to implant.	Doctor inserts IUD in uterus at Doctor's office. Patient checks periodically to see if IUD is still in place first year. Doctor removes IUD if pregnancy desired.	Cost of office call and follow-up examination. In reality doctors charge varying amounts. A one-time fee of $25 is reasonable.	Yes

Methods of Birth Control *(continued)*

CONTRACEPTIVE	RATING*	TYPE OF CONTROL	PROCEDURE	APPROXIMATE COST	DOCTOR INVOLVED?
Condom	17.9 (theoretic rate is 2.6)	Mechanical barrier worn by man.	Worn on erect penis. Should be used during all times penis is in vagina, including foreplay, and removed before penis loses rigidity for increased effectiveness.	\$.75 to \$1.80 for 3; \$1.75 to \$6.75 a dozen, depending upon type.	No. Choice of many kinds at drugstore.
Diaphragm	17.9	Mechanical barrier worn by woman.	Fitted by doctor who will instruct how to insert it. Covers the cervix of the uterus. Used only with special jelly or cream. May be inserted as long as 6 hours before intercourse and *must* remain in place 6 hours after intercourse. New fitting necessary after birth of each baby.	Physicians' fee for fitting & diaphragm; about \$5.00; 20 applications of cream or jelly about \$3.50.	Yes. A doctor must fit diaphragm properly.
Foam	10-30 (FDA rating 28.3)	Chemical (spermacide) and mechanical barrier.	Insert *two* applicators as directed into vagina under cervix not more than an hour before intercourse. Don't walk around before intercourse.	\$3.00 or more for 20 applications	No. Buy at drugstore without prescription.

Methods of Birth Control *(continued)*

CONTRACEPTIVE	RATING*	TYPE OF CONTROL	PROCEDURE	APPROXIMATE COST	DOCTOR INVOLVED?
Creams & Jelly	20-40 Unreliable	Chemical & Mechanical	Inserted as directed on package shortly before intercourse.		No. Buy at drugstore.
Foaming Vaginal Tablets	20-40 Unreliable	Chemical & Mechanical	Tablet is inserted into vagina under cervix. Waiting period of 10 minutes required for tablet to dissolve and foam up. Some secretion must be present to dissolve tablet.		No.
Rhythm	20-40 Unreliable	No intercourse during time pregnancy can occur.	If intercourse is avoided 3 days before and 3 days after ovulation, theoretically pregnancy should not occur. Virus infection or emotional disturbance can cause egg to be released, however.	Nothing (except cost of unplanned babies!)	Yes.

*Rating signifies the number of women out of 100 women using the particular method who will probably be pregnant at the end of one year. As an example, 17.9 women out of 100 women for whom the condom was the contraceptive choice will be pregnant at the end of one year. They may be pregnant because the condom was not put on until just before orgasm or because the condom was not removed before the penis lost its rigidity, allowing some sperms to escape around the edges, or because the condom was not held on while withdrawing. Seldom is the failure due to a faulty condom any more.

Post-coital Douche - Very unreliable due to the fact that some sperms have entered the *uterus* within 90 seconds after ejaculation. The douche only washes sperms out of the *vagina*, not out of the uterus.

Abortion is a method of contraception gaining acceptance in many countries as a method where other methods have failed. In the United States, however, though attitudes and laws are changing, this is often not a legal method. In California the law was liberalized in 1969 to allow legal abortion where the pregnancy would gravely impair the physical or mental health of the mother or where the pregnancy resulted from rape or incest. In 1970 a U.S. Court of Appeals ruled that it is unconstitutional to deprive a woman of the right to determine the fate of her own body. This may reinstate abortion as an option for all American women.

Bibliography and Suggested Readings

BIBLIOGRAPHY

Gordon, Arthur: "Louisiana's Quiet Revolution in Family Planning," *Today's Health*, 48, 1970.

Jones, Kenneth L. Shainberg, Louis W., and Byer, Curtis O.: *Environmental Health*, Harper and Row, Publishers, Inc., New York, pp. 37-66.

Monahan, Thomas P.: "Premarital Pregnancy in the U.S.," *Eugenics Quarterly*, 7, 1960, pp. 133-147.

Phillips, Nancy: "The Prevalence of Surgical Sterilization in a Suburban Population," *Demography*, 8, No. 2, May, 1971, pp. 261-270.

U.S. Advisory Committee on Obstetrics and Gynecology: *Second Report on the Oral Contraceptives*, Washington, D.C., U.S. Government Printing Office, 1969.

Westoff, Leslie Aldridge, and Westoff, Charles F.: *From Now to Zero-Fertility, Contraception and Abortion in America*, Second Edition, Little, Brown & Company, Boston, 1971.

Whelptom, P. K., Campbell, A. A., and Patterson, J. E.: *Fertility and Family Planning in the U.S.*, Princeton University Press, New Jersey, 1966.

SUGGESTED READINGS

Kovar, Mary Grace: "Interval Between First Marriage and Legitimate First Birth in the U.S. 1964-1966," *Monthly Vital Statistics Report*, 18, U.S. Department of Health, Education and Welfare, 1970.

Mead, Margaret: "Marriage in Two Steps," *Redbook Magazine*, Published by McCall Corporation, New York, July, 1966.

Mead, Margaret: "New Designs in Family Living," *Redbook Magazine*, Published by McCall Corporation, New York, October, 1970.

Otto, Herbert A., ed.: *The Family in Search of a Future—Alternate Models for Moderns*, Appleton-Century-Crofts, (An Affiliate of the Educational Division of Meredith Corporation), New York, 1970.

Otto, Herbert A.: "Has Monogamy Failed?" *Saturday Review*, April 25, 1970.

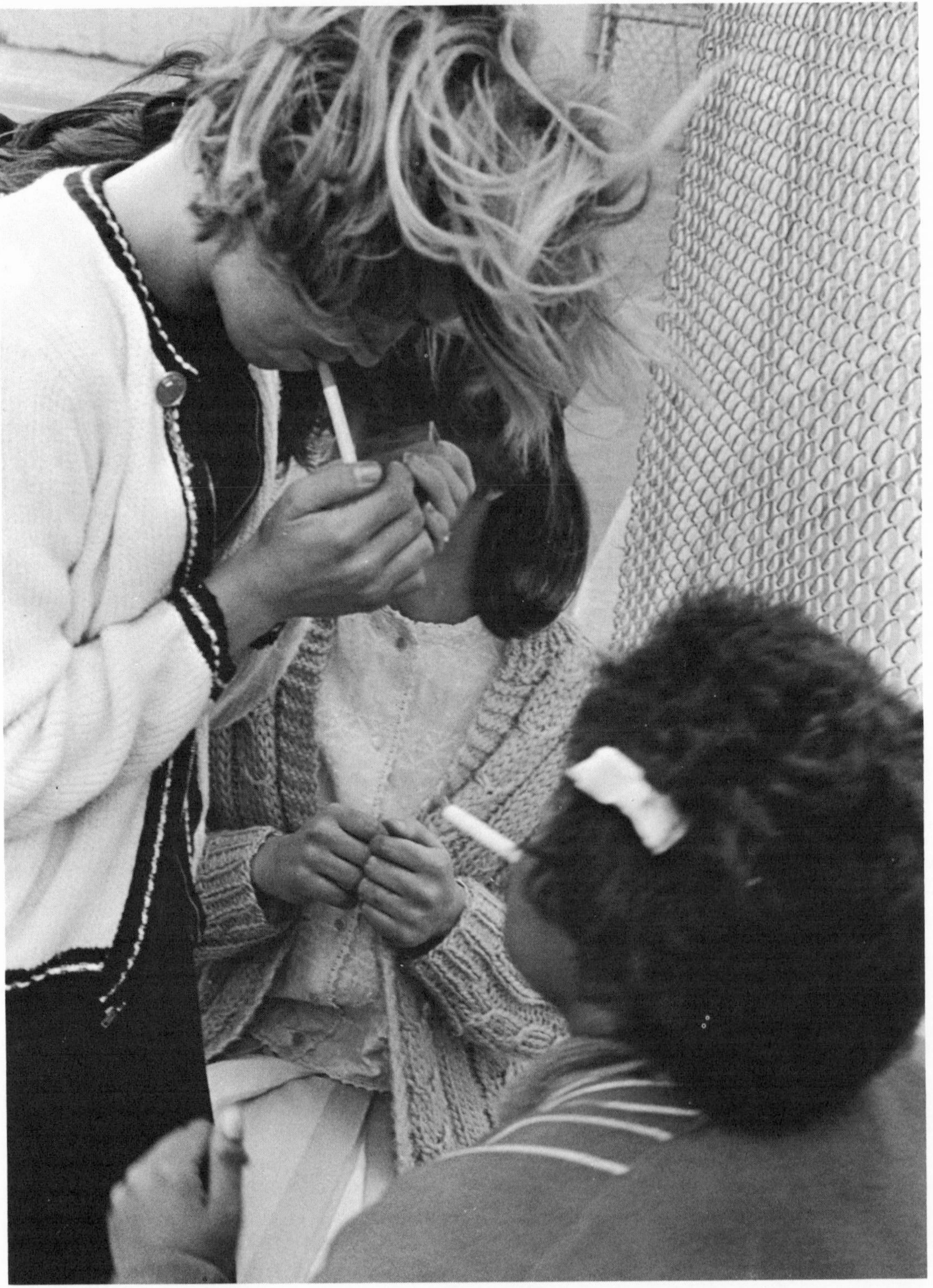

UNIT 3

Drug Use and Abuse

We live in a drug-oriented society. It is well known to all of us, from watching TV, listening to radio, looking at advertisements on billboards along the highway and in all magazines, walking into a drug or liquor store, and talking with our fellow citizens, that there is a drug to cure every malady and enhance every attribute! One can drive or study all night on No-doz or amphetamines; become president of the PTA or vice president of the company on Compoz; become an exciting romantic spouse on Vivarin; win the football game on amphetamines; or use alcohol for all eventualities. "Relief is just a swallow away!"

With a bit of research and thought it becomes apparent that the greatest drug pushers in the society are the legitimate drug industries. The alcohol, tobacco and over-the-counter pseudo-sedative industries jointly spend more than $2,000,000 a day in the United States alone to promote as much drug use as possible (Dr. Fort, "A Rational Approach to Pot"). Drug companies spend a large portion of their income for employing psychologists and psychiatrists to research and suggest ways of subtly and overtly appealing to our psychological needs and fears. They do this by advertising, design of package, and displaying their products in the right place in the right way. There are many agencies whose business consists totally of such research.

As you drive down the highway or through the city, figure out the ratio of alcohol and cigarette billboards to those advertising other products. Take a Christmas issue of Life magazine and tear out every page with at least a half page ad for alcohol and cigarettes. What per cent of the magazine is still intact? It is important to note that there are over 6,000,000 alcoholics in the United States, that alcohol is involved in at least half of the 53,000 annual automobile accident deaths, that alcohol is addicting, and that it causes cirrhosis of the liver and brain damage to alcoholics. Furthermore, we should realize that drugs in cigarettes indisputedly cause death due to cancer of the lungs, heart disease and emphysema, and are a factor in many other diseases. We certainly can't dispute the maleficence of the heroin pusher, although we've become much more concerned about him now that middle class white youths have been engineered into using this drug (Dr. David Smith, "The Year of the Middle-Class Junkie"). Let's take recognizance that it is the legal socially accepted pushers who affect by far the most lives and cause the most deaths.

Drug use in the United States is so clouded with emotionalism it is difficult to be objective. Every segment of the society has its group of drugs it favors and another group it disparages. The favorite drugs of the groups in positions of law and policy-making power are generally socially accepted and legal to "push." It does not follow that the safest to use are necessarily the most legal and the more dangerous the more illegal. Even two drugs with the same legal status are inconsistently enforced by the police and judged in the courts. For example, in California each of the three following offenses is a misdemeanor: using or being under the influence of marijuana, selling cigarettes to anyone under age 18, possession of alcohol by a minor. Consider the variance in legal prosecution for the three offenses.

Even the government of the United States is inconsistent in its treatment of tobacco; the United States Department of Agriculture subsidizes tobacco growers while the United States Health Department warns against its dangers due to cancer and heart disease!

If a person feels that drugs have no value in his life and chooses not to knowingly use Aspirin, Compoz, Excedrin, Nytol, Vivarin, alcohol, marijuana, barbiturates, tranquilizers, or any other drug, he is still an unwitting drug user.

Over 700 chemicals have been approved (of which about 550 have been tested) for addition to our foods as preservatives, coloring agents, flavoring agents, nutrient supplements, emulsifiers, stabilizers, and thickeners. These include such chemicals as formaldehyde in milk, boric acid or borax in codfish and whole eggs, and sex hormones to increase growth in beef. There are also a myriad number of unintentional chemical additives such as DDT and other pesticides, and nitrates from fertilizers.

Used wisely, drugs can be a marvelous benefit to health. Very few would dispute the beneficial and humanitarian effects of penicillin, or of stimulant and depressant drugs that reduce the anguish of mental patients. Even with these, there are abuses; unnecessary and excessive use of penicillin has allowed emergence of a dominant population of germ organisms that are immune to penicillin so it is no longer as effective in treatment, and too often mental patients in our state hospitals are kept "managable" with sedatives and stimulants rather than being given the psychotherapy they need. It is a common practice for doctors to give a prescription for a drug when psychological counselling is the basic need or, given time, the problem would clear up by itself. There are many rasons for this, among them are the short amount of time doctors are able to spend with their many patients and the fantastic proliferation of therapeutic drugs so that doctors cannot know all of them but must take the drug companies' word. Another important factor is that doctors are just people like the rest of us and are also susceptible to the psychological research and its implementation by the motivation research psychologists.

There are also a number of doctors whose greed for money is an important motive in prescribing pills. A federal senate sub-committee heard testimony of a millionnaire "fat doctor" who had been paid monthly commissions of $1200 by a pharmaceutical firm for advising doctors on how to prescribe its diet pills. A doctor who attended the company's "obesity symposium" testified the assembled doctors were told they should be making at least $100,000 a year from their diet program. "If you did not make this kind of money then they would send out a trouble shooter to your office to show you where you were making your mistakes and correct the problem," they were told (*Newsweek,* Feb. 6, 1970). The vast majority of doctors sincerely try to make their diagnosis and treatments in the best interests of their patients. The point is that *no* segment of the society is immune to potential drug abuse.

Americans have come to rely on a chemical solution for every ill imagined or real. It is time we individually examine our drug-using philosophy and habits. These questions may be of value:

What drugs am I using both purposely and unthinkingly?

Is my use of this drug the result of my own independent choice or am I the victim of the brainwashing of the Madison Avenue pushers and their 'motivation research' psychologists or of my pusher-friends who have a vested economic or ego interest in added consumption of their drugs?

What actual needs do these drugs (from aspirin on) fill for me as a person attempting to become a self-actualized and fully functioning human?

Is the need for which I'm taking this drug related to doubts I have about my value as an individual or about my relation to my environment? Would some of the "Human Potential" involvements (Unit I) do a more thorough job with fewer harmful side effects?

Dr. Fort's article tries to put the problem of marijuana in a more reasonable perspective. The other articles survey some particular newly emergent aspects of drug use. The last article tells us of yet another value system conflict.

1 Pot: A Rational Approach

by Joel Fort, M.D.

A leading authority on psychopharmacology calls for a lifting of legal prohibitions and punishments relating to marijuana—and explains why.

There are an estimated 10,000,000 Americans who smoke marijuana either regularly or occasionally, and they have very obvious reasons for wishing that pot were treated more sensibly by the law. As one of the 190,000,000 who have never smoked marijuana, I also favor the removal of grass from the criminal laws, but for less personal reasons. It is my considered opinion, after studying drug use and drug laws in 30 nations and dealing with drug-abuse problems professionally for 15 years, that the present marijuana statutes in America not only are bad laws for the offending minority but are bad for the vast majority of us who have never lit a marijuana cigarette and never will.

That some changes in these laws are coming in the near future is virtually certain, but it is not at all sure that the changes will be improvements.

On May 19, 1969, the U.S. Supreme Court, in an 8-0 vote, declared that the Marijuana Tax Act of 1937 was unconstitutional. This decision delighted the defendant, Timothy Leary, and was no surprise at all to lawyers who specialize in the fine points of constitutional law. It had long been recognized that the Marijuana Tax Act was "vulnerable"—a polite term meaning that the law had been hastily drawn, rashly considered and railroaded through Congress in a mood of old-maidish terror that spent no time on the niceties of the Bill of Rights, scientific fact or common sense.

Celebrations by marijuanaphiles and lamentations by marijuanaphobes, however, are both premature. The Court, while throwing out this one inept piece of legislation, specifically declared that Congress has the right to pass laws governing the use, sale and possession of this drug (provided these laws stay within the perimeter of the Constitution). And, of course, state laws against pot, which are often far harsher than the Federal law, still remain in effect.

There were two defects found by the Supreme Court in the Federal anti-marijuana law—a section that requires the suspect to pay a tax on the drug, thus incriminating himself, in violation of the Fifth Amendment; and a section that assumes (rather than requiring proof) that a person with foreign-grown marijuana in his possession knows it is smuggled. These provisions were perversions of traditional American jurisprudence, no less than the remaining parts of the law that are bound to fall when challenged before the Supreme Court. These forthcoming decisions will, inevitably, affect the anti-marijuana laws of the individual states as well. However, the striking down of the old laws does not guarantee that the new ones will be more enlightened; it merely invites more carefully drawn statutes that are less vulnerable to judicial review. In fact, in a message to Congress, President Nixon specifically demanded harsher penalties for marijuana convictions. But every sane and fair-minded person must be seriously concerned that the new laws are more just and more in harmony with known fact than the old ones. In my opinion, such new laws must treat marijuana no more harshly than alcohol is presently treated.

It is ironic that our present pot laws are upheld chiefly by the older generation, and flouted and condemned by the young; for it is the senior generation that should understand the issue most clearly, having lived through the era of alcohol prohibition. They saw with their own eyes that the entire nation—not just the drinkers and the sellers of liquor—suffered violent moral and mental harm from that particular outbreak of armed and rampant puritanism. They should certainly remember that attempts to legislate morality result only in widespread disresepct for law, new markets and new profits for gangsters, increased violence and such wholesale bribery and corruption that the Government itself becomes a greater object of contempt than the criminal class. Above all, they should be able to see the parallel between the lawless Twenties and the anarchic Sixties and realize that both were produced by bad laws—laws that had no right to exist in the first place.

"Bad law," it has been said, "is the worst form of tyranny." An open tyranny breeds open rebellion, and the issues are clear-cut; bad law, in an otherwise democratic nation, provokes a kind of cultural nihilism in which good and evil become hopelessly confused and the rebel, instead of formulating a single precise program, takes a perverse delight in anything and everything that will shock, startle, perplex, anger, baffle and offend the establishment. Thus it was during alcohol prohibition and thus it is under marijuana prohibition. The parallel is not obvious only because there were already millions of whiskey drinkers when the Volstead Act became law in 1919, leading to immediate flouting of "law and order" by vast hordes—whereas the use of marijuana did not become extensive until the early 1950s, more than 13 years after the Government banned pot in 1937. But the results, despite the delay, are the same: We have bred a generation of psychological rebels.

Banning marijuana not only perpetuates the rebelliousness of the young, but it also establishes a frightening precedent, under which puritanical bias is more important to our legislators than experimentally determined fact—something every scientist must dread. Dr. Philip Handler, board chairman of the National Science Foundation, bluntly told a House subcommittee investigating drug laws, "It is our puritan ethics . . . . rather than science" that say we should not smoke marijuana.

Consider the most recent study of the effects of marijuana, conducted under careful laboratory conditions and reported in *Science.* This is the research performed by Drs. Norman E. Zinberg and Andrew T. Weil at Boston University in 1968. This study was "double-blind"; that is, neither the subjects nor the researchers knew, during a given session, whether the product being smoked was real marijuana (from the female Cannabis plant) or an inactive placebo (from the male Cannabis plant). Thus, both suggestibility by the subjects and bias by the experimenters were kept to the scientific minimum. The results were:

1. Marijuana causes a moderate increase in heartbeat rate, some redness of the eyes and virtually no other physical effects. Contrary to the belief of both users and policemen, pot does not dilate the pupils—this myth apparently derives from the tradition of smoking Cannabis in a darkened room; it is the darkness that dilates the pupils.

2. Pot does not affect the blood-sugar level, as alcohol does, nor cause abnormal reactions of the involuntary muscles, as LSD often does, nor produce any effects likely to be somatically damaging. In the words of Zinberg and Weil, "The significance of this near absence of physical effects is twofold. First, it demonstrates once again the uniqueness of hemp among psychoactive drugs, most of which strongly affect the body as well as the mind. . . Second, it makes it unlikely that marijuana has any seriously detrimental physical effects in either short-term or long-term usage."

3. As sociologist Howard Becker pointed out long ago, on the basis of interviews with users, the marijuana "high" is a learned experience. Subjects who had never had Cannabis before simply did not get a "buzz" and reported very minimal subjective reactions, even while physically "loaded" with very high doses, while experienced users were easily turned on.

4. The hypothesis about "set and setting" strongly influencing drug reactions was confirmed. The pharmacological properties of a psychoactive drug are only one factor in a subject's response; equally important—perhaps more important—are the set (his expectations and personality type) and the setting (the total emotional mood of the environment and persons in it).

5. Both inexperienced subjects and longtime users did equally well on some tests for concentration and mental stability, even while they were on very high doses. On tests requiring a higher ability to focus attention, the inexperienced users did show some temporary mental impairment, but the veterans sailed right on, as if they were not high at all. In short, experienced potheads, do not have even a temporary lowering of the intelligence while they are high, much less a permanent mental impairment.

6. On some tests, the experienced users scored even higher while stoned

than they did when tested without any drug.

7. Not only alcohol but even tobacco has more adverse effects on the body than marijuana does.

As Zinberg and Weil noted sardonically in a later article in *The New York Times Magazine*, there is a vicious circle operating in relation to marijuana: "Administrators of scientific and Government institutions feel that marijuana is dangerous. Because it is dangerous, they are reluctant to allow (research) to be done on it. Because no work is done, people continue to think of it as dangerous. We hope that our own study has significantly weakened this "trend."

One slight sign that the trend may have been weakened was the appearance last June of a study by the Bureau of Motor Vehicles in the state of Washington concerning the effects of Cannabis on driving ability. Using driving-traffic simulators, not only did the study find that marijuana has less adverse effect on driving than alcohol—which many investigators have long suspected, but also, as in the Boston study, the evidence indicated that the only detrimental effect is on inexperienced users. Veteran potheads behave behind the wheel as if they were not drugged at all.

In short, we seem to have a drug here that makes many users very euphoric and happy—high—without doing any of the damage done by alcohol, narcotics, barbiturates, amphetamines or even tobacco.

But we didn't have to wait until 1968 to learn that pot is relatively harmless. Some research has been done in the past, in spite of the vicious circle mentioned by Zinberg and Weil. As far back as 1942, the mayor of New York City, Fiorello La Guardia, alarmed by sensational press stories about "the killer drug, marijuana" that was allegedly driving people to rape and murder, appointed a commission to investigate the pot problem in his city. The commission was made up of 31 eminent physicians, psychiatrists, psychologists, etc., and six officers from the city's narcotics bureau. If there was any bias in that study, it must have been directed against marijuana, considering the presence of the narcotics officers, not to mention psychiatrists and M.D.s, who were then, as now, rather conservative groups. Nevertheless, after two years of hard study, including psychological and medical examinations of users, electroencephalograms to examine for brain damage, sociological digging into the behavior patterns associated with marijuana use and intelligence tests on confirmed potheads, the commission concluded:

> Those who have been smoking marijuana for a period of years showed no mental or physical deterioration which may be attributed to the drug . . . . Marijuana is not a drug of addiction, comparable to morphine . . . . Marijuana does not lead to morphine or heroin or cocaine addiction . . . Marijuana is not the determining factor in the commission of major crimes . . . The publicity concerning the catastrophic effects of marijuana smoking in New York City is unfounded.

Even earlier, a study of marijuana use in the Panama Canal Zone was undertaken by a notably conservative body, the United States Army. Published in 1925, the study concluded, "There is no evidence that marijuana as grown here is a habit-forming drug" and that "Delinquencies due to marijuana smoking which result in trial by military court are negligible in number when compared with delinquencies resulting from the use of alcoholic drinks which also may be classed as stimulants or intoxicants."

What may be the classic study in the whole field goes back further: to the 1893-1894 report of the seven-member Indian Hemp Drug Commission that received evidence from 1193 witnesses from all regions of the country (then including Burma and Pakistan), professionals and laymen Indians and British, most of whom were required to answer in writing seven comprehensive questions covering most aspects of the subject. The commission found that there was no connection between the use of marijuana and "social and moral evils" such as crime, violence or bad character. It also concluded that occasional and moderate use may be beneficial; that moderate use is attended by no injurious physical, mental or other effects; and that moderate use is the rule: "It has been the most striking feature of this inquiry to find out how little the effects of hemp drugs have intruded themselves on observation. The large numbers of witnesses of all classes who profess never to have seen them, the very few witnesses who could so recall a case to give any definite account of it and the manner in which a large proportion of these cases broke down on the first attempt to examine them are facts which combine to show most clearly how little injury society has hitherto sustained from hemp drugs." This conclusion is all the more remarkable when one realizes that the pattern of use in India included far more potent forms and doses of Cannabis than are presently used in the United States. The commission, in its conclusion, stated:

> Total prohibition of the hemp drugs is neither necessary nor expedient in consideration of their ascertained effects, of the prevalence of the habit of using them, of the social or religious feelings on the subject and of the possibility of its driving the consumers to have recourse to other stimulants (alcohol) or narcotics which may be more deleterious.

Ever since there have been attempts to study marijuana scientifically, every major investigation has arrived at, substantially, the same conclusions, and these directly contradict the mythology of the Federal Bureau of Narcotics. In contrast with the above facts, consider the following advertisement, circulated before the passage of the 1937 Federal anti-marijuana law:

> Beware! Young and Old—People in All Walks of Life! This (picture of a marijuana cigarette) may be handed you by the friendly stranger. It contains the Killer Drug "Marijuana"—a powerful narcotic in which lurks Murder! Insanity! Death!

Such propaganda was widely disseminated in the mid-1930's, and it was responsible for stampeding Congress into the passage of a law unique in all American history in the extent to which it is based on sheer ignorance and misinformation.

Few people realize how recent anti-marijuana legislation is. Pot was widely used as a folk medicine in the 19th Century. Its recreational use in this country began in the early 1900's with Mexican laborers in the Southwest, spread to Mexican Americans and Negroes in the South and then the North, and then moved from rural to urban areas. In terms of public reaction and social policy, little attention was paid to pot until the mid-1930's (although some generally unenforced state laws existed before then). At that time, a group of former alcohol-prohibition agents headed by Harry J. Anslinger, who became head of the Federal Bureau of Narcotics, began issuing statements to the public (via a cooperative press) claiming that marijuana caused crime, violence, assassination, insanity, release of anti-social inhibitions, mental deterioration and numerous other onerous activities.

In what became a model for future federal and state legislative action on marijuana, Congressional hearings were held in 1937 on the Marijuana Tax Act. No medical, scientific or sociological evidence was sought or heard; no alternatives to criminalizing users and sellers were considered; and the major attention was given to the oilseed, birdseed and paint industries' need for unrestrained access to the hemp plant from which marijuana comes. A U.S. Treasury Department witness began his testimony by stating flatly that "Marijuana is being used extensively by high school children in cigarettes with deadly effect," and went on to introduce as further "evidence" an editorial from a Washington newspaper supposedly quoting the American Medical Association as having stated in its journal that marijuana use was one of the problems of greatest menace in the United States. Fortunately for historical analysis, a Dr. Woodward, serving as legislative counsel for the American Medical Association, was present to point out that the statement in question was by Anslinger and had only been reported in the A.M.A. Journal.

Dr. Woodward deserves a posthumous accolade for his singlehanded heroic efforts to introduce reason and sanity to the hearing. Most importantly, the doctor (who was also a lawyer) criticized the Congressmen for proposing a law that would interfere with future medical uses of Cannabis and pointed out that no one from the Bureau of Prisons had been produced to show the number of prisoners "addicted" to marijuana, no one from the Children's Bureau or Office of Education to show the nature and extent of the "habit" among children and no one from the Division of Mental Hygiene or the Division of Pharmacology of the Public Health Service to give "direct and primary evidence rather than indirect and hearsay evidence." Saying that he assumed it was true that a certain amount of "narcotic addiction" existed, since "the newspapers have called attention to it so prominently that there must be some grounds for their statements," he concluded that the particular type of statute under consideration was neither necessary nor desirable. The Congressmen totally ignored the content of Dr. Woodward's testimony and attacked his character, qualifications, experience and relationship to the American Medical Association, all of which were impeccable. He was then forced to admit that he could not say with certainty that no problem existed. Finally, his testimony was brought to a halt with the warning, "You are not cooperative in this. If you want to advise us on legislation, you ought to come here with some constructive proposals rather than criticism, rather than trying to throw obstacles in the way of something that the Federal Government is trying to do."

A similar but shorter hearing was held in the Senate, where Anslinger presented anecdotal "evidence" that marijuana caused murder, rape and insanity.

Thus, the Marijuana Tax Act of 1937 was passed—and out of it grew a welter of state laws that were, in many cases, even more hastily ill conceived.

The present Federal laws impose a two-to-ten year sentence for a first conviction for possessing even a small amount of marijuana, five to twenty years for a second conviction and ten to forty for a third. If Congress is not forced to recognize scientific fact and basic civil liberties, these penalties will be retained when the new Federal law is written without the sections declared invalid in the Leary case. The usual discretion that judges are given to grant probation or suspended sentences for real crimes is taken from them by this (and state) law as is the opportunity for parole. For sale or "dissemination," no matter how small the quantity of marijuana involved, and even if the dissemination is a gift between friends, the Federal penalty for first-offense conviction is five to twenty years; for a second offense, it's ten to forty.

The state laws, as I stated, are even hairier. Here are two real, and recent cases: In Texas, Richard Dorsey, a shoe-shine-stand operator in a bowling alley, sold a matchbox full of marijuana (considerably less than an ounce) to a Dallas undercover policeman, for five dollars. His sentence: 50 years.

In Michigan, for selling five dollars' worth of grass to another police agent, Larry Belcher was sentenced to 20 to 30 years in prison. This case is worth noting as an example of how the marijuana laws actually function in many instances. Belcher is the only individual in Grand Traverse County to receive this sentence in the past two years; 25 other marijuana arrestees were all placed on probation within that time. Belcher, it appears, was the author of a column called "Dope-O-Scope" in a local underground newspaper and had presented there some of the same scientific facts incorporated into this article. People who publicly oppose the marijuana laws and marijuana mythology of our narcotics police have an unusually high arrest record.

There is no consistency in these laws from state to state. Until 1968, South Dakota had the nation's lowest penalty for first-offense possession—90 days (it has since been raised to two to five years); however, if you crossed the state line to North Dakota, the picture changed abruptly. North Dakota had (and still has) the nation's highest penalty for first-offense possession—99 years at hard labor. In New York state, in spite of the revelatory work of the La Guardia commission, the penalties have increased since the Forties. Today, in that state, selling or transferring marijuana to anyone under 21 carries a penalty of one to 25 years, even if the transfer is by somebody who is also under 21 and is a gift to a friend. (The state legislature recently tried to raise this penalty to 15 years to life, but Governor Rockefeller vetoed the bill.) In Louisiana, a minor selling to a minor is subject to five to fifteen years' imprisonment, while an adult selling to a minor may receive the death penalty. Finally, in Georgia, the penalty for a first conviction for selling to a minor is life imprisonment. If the offender is paroled or his sentence suspended, and he is convicted again, he can be sentenced to death.

The barbarity of such penalties in relation to pot's relative harmlessness is even beginning to be recognized in Washington, despite incessant and quite unscientific efforts to maintain the old mythology, emanating from the Federal Bureau of Narcotics. In 1963, President Kennedy's Advisory Commission on Narcotic and Drug Abuse called into question some of the prevailing beliefs about marijuana and recommended lighter sentences for possession. In 1967, President Johnson's Commission on Law Enforcement and the Administration of Justice took a similar view, recommending more flexible penalties; more significantly, it stated that marijuana has virtually nothing in common with true narcotics or opiates—the first time that fact was publicly admitted by a U.S. Government agency. And in 1967, Dr. James Goddard, while commissioner of the U.S. Food and Drug Administration, was quoted as saying that it would disturb him less if his teenage daughter smoked one marijuana cigarette than if she drank an alcoholic beverage. (Faced with a predictable outcry from conservatives in Congress,

Goddard said he had been misquoted—but quite honestly added that the known facts did not support the opinion that marijuana is more dangerous than alcohol.)

Not only is marijuana comparatively harmless on the face of all the evidence but there are even reasons to believe it may be beneficial in some cases. In many countries, Cannabis has been used medicinally for as long as 5000 years and is regarded as a sovereign remedy for a variety of ills. There are references to medicinal uses of marijuana in American medical journals (mostly of the 19th Century) where doctors reported it as useful as an analgesic, appetite stimulant, anti-spasmodic, anti-depressant, tranquilizer, anti-asthmatic, topical anesthetic, child-birth analgesic and antibiotic. My own investigations in areas of the world where this folk medicine still flourishes and my study of 20th Century scientific literature lead me to believe that marijuana would be useful for treating depression, loss of appetite, high blood pressure, anxiety and migraine.

An English psychiatrist who employed marijuana in the therapy of depressive patients, Dr. George T. Stockings, concluded that it "might be more effective than any tranquilizer now in use." Dr. Robert Walton of the University of Mississippi has also suggested its use for certain gynecological and menstrual problems and in easing childbirth. We should not let lingering puritanical prejudices prevent us from investigating these areas further. As Dr. Tod Mikuriya, a psychiatrist formerly associated with the National Institute of Mental Health, notes, "The fact that a drug has a recreational history should not blind us to its possible other uses. Morton was the first to use ether publicly for anesthesia after observing medical students at 'ether frolics' in 1846." While such speculations about the benefits of pot must await further research before final answer is given, there can be no doubt that a grave injustice has been suffered by those currently in prison because of laws passed when the drug was believed to incite crime and madness.

Even the Federal Bureau of Narcotics and its propagandists have largely given up the "steppingstone theory" (that marijuana smoking leads to use of addictive drugs) and the "degeneracy theory" (that it leads to crime or "bad character"). They have recently rallied around the oldest, and most discredited, canard of all—the legend that marijuana causes insanity. To shore up this crumbling myth, they cite recent research at the Addiction Research Center in Lexington, Kentucky, where 30 former opiate addicts were given high doses of synthetic THC (the active ingredient in marijuana) or concentrated Cannabis extract. Most of the subjects showed marked perceptual changes, which the experimenter chose to describe as "hallucinations" and "psychotic reactions." This, of course, merely confirms a basic axiom of pharmacology; i.e., with increasing doses of any drug, different and more dangerous responses will occur; you could obtain some spectacularly adverse reactions with horse doctors' doses of aspirin, coffee or even orange juice. (With ordinary doses of THC or marjuana, the subject experienced the same "high" found in normal social marijuana smoking.)

A more serious defect in this research lies in the loaded terminology with which the experimenter, Dr. Harris Isbell, reported his results. Psychiatrist Thomas Szasz, a crusader for reform in the mental health field, points out that a "psychotic reaction" is not something in an individual, Mr. A, like cancer; rather, it is a label that a second individual, Mr. B (more often, Dr. B), pins on Mr. A. The fact is that the subjects experienced perceptual changes; it is not a fact but merely an opinion whether one wants to call these changes "consciousness expansion" and "transcendence of the ego" (with Timothy Leary) or "hallucinations" and "psychotic reactions" (with Dr. Isbell).

Sociologist Howard Becker—the observer who first noted the effect of "learning" on the marijuana experience—has researched medical literature from the early 1930s to the present in search of reported cases of "marijuana psychosis." He found none after 1940, a remarkable fact, considering the pyramiding acceleration of marijuana use during the Forties, Fifties and Sixties. Becker concluded that persons who were diagnosed as "marijuana psychotics" in the Thirties were simply anxious and disoriented because they hadn't learned yet how to use the drug. Dr. Isbell's subjects, almost certainly, were not advised about the effects of the drug; and his experiment is really just another proof of the effect of "set and setting" as well as high doses on drug experience.

A 1946 study examined 310 persons who had been using marijuana for an average of seven years each. There was no record of mental-hospital commitment among any of them.

The marijuanaphobes also cite studies from the Near East to prove that marijuana is associated with psychosis. In the first place, many of the people in these studies smoked hashish, not marijuana; and while hashish is derived from the same plant, Cannabis sativa, it is otherwise a considerably stronger form of the drug. One might compare the two Cannabis drugs with two alcohol drugs as follows: Smoking a pipe of hashish is equivalent to drinking a fifth of vodka; smoking the same pipe of marijuana is about like drinking a bottle of beer. However, the studies themselves do not deserve such careful rebuttal; they are scientifically worthless. They prove only that, in countries where most of the population regularly use Cannabis, many of the patients in mental hospitals also have a history of Cannabis use. Usually the proportion of users in the institution is less than that in the general population, leading to a possible conclusion that it is psychologically beneficial. In fact, however, there are no scientifically valid statistics or records kept at these facilities. The testimony turns out, on examination, to be impressionistic and anecdotal rather than scientific and precise. The diagnosis of psychosis and its attribution to Cannabis is often made by a ward attendant. In short, we are faced with the kind of "evidence" that the Indian Hemp Drug Commission discarded in 1893. I have visited the mental hospitals of several of the countries involved in the "Cannabis psychosis" and none of the record keeping involved meets the minimum requirements demanded of freshman scientific reports in American colleges.

Perhaps the last bastion of marijuanaphobia is the argument by uncertainty. "Who knows?" this line goes. "Maybe in the future, marijuana might be discovered, by further research, to have dangerous side effects that haven't been noted yet." This argument, of course, is unanswerable; but it applies equally well to such diverse objects as diet pills and bubble gum. One cannot prove that the future will not discover new things; but does such a fact—science's lack of clairvoyance—justify our present marijuana laws? It clearly does not. No drug, including marijuana, will ever be found to be totally harmless; and no drug, particularly marijuana, will ever be found to be as dangerous as the hydrogen bomb (once claimed by Anslinger). Social policy should not be determined by this anyway. The possible risks should be dealt with by education. What is unacceptable is locking a man up for 99 years for possessing something of far less proven danger than tobacco, alcohol, automobiles and guns.

Instead of decreasing marijuana usage, our present laws have created the contempt for Government about which I spoke earlier. In addition to continuing to disobey the law, hordes of young people have begun to flout it publicly. There have been smoke-ins—masses who gather in a public park, where those in the inner core of the group light up, while the outer perimeter obstruct and slow down the police until the evidence is consumed—at Berkeley, in Boston and elsewhere. Planting marijuana in conspicuous places has become a fad; among the notable seedings have been the center strip of Park Avenue in New York City, the lawn in front of a police station in ultrarespectable Westchester County, the UN Building and (twice recently) in front of the state capitol in Austin, Texas.

But the American marijuana tragedy is even worse than I have indicated. Like other crimes-without-victims, pot smoking is a private activity and involves no harm to anyone else. Remember: The police do not have to engage in cloak-and-dagger activities to find out if there have been any banks or grocery stores robbed lately—the bankers and store owners (the victims) call them immediately. But since there is no victim in the "crime" of smoking marijuana, nobody is going to call the police to report it—except, very rarely, a neighbor who finds the evidence. Hence, the entire apparatus of the police state comes into existence as soon as we attempt to enforce anti-grass legislation; and by the nature of such legislation, totalitarian results must ensue. We cannot police the private lives of the citizenry without invading their privacy; this is an axiom.

That a man's home is his castle has long been a basic principle of Anglo-American jurisprudence, and some of us can still recall the near poetry of the great oration by William Pitt in which he says, "The poorest man may in his cottage bid defiance to the force of the Crown. It may be frail, its roof may shake; the wind may blow through it; the storms may enter; the rain may enter; but the King of England cannot enter—all his forces dare not cross the threshold of the ruined tenement!" This principle goes back to the Magna Charta and is firmly entrenched in the Fourth Amendment to our own Constitution guaranteeing the people "the right . . . to be secure in their persons, houses, papers and effects, against unreasonable searches and seizures."

This liberation tradition is a great hindrance to the police when they attempt to enforce sumptuary laws—laws concerning the private morals of the citizens. And, in fact, the enforcement of the marijuana law requires pernicious police behavior.

For instance, the *Chicago Sun-Times* told, in 1967, how the police of that city obtain search warrants for use in legalizing raids that otherwise would be mere "fishing expeditions"—intolerable to any American court. In dealing with the organized-crime cartel usually called "the Syndicate," the police have obtained from the courts the right to use what are called "blank warrants"—warrants in which the witness who alleges he has seen the crime is permitted to sign a false name. This is supposedly necessary to protect informers against the wrath of the reputedly all-seeing and all-powerful Syndicate. Once this dangerous precedent was set, the police began applying it to marijuana users as well. As the *Sun-Times* noted:

> Those methods are dubious . . . We refer to the method of obtaining search warrants. The informer signs a search-warrant complaint, with an assumed name, alleging perhaps that he bought illicit drugs from a certain person, at a

certain place. The police do not have to disclose the name of the informer or the time when the drugs were bought. There is also a device known as constructive possession: The police can arrest anybody found in the vicinity of prohibited drugs, whether he's an innocent visitor or the real culprit. The frameup is easy. Plant the drugs, get the search warrant, grab everybody in sight. It could happen to you and you'd never have the right to face your accuser.

William Braden, a *Sun-Times* reporter, also uncovered one informer, a heroin addict, who admitted signing dozens of such warrants without the names of the accused on them. The narcotics squad could then type in the name of any individual whose apartment they wanted to raid and it would be perfectly "legal" in form—but a terrifying distance in spirit from the actual meaning of the Constitution. Such raids, of course, violate the Sixth Amendment—guaranteeing the right "to be confronted with the witnesses" against you—as well as the Fourth (no "unreasonable searches"); and they occur everywhere in the nation.

Most of us never hear of such things, because reporters routinely print the police version of the raid, without interviewing the arrested "dope fiends." It is also standard practice for the police to multiply the quantity of drugs seized in such a raid by a factor of two (and the price by a factor of ten) when giving the news to the press. This makes for impressive headlines; it also contributes to the growing tendency toward "trial by newspaper," which worries civil libertarians.

Some types of entrapment are regarded as legal in America today—although some still are not. In my own opinion, all forms of entrapment are profoundly immoral, whether technically legal or illegal; but my opinion is, perhaps, immaterial. The results of this practice, however, are truly deplorable from the point of view of anyone who has any lingering affection for the spirit of the Bill of Rights.

Here is a specific case: John Sinclair, a poet, leader of the Ann Arbor hippie community and manager of a rock group called MC-5, became friendly, around October 1966, with Vahan Kapagian and Jane Mumford, who presented themselves to him as members of the hippie-artist-mystic subculture that exists in all of our large cities. Over a period of two months, they worked to secure his confidence and friendship and several times asked him to get them some marijuana. Finally, on December 22, Sinclair, apparently feeling that he could now trust them, gave two marijuana cigarettes to Miss Mumford—one for her and one for Kapagian. He was immediately arrested; his "friends" were police undercover agents.

Sinclair has been convicted of both "possessing" and "dispensing" marijuana and faces a minimum of 20 years under each statute, and a maximum of life for the sale. If his appeal is not upheld, the very smallest sentence he could receive is 40 years. As his lawyers pointed out in his appeal, "The minimum sentence to which (Sinclair) is subject to imprisonment is 20 times greater than the minimum to which a person may be imprisoned (in Michigan) for such crimes as rape, robbery, arson, kidnapping or second-degree murder. It is more than 20 times greater than the minimum sentence of imprisonment for any other offense in Michigan law, except first-degree murder."

That illegal wire tapping has also been wisely used by the narcotics police was an open secret for years; now it is no secret at all—and not illegal, either. The 1968 Omnibus Crime Bill authorizes such wire tapping for suspected marijuana users.

Since this usage has spread to all classes and all educational levels, such suspicion can be directed at virtually anyone (after all, the nephew and the brother of one of President Nixon's closest friends were recently busted on pot charges); thus, almost any American can now have his phone tapped legally. Considering the elastic interpretation police usually give to such Congressional authorization, an anonymous tip by any crank in your neighborhood would probably be enough to get a tap on your phone by tomorrow morning. Why not? As *Chicago Daily News* columnist Mike Royko recently wrote, "There is a democratic principle in injustice. If enough people support it, they'll all get it."

With the doctrine of "constructive possession," anyone who has a pot-smoking friend is subject to marijuana laws if he walks into the friend's house at the wrong time. In California two years ago, a woman was sentenced to sterilization for being in the same room with a man who was smoking grass. The fact that a higher court overturned this sentence does not lessen its frightening implications.

And a new wrinkle has been added. According to a story in the *San Francisco Chronicle* last June 20, the Government is planning "an unpleasant surprise for marijuana smokers—'sick pot.' " The article goes on to explain how an unspecified chemical can be sprayed on Mexican marijuana fields from a helicopter, whereupon "just a puff or two produces uncontrollable vomiting that not even the most dedicated smoker could ignore."

This, I submit, could have come from the morbid fantasy of Kafka, Burroughs or Orwell. The Government, in its holy war against a relatively harmless drug, is deliberately creating a very harmful drug. Nor is the *Chronicle* story something dreamed up by a sensation-mongering reporter. A call to the Justice Department in Washington has confirmed that this plan has been discussed and may go into operation in the near future.

Consider, now, the actual social background in which this crusade against Cannabis is being waged. America is not the Victorian garden it pretends to be; we are, in fact, a drug-prone nation. Parents and other adults after whom children model their behavior teach them that every time one relates to other human beings, whether at a wedding or at a funeral, and every time one has a pain, problem or trouble, it is necessary or desirable to pop a pill, drink a cocktail or smoke a cigarette. The alcohol, tobacco and over-the-counter pseudo-"sedative" industries jointly spend more than $2,000,000 a day in the United States alone to promote as much drug use as possible.

The average "straight" adult consumes three to five mind-altering drugs a day, beginning with the stimulant caffeine in coffee, tea or Coca-Cola, going on to include alcohol and nicotine, often a tranquilizer, not uncommonly a sleeping pill at night and sometimes an amphetamine the next morning to overcome the effects of the sedative taken the evening before.

We have 80,000,000 users of alcohol in this country, including 6,000,000 alcoholics; 50,000,000 users of tobacco cigarettes, 25,000,000 to 30,000,000 users of sedatives, stimulants and tranquilizers; and hundreds of thousands of users of consciousness alterers that range from heroin and LSD to cough syrup, glue, nutmet and catnip—all in addition to marijuana use.

Drs. Manheimer and Mellinger, surveying California adults over 21, found that 51 per cent had at some time used sedatives, stimulants or tranquilizers (17 per cent had taken these drugs frequently) and 13 per cent had at some time used marijuana.

Further underlining the extent of use of the prescription drugs is the estimate from the National Prescription Audit that 175,000,000 prescriptions for sedatives, stimulants and tranquilizers were filled in 1968. Also enough barbiturates (Nembutal, Seconal, phenobarbital) alone are manufactured to provide 25 to 30 average doses per year for every man, woman and child in this country.

In the light of this total drug picture, the persecution of potheads seems to be a species of what anthropologists call "scapegoatism"—the selection of one minority group to be punished for the sins of the whole population, whose guilt is vicariously extirpated in the punishment of the symbolic sacrificial victims.

Meanwhile, my criticisms—and those of increasing numbers of writers, scientific and popular—continue to bounce off the iron walls of prejudice that seem to surround Congress and state legislatures. It is quite possible that our new, post-Leary pot laws will be as bad as the old ones. If there is any improvement, it is likely to come, once again, from the courts.

Several legal challenges to our anti-pot mania are, in fact, working their way upward toward the Supreme Court, and the issues they raise are potentially even more significant than those involved in the Leary case.

First is the challenge raised by attorney Joseph Oteri in his defense of two Boston University students. Oteri's case cites the equal-protection clause of the Constitution—grass is less harmful than booze, so you can't outlaw one without the other. He also argues that the marijuana statute is irrational and arbitrary and an invalid exercise of police power because pot is harmless and wrongly defined as a narcotic, when it is, technically, not a narcotic. This is not mere hairsplitting. It is impossible, under law, to hang a man for murder if his actual crime was stealing hubcaps; it should be equally impossible to convict him of "possession of a narcotic" if he was not in possession of a narcotic but of a drug belonging to an entirely different chemical family.

And marijuana, decidedly, is not a narcotic—although just what it should be called is something of a mystery. The tendency these days is to call it a "mild psychedelic," with the emphasis on mild; this is encouraged both by the Tim Leary crowd—to whom psychedelic is a good word, denoting peace, ecstasy, non-violent revolution, union with God and the end of all neurotic hang-ups of Western man—and by those to whom psychedelic is a monster word denoting hallucinations, insanity, suicide and chaos. I doubt the psychedelic label very much and think it is as off base as narcotic. Since marijuana has very little in common with LSD and the true psychedelics, but much in common with alcohol and other sedatives, and a certain similarity also to amphetamine and other stimulants, I prefer to call it a sedative-stimulant as it is classified by Dr. Frederick Meyers, who also notes its resemblance to laughing gas (nitrous oxide). Dr. Leo Hollister finds enough resemblance to LSD to call it a sedative- hypnotic-psychedelic. *Goodman and Gilman*, the orthodox pharmacological reference, dodges the issue entirely by listing marijuana as a "miscellaneous" drug. In any case, it is not a narcotic, and anyone arrested for having a narcotic in his possession when he actually has marijuana definitely is being charged with a crime he hasn't committed.

A second challenge, raised by Oteri and also being pressed by two Michigan attorneys, is based on the prohibition of "cruel and unusual punishments" in the Eighth Amendment. The courts have held, in the past, that a law can be struck down if the punishments it requires are cruel and unusual in comparison with the penalties in the same state for similar or related crimes. For instance, the statute against chicken stealing was made quite harsh in the early days of Oklahoma, apparently because the offense was common and provoked great public indignation. As a result, a man named Skinner was threatened with the punishment of sterilization under one section of this law. He appealed to the Supreme Court, which struck down the Oklahoma statute because similarly harsh penalties were not provided for other forms of theft. Obviously, in the states where the penalty for possession of marijuana is higher than the penalty for armed robbery, rape, second-degree murder, etc., the law is vulnerable to legal attack as cruel and unusual.

There is also the "zone of privacy" argument, originally stated in the Connecticut birth-control decision and more recently invoked by the Kentucky supreme court, in striking down a local (Barbourville, Kentucky) ordinance making it a crime to smoke tobacco cigarettes. The court ruled that "The city . . . . may not unreasonably interfere with the right of the citizen to determine for himself such personal matters." The zone of privacy was also cited by the U.S. Supreme Court in invalidating the Georgia law against possession (not sale) of pornography.

The drug police and their legislative allies have been experimenting with our liberties for a long time now. The Leary decision, however, shows that it is not too late to reverse the trend, and the issues raised by the constitutional questions discussed above show how the erosion of our liberties can, indeed, be reversed.

A compelling medical, sociological and philosophical case exists for the full legalization of marijuana, particularly if legislation is the only alternative to the present criminalization of users. But an even more substantial case exists for ending all criminal penalties for possession or use of the drug, while still exercising some caution. I would recommend, for example, that to prevent the sale of dangerously adulterated forms of the drug, marijuana be produced under Federal supervision, as alcohol is. Furthermore, sellers of the drug should be licensed, and they should be prohibited from selling to minors. If there are infractions of these laws, the penalties should be directed at the seller, not the user. I would also strongly recommend that all advertising and promotion of marijuana be prohibited, and that packages of the drug carry the warning: CAUTION: MARIJUANA MAY BE HARMFUL TO YOUR HEALTH.

If marijuana were to be legalized, what would happen? According to the marijuanaphobes, the weed will spread into every American home; people will become lazy and sluggish, sit around all day in a drugged stupor and talk philosophy when they talk at all; we will sink into the "backward" state of the Near Eastern and Asian nations.

There are good, hard scientific reasons for doubting this gloomy prognostication.

1. Most Americans have already found their drug of choice—alcohol—and there is more conditioning involved in such preferences than most people realize. The average American heads straight for the bar when he feels the impulse to relax; a change in the laws will not change this conditioned reflex. When the Catholic Church allowed its members to eat meat on Friday, the majority went right on following the conditioned channel that told them, "Friday is fish day."

2. Of the small minority that will try pot (after it is legalized) in search of a new kick, most will be vastly disappointed, since (a) it doesn't live up to its sensational publicity, largely given to it by the Federal

Narcotics Bureau; and (b) the "high" depends, as we have indicated, not only on set and setting but, unlike alcohol, on learning.

This involves conditioning and the relationship of the actual chemistry of the two drugs to the total Gestalt of our culture. What pot actually does—outside mythology—is produce a state midway between euphoria and drowsiness, like a mild alcohol high; accelerate and sharpen the thoughts (at least in the subjective impression of the user), like an amphetamine; and intensify sound and color perception, although not nearly as much as a true psychedelic. It can also enhance sexual experience, but not create it—contrary to Mr. Anslinger, pot is not an aphrodisiac. It is, in short, the drug of preference for creative and contemplative types—or, at least, people with a certain streak of that tendency in their personality. Alcohol, on the other hand, depresses the forebrain, relaxes inhibitions, produces euphoria and drowsiness and, while depleting some functions, such as speech and walking, does not draw one into the mixture of sensuality and introspection created by pot. It is the drug of preference for aggressive and extroverted types. Therefore, the picture of pot spreading everywhere and changing our culture is sociologically putting the cart before the horse; our society would first have to change basically before pot could spread everywhere.

3. Even if, against all likelihood, marijuana were to sweep the country, this would not have dire consequences. Marijuana has no specifically anti-machine property in it; it would not make our technology go away, like a wave of an evil sorcerer's hand. Nor does it dull the mental faculties, as we have seen in reviewing the scientific evidence. (I might add, here, that the highest honor students at certain Ivy League colleges are frequently pot users, and one study at Yale found more marijuana smokers at the top of the class than at the bottom.)

4. Finally, the whole specter of American sinking into backwardness due to pot is based upon totally false anthropological concepts. The Near East is not tribal, preindustrial, superstitious, and so forth, merely because Mohammed banned alcohol in the Koran but forgot to exclude Cannabis drugs also; a whole complex of historical and cultural factors is involved, not the least of which is the continuous intervention of Western imperialism from the Crusades onward. Other factors are the rigid structure of the Islamic religion and the lack of a scientific minority that can effectively challenge these dogmas; the Western world was equally backward—please note—where the Christian religion was not open to scientific dissent and criticism. Backwardness is a relative concept, and, although pot has been used in the Arabic countries for millenniums, they have several times been ahead of the West in basic science (the most famous example being their invention of algebra). The populations of these nations are not "lazy" due to marijuana nor to any other cause; they are merely underemployed by a feudalistic economic system. The ones lucky enough to find work usually toil for longer hours, in a hotter sun, than most Americans would find bearable.

Thus, treating marijuana in a sane and rational way presents no threat to our society, whereas continuing the present hysteria will alienate increasing numbers of the young while accelerating the drift toward a police state. I take no pleasure in the spread of even so mild a drug as marijuana, and I am sure (personally, not scientifically) that in a truly open, libertarian and decent society, nobody would be inclined to any kind of drug use. While I agree with the psychedelic generation about the absurdity and injustice of our criminal laws relating to drugs, I am not an apostle of the "turn on, tune in, drop out" mystique. I recognize that drugs can be an evasion of responsibility, and that there is no simple chemical solution to all the psychic, social and political problems of our time. My own program would be: Turn on to the life around you, tune in to knowledge and feeling, and drop in to changing the world for the better. If that course could prevail, the adventurous young, no longer haunted by the anxiety and anomie of the present system, would probably discover that love, comradeship, music, the arts, sex, meaningful work, alertness, self-discipline, real education (which is a lifelong task) and plain hard thought are bigger, better and more permanent highs than any chemical can produce.

But meanwhile, I must protest—I will continue to protest—against the bureaucrat who stands with cocktail in one hand and cigarette in the other and cries out that the innocent recreation of pot smoking is the major problem facing our society, one that can be solved only by raising the penalty to castration for the first offense and death for the second. He would be doing the young people—and all the rest of us—a true favor if he forgot about marijuana for a while and thought, a few minutes a day, about such real problems as racism, poverty, starvation, air pollution and our stumbling progress toward World War Three and the end of life on earth.

It is an irony of our time that our beloved George Washington would be a criminal today, for he grew hemp at Mount Vernon, and his diary entries, dealing specifically with separating the female plants from the male before pollination, show that he was not harvesting it for rope. The segregation of the plants by sex is only necessary if you intend to extract "the killer drug, marijuana" from the female plants.

Of course, we have no absolute evidence that George turned on. More likely, he was using marijuana as many Americans in that age used it: as a medicine for bronchitis, chest colds and other respiratory ailments. (Pot's euphoric qualities were not well known outside the East in those days.) But can you imagine General Washington trying to explain to an agent of the Federal Narcotics Bureau, "I was only smoking it to clear up my lumbago?" It would never work; he would land in prison, perhaps for as long as 40 years. He would be sharing the same cruel fate as several thousand other harmless Americans today. As it says in the book of Job, "From the dust the dying groan, and the souls of the wounded cry out."

2 The Year of the Middle Class Junkie

by David J. Bentel, D. Crim
and David E. Smith, M.D.

Heroin, recent newspaper headlines proclaim, is no longer limited to the "lower classes," but is now infecting the sons and daughters of respectable, well-to-do citizens of middle and upper class America.

This alarm about heroin now being sounded across the country does not emanate from concern about the long standing drug abuse problems in racial ghettos, but rather is a result of "dope" infiltrating white youth in "good" neighborhoods.

Patterns of narcotic use now dominant in the well-known psychedelic communities of Greenwich Village, New York and the Haight-Ashbury district of San Francisco, are "rippling out" to such diverse communities as Palo Alto, California; Ann Arbor, Michigan; Phoenix, Arizona; Grinnell, Iowa; and Bar Harbor, Maine, to name just a few.

This Is The Year

1971 has become the year of the Middle-Class Junkie. Shocked, distraught, unbelieving parents who discover that their son or daughter

SOURCE: Reprinted from the April 1971 issue of *California's Health*. Dr. Bentel is co-director University of California Drug Abuse Information Project, and Dr. Smith is founder and Medical Director Haight-Ashbury Free Clinic and Co-director University of California Drug Abuse Information Project.

is a heroin addict are demanding government and community response to deal with the crisis. Chiefs of police, judges, school superintendents, principals, and politicians are being put on the spot to "do something now."

Investigations reveal that young, teenage white kids, just like the kids in the ghetto slums, rob, steal and prostitute—"hustle"—on the streets to support drug habits of $25, $50 and even $150 a day.

An 18-year-old son of a well-to-do Mill Valley resident committed 376 burglaries of local homes to support his $150 a day habit which required that he steal and "fence" $500 to $600 a day worth of merchandise. Selling drugs to other kids in school is another common way to finance a drug habit. In some high schools, the boys' lavatory is called "the drug store" because of the volume of illicit business done between classes.

New Breed

The "new breed" of heroin addicts, noted in the San Francisco *Chronicle* on November 18, 1969, marks a drastic new phase in youthful drug abuse.

In New York City alone, out of an estimated 100,000 current heroin addicts, over 1,000 deaths due to drug overdose occurred last year. In the 15- to 35-year old group, heroin overdoses is the leading cause of death in Manhattan.

Police in most of the larger cities agree generally that almost 50 per cent of all property crimes are committed by young heroin addicts desperate to get enough cash together to make their "connection." This recent move to heroin, however, is only part of a much broader, constantly shifting drug scene.

Drug use, in general, and among adolescents heroin use, in particular, have steadily increased in the last five years despite repeated assurances by State and federal officials that this was just a passing phenomenon. We predict that the majority of school age youth across the whole country will experiment with some type of illegal drug before they reach high school graduation.

The only thing constant about the "drug scene" is that it constantly changes, and chances are good that it'll get a lot worse before it starts to get better.

The classic "nickel bag" of heroin, a plastic bag or rubber balloon which sells on the street for $5 to $15, and contains about 3 per cent heroin bulked up with milk sugar, quinine, or any other white crystalling powder additive which looks like heroin—including household cleanser or strychnine—is no longer the exclusive merchandise of the ghetto dweller.

Hook the Whites!

One black mother, quoted in a recent *Ebony Magazine* article titled, "Blacks Declare War on Dope," exclaimed: "The best news I've heard in a long time is that more white kids are getting hooked on heroin. You know the best way to deal with the dope problem? Get as many white kids hooked on it as possible! Then maybe the government will do something about the dope problem."

Ghetto youths, Blacks, Mexican-Americans, and Puerto Ricans, some minority leaders feel, have too long been the easy prey for rich white drug pushers who have exploited them with diluted dope. Ghetto dwellers bought heroin to diminish the acute pain of living in an almost escape-proof trap of poverty, racism and despair. The long-standing traffic in heroin they now see as a conspiracy by whites to keep them dependent and "nodding on the street corner" instead of organizing militantly for their rights.

Heroin Addiction

Heroin, although not the most chemically destructive of the currently abused illegal drugs (barbiturates cause more severe addiction, and amphetamines are more acutely destructive to the central nervous system) is the worst type of compulsive drug abuse pattern in which to be involved. Once you're "on it," you crave it—even "garbage" heroin that has been "cut" (diluted) by a dozen or more "middlemen." Unless a kid is independently wealthy, he's going to have to steal or hustle in some illegal way which means his whole life-style is typically involved in a criminal process.

Old Story—New Chapter

But why, after almost a century, has drug abuse and especially the most destructive form of such abuse, heroin use, become a drug syndrome? Why the middle class heroin scene?

Stories of heroin smugglers, "smack" and depraved "junkies" are old and well known. "Dope" has been around since the Civil War. By 1863, scarcely 20 years after the development of the hypodermic needle, estimates of addiction in the U.S. ran as high as four per cent of the total population.

While civil war casualties were sedated with morphine, country stores sold crude elixirs and other cure-claiming remedies that owed their therapeutic properties only to a high alcohol content with an opium base of 5 or even 10 per cent. After the Harrison Narcotic Act was passed in 1914, the criminal underworld heroin smuggling chains developed. Gum opium from Turkey and the Orient was taken to Marseilles and other French port towns and refined into heroin.

Smuggled to New York and New Orleans in freighters, pure heroin was cut and distributed to middlemen pushers who moved it down the distribution line to street level dealers, most of whom sold the drug to support their own habits.

Heroin Myth vs. Reality

Everyone knows of the monster "dope fiend," an arch-criminal whose vicious and depraved crimes make him a sex maniac and public enemy number one.

The lurid sensationalism which created the myths of the dope fiend in the first place has recently given way to more factual reporting of contemporary drug problems which includes scientific studies by scholars such as Isador Chein and associates who studied heroin addiction in New York for over a decade.

Chronic addiction, they found, was more a product of the conditions of inner city ghetto life than of the chemistry of the drugs themselves. Junkies were most often living in slums or areas of high usage distinguished by impoverished families and high concentrations of discriminated-against minorities including recent immigrant groups. Such communities produced higher than normal numbers of disrupted families and other forms of human misery.

Chein, in his classic book, *The Road to H*, found heroin users for the most part to be delinquent minority kids from 16 to 21 years of age who "suffer deep rooted major personality disorders." The ghetto drug-using community, he notes, is one "in which there is a relative breakdown in the fabric of human relationships . . . (where) the individual feels essentially standing alone against the world (where) the values of society have only negative significance for him, for living up to them can only protect him from an additional burden of trouble rather than provide him with the missing satisfactions of living."

No One Type

Today it can no longer be stated categorically that there is just one type of person who gets involved with illegal drugs, including heroin.

Any drug pattern is a complex interaction between chemical, personality and social environment. The amount of use, the style of use, and the effect achieved at one particular time and place, are dramatically influenced by the user's attitude and personal environment.

Dr. George Gay, Chief of the Haight-Ashbury Medical Clinic's drug detoxification section, feels that perhaps affluent white youths use heroin for many of the same psychological reasons as do ghetto blacks—alienation and despair. Gay points out that the optimism and love manifested by the country's hippie population, exemplified in what is now nostalgically referred to as the Summer of Love of 1967 in San Francisco, have vanished. There are now mostly hate, paranoia, and disillusionment among the already alienated young.

During that summer, thousands of young persons from all over the United States flocked to the "Haight" to "turn on" with psychedelic drugs, share each other's companionship and also to express a happy, carefree, uninhibited hippie philosophy. But from the time of their arrival, they were harrassed by violence and exploitation.

Love Dies in Haight

A lot of bad things happened to the bearded, beaded flower children of psychedelia. They were robbed, raped, hassled and arrested until they either left the "scene" or successfully adapted to the destructive criminal life style of the street.

Many of them were exploited by the maurauding bands of street toughs who also came on the scene to get what they could. The old criminals and the street kids called these middle class white kids "fresh meat" because they were so unprepared, naive, and gullible. Thousands of upper and middle class white kids had come to an area that they had neither understanding of, nor cultural framework for, and they consequently got involved in destructive and tragic life styles.

The new white heroin addicts had no basis or experience for survival in the drug ghetto. And the Summer of Love turned to depression, violence and a tragic end for many.

"It got too heavy . . ."

The result was that the drug-using styles underwent radical transformation. The flower children who didn't make it out of the Haight to a peaceful counter culture commune or back home, often went from mystical drug use to compulsive drug use. But as one hip girl explained:

> "I used to turn on with our own group . . . we all dug each other and it was a pretty groovy experience. But after awhile it got too heavy. All these people I had never seen before started coming over and crashing and I started getting paranoid. All the good vibrations that we had built up together got lost . . . everybody was getting hassled. One chick living with us got ripped off a couple of times and I just said to myself, forget this, I'm going to split. So my 'old man' and I took off, which was pretty sad . . . that's the story with lots of the people who used to live around here."

The many arrests or threats of them, the cheating and exploitation which developed around the illegal drug traffic, and the heavy violence which scarred the district with something like 44 murders in two and a half years fostered even more "bad trips" and generated feelings of distrust and depression.

The early psychedelic community was almost exclusively involved with marijuana and LSD. But with the continued influx of thousands of teenie-boppers and would-be hippies, an almost frantic compulsion developed to "get it on" with almost any type of chemical which could be swallowed or injected.

Unknown

Drug experimentation became dramatically indiscriminate. Kids acting the role of pushers on the street were passing out or selling all kinds, colors, and types of pills or capsules. Most who thought they knew what they were taking were wrong, because the pills—when analyzed by the State narcotics labs—contained something other than what they were sold as.

The results were typically "bad trips," sickness, sometimes even death. And coupled with the dangerous, violent social environment, the result was typically a general but steady physical and mental deterioration of the street habitue.

As young people came and left the community, a "settling out" process occurred. Those who didn't leave, but settled out to the bottom of the culture, were the sicker, more disturbed.

New Community Failures

Those who couldn't even make it as hippies, who were outcasts even within an outcast society, formed their own unique drug-using community and were probably responsible for the first major, youth "speed scene" in the United States. To counteract acute depression and to get relief from the aftermath of bad trips, they started injecting amphetamines.

Shooting "speed" allows a depressed user, who has a negative self image to become hyperactive, excited, happy and optimistic for a while. One might say that he even becomes frantically successful. He can do lots of things which he couldn't in his previous depressed, lethargic state. He can also act out violently and irrationally in a paranoid fashion.

The high dose amphetamine abuser injects himself many times a day with increasing doses of the easily obtained, cheap, black market methamphetamine. He will stay up for several days and nights in a row, continuously on the go, hardly eating and never sleeping. But this all ends abruptly in the "crash" which leaves the user physically and mentally exhausted and even more acutely depressed than before.

To get back up, he has a compulsion to "shoot up" again in even larger doses. What follows is a series of back-to-back speed cycles which eventually end with the sufferer in a state of extreme mental and physical collapse—sometimes near death.

Iron the "Wrinkles"

To escape from the grasp of speed, the user ultimately seeks relief from paranoia anxiety and insomnia by using a "downer" or depressant to soothe his frayed nerves and "iron out all the wrinkles." Although he may use barbiturates initially, he soon finds that the best downer on the illegal market is heroin. Amphetamine abuse then, has become a new road to H.

Heroin use to many, however, seems almost a death wish. Perhaps it's even a symbolic substitution for suicide. The new style heroin users, Dr. Gay feels, are sick because their lives and their world are sick, in spite of affluence. They are almost totally alienated from the rest of America. They no longer identify with or trust society or even see much good in it. They feel that they have been betrayed and deserted by their parents, their teachers and their society. So they drop out, sometimes literally. Heroin, they feel, is their best or perhaps only path of escape.

The Adolescence Trial

To buy, sell, possess or use illegal drugs is a criminal offense. Chances are high of eventual imprisonment and further character destruction because of group pressure from older, hardened criminals. This is true even if the user never reaches the point of self-destruction through drug use alone.

Although the popular "stepping stone theory" that marijuana smoking leads to heroin has been discredited by most analytical persons, there is substance in the contention that persons introduced into an illegal, criminal underground to buy or sell one drug will soon be exposed to the opportunity to try others, "smack" included.

The initial motivations for trying illegal drugs are not pathological so much as they are social. Drugs are the current "in" thing with the kids. Everybody has heard about them, some have tried them, but all are curious. The average kids from good families who experiment with drugs are not mentally ill, but rather going through the normal process of adolescent turmoil.

Drug use is an excellent way of rebelling because the conventional morality considers it "so bad." Every adolescent in this country may go through a process of rebellion and turmoil while growing up, during which time he is strongly oriented to finding a coherent identity and a social group to which he can belong.

Wanting to do what the group does, to be accepted, and to be established with his peers, separate from his family, are of paramount importance. The emerging adult is struggling for a sense of self and individual worth.

End of the Tunnel

If during this period he contacts or engages those persons who are deeply involved in the drug culture, the social and psychological dynamics may be present for the person first to experiment, and then later to become compulsively involved with dangerous drugs. Once the kid is really into heroin, the light at the end of the tunnel becomes dimmer and dimmer.

There are, of course, other predisposing factors to heroin dependence. Some users even from childhood had serious and well-established personality pathology, often caused by trauma, unhappiness, violence and neglect in the home. These people were "made for heroin" as some of them admit. They were waiting all their lives for heroin to "find them."

Still, some radical redefinition must occur in contemporary theories of drug dependence, because many thousands of recent converts to heroin might never have gotten started had there not been powerful external social pressures for them to do so.

In addition, the most critical moderating influence for young people—that institution which helped moderate previous generations in their adolescence, the American family—has degraded badly. The cohesiveness of the family structure has been eroded and compromised by external forces and demands. Contemporary patterns of youthful drug abuse are predictive of increasing social pathology, and foretell drastic changes to come in the direction and quality of American life.

Drug use and abuse have multiple causes and consequences, and can only be moderated by a multiple modality, community-oriented approach.

Drug Education—Balanced

For drug education to be an effective preventive in nature, it must occur before the age of actual drug experimentation. Too-structured a program either within the family or in education tends to create artificiality. It becomes, to the young person, irrelevant and more of the same old adult propaganda.

Any valid community-based approach must be a balanced effort between law enforcement, research, education and treatment. Administration of such a program or series of programs cannot simply be turned over to health or education "professionals," but has to have active backing as well as the participation of the legal and educational establishment, influential citizens and participation by young people from communities in which the problem first developed.

The kids must be part of the solution rather than just part of the problem.

Tailor-Made

Effective education for drug abuse prevention has to be tailor-made to the community where it is to be applied. A big city clinic service may be completely ineffective in a small rural setting.

Each approach must be sophisticated and highly selective as well as completely community based.

Also it must *not* be a one shot, chemically-oriented, law enforcement, scare tactic process.

Communication

Most successes in prevention have been achieved not through didactic presentation, that is, an expert or a teacher standing in front of a group and lecturing, but through honest, small group interaction and discussion. Such groups must include kids, parents, teachers, counselors and other community representatives, including local law enforcement.

It is constantly surprising how little real communication or understanding exists between many parents and their own children whom they claim to love. A well-to-do mother, proud of her involvement in many community service projects, may give more attention and understanding to the family's pet poodles than to her own son or daughter. One mother voiced the sentiments of many, stating:

> "I told my kids if I ever caught'em fooling around with drugs—if they ever got into that kind of trouble—they could just pack their bags and get the hell out. They've had it as far as I'm concerned. I won't have any part of it."

Tremendous Gap

There is a tremendous information gap between parent and drug-using child. An inverse relationship seems to exist: the higher up the status ladder—the more prestigious or affluent the parents—the less they seem to know about what their kids spend their time doing.

They typically lament afterwards, "I just can't understand what went wrong. We did everything we could for our kids, gave them everything they ever wanted. I just don't, for the life of me, understand how they could have gone and done what they did."

The upper or middle-class parent is more and more out of touch with his offspring in the same way as the parent in the lower socio-economic strata, where both husband and wife work all day and let the kids run the streets after school without parental supervision.

The upper-class parent, like the lower, may not even realize for months that his kid is chronically addicted to heroin. He may only find out after his child's behavior and life patterns have so deteriorated that the youth's waking hours are spent on a bizarre, compulsive search for the next fix.

Parental Response

Typically at that point, parental reactions will be irrational, emotional, full of hostility and misgivings, but certainly counter-productive to any possible therapeutic solution to the problem.

Community drug treatment programs often employ young, experienced ex-drug users on whom the needy can rely for treatment and advice. Many of the free clinics have gained widespread acceptance because they are non-judgmental and have voluntary access to the existing drug population.

It is destructive to the child and to society to arrest and send to detention centers or institutions those who have used or abused illegal drugs. This may be necessary only when a drug pattern is acutely destructive or where the young person is so disturbed that institutional treatment is needed to protect him and society. But treatment involves a caring, informal, community approach with active participation of all community agencies, including the immediate family of the abuser.

Treatment of heroin addiction has recently become polarized into camps with advocates of two different treatment approaches: methadone, the chemical approach, and the third community therapeutic approach. Both see the addict as sick rather than criminal, but differ in their approach to the illness.

Methadone Treatment

Methadone is a long acting, orally active narcotic which was employed initially as a viable treatment modality by Dole and Nyswander in New York. Its use is strongly advocated by those who see heroin abuse primarily as a metabolic disease requiring replacement therapy with a less destructive drug.

Studies in fact have demonstrated a high heroin-free, crime-free rate, with daily oral doses of methadone.

Users report diminished interest in drugs themselves and in the people who gravitated around the drug-using life. Many are able to go to work for the first time in years and also marry and raise families. The "rush" and the "high" are not experienced by the user once a maintenance level dose of methadone is established.[1]

Non-drug therapeutic groups like Synanon, however, are opposed to methadone which they claim is just another drug crutch to carry a drug-dependent personality. In spite of the fact that methadone programs have a high success rate, those of a more psychotherapeutic bent insist on changing the user's drug-using style of life, social environment and ways of dealing with himself and others by non-drug means.

Many drug treatment specialists are convinced that Synanon and Synanon-like groups are the solution to drug addiction. Such programs typically offer a living-in community such as "The Family" at Mendocino State Hospital in California.

Treatment specialists often turn out to be ex-users themselves who insist on embarrassingly frank personal intercommuni-

[1] A review of California Methadone Maintenance Programs can be found in the Fourth Annual UC Drug Abuse Information report, available through the University of California—San Francisco, Department of Pharmacology.

cations. Within the therapeutic community, there is intense verbal attacking of personal habits and character traits which are "drug-oriented." Treating means group focusing on habits, traits, and emotions that drive the addict to drugs.

Face the Truth

"I know the junkie mind, man, I'm an ex-user myself. The junkie uses every kind of trick—he lies, he steals, he even lies to himself. We make our people face the worst thing for them, man, the truth. We make them look at the life they are living, what they are doing to other people and especially to themselves. The truth, really hurts, baby, and we rub it in."

Within the therapeutic community there is honesty, openness and truthfulness about interpersonal realtionships which help the sick and the alienated get back to normalcy as well as coherent social functioning.

Yet the key to the therapeutic community, besides just living away from drug-using groups, is the group encounter, variously called Synanon game, attack therapy or just encounter group. The process involves selecting one group-member after another, using newer members, for accusation and direct confrontation. Lying and rationalization manipulation, the favorite interpersonal gambits of the doper, are ruthlessly attacked and dissected.

The subject of a group "haircut" is told to "come clean" or else! The therapeutic communities move residents through "phases" during which they are expected to undergo radical behavioral and attitudinal transformation. Finally the rebuilt ex-addict is re-exposed to the outside community and eventually re-established.

Such "reality" type therapy is considered to reach the underlying motivational level which creates the need, the weakness for drugs in the first place. Therapeutic communities have sprung up all over the United States and have become a major treatment modality along with methadone.

Little Support

Unfortunately, these projects usually receive very little financial support and are severely limited in capacity to handle the thousands of new young addicts who are being "born" on the streets every month. Fortunately, however, there is evidence of a slow shift in the attitude of the general public and the official agencies toward drug problems. There is a gradual but beneficial shift in attitudes regarding education and treatment.

For only when the dominant culture accepts a combination social and health-care model of drug addiction, and rejects the prevailing criminal-punishment rationale, can progress be made toward resolving middle-class heroin addiction and the broader problems of America's Drug Epidemic.

How Safe is Aspirin? 3

Acetylsalicylic acid—better known as aspirin—is a true miracle drug. It works wonders, relieving everything from the throb of a hangover to the ache of a sprained ankle; it can lower the fever of a common cold or flu and—more effectively than cortisone—reduce the inflammation of rheumatoid arthritis. It is cheap; Americans alone swallow some 16 billion aspirin tablets a year, plus buffered compounds that contain aspirin as a principal ingredient. And it remains a mystery; though considered safe enough to be sold without a prescription, no one knows precisely how aspirin performs all its wondrous tasks. Last week researchers from Scripps Clinic and Research Foundation in La Jolla, California, took away some of the mystery—but raised some disturbing questions about aspirin's beneficence.

Doctors Richard S. Farr, R. Neal Pinckard and David Hawkins told the annual meeting of the Federation of American Societies for Experimental Biology in Atlantic City that aspirin alters serum albumin, the main protein in the blood plasma. While studying the blood of rheumatoid arthritis patients, the Scripps team found that the patients' serum albumin had a tendency to combine chemically with a substance called acetrizoate. At first, Farr and his associates suspected that the abnormal albumin was a result of the arthritis itself. But later they learned that the abnormality was most prevalent in patients taking aspirin.

Tag: To find how aspirin altered the blood protein, the researchers tagged different parts of the acetylsalicylic-acid molecule with a radio carbon. Then they mixed each of the labeled compounds with serum albumin. They found that the "acetyl group" within the drug combined with albumin and produced the chemical change they had observed. The "salicylate group" had no such effect on serum albumin.

Moreover, the California investigators have found that aspirin seems to "acetylate" other important substances beside albumin—in the test tube. These include gamma globulin, hormones and the genetic material, DNA.

Farr is not urging anyone to throw out aspirin bottles. Indeed, he points out, the ability of the acetyl group to combine with body chemicals could help explain why aspirin is a better pain reliever than sodium salicylate, a related compound that doesn't have an acetyl group. On the other hand, he notes, the acetyl group might account for some of aspirin's known side-effects—including allergies—that occur in two out of every thousand aspirin users. And, if it turns out that aspirin also may be harming the genetic material, medicine may have to look for another miracle pain reliever.

Phenobarbital Technique for Treatment of Barbiturate Dependence

4

by David E. Smith, and
Donald R. Wesson, M.D.

A technique for withdrawal of patients physically dependent upon barbiturates and other sedative-hypnotics is described. The technique

SOURCE: Printed by permission of David E. Smith. Originally printed by *Arch Gen Psychiat*/Vol 24, Jan. 1971. Accepted for publication March 16, 1970, from the Department of Pharmacology, San Francisco Medical Center, and the Haight-Ashbury Free Clinic (Dr. Smith), and the Department of Psychiatry, San Francisco General Hospital (Dr. Wesson), San Francisco. Reprint requests to Department of Pharmacology, San Francisco Medical Center, University of California, San Francisco 94122 (Dr. Smith).

involves substituting phenobarbital, a long-acting barbiturate, for the addicting agent and subsequent withdrawal of the phenobarbital. The longer action of phenobarbital provides a more constant barbiturate blood level than the shorter-acting barbiturates which are the classical withdrawal agents. The more constant blood level allows the safe utilization of smaller daily doses of barbiturates during withdrawal.

When barbiturates were first introduced into medical practice, their ability to produce physical dependence was not immediately recognized. Later, a definite withdrawal syndrome was described. It usually included a progression of symptoms such as muscular weakness, systolic postural hypotension, nausea, insomnia, major motor seizures, hyperpyrexia, and, in some cases, death. Also occurring in some cases—usually on the third to seventh day of withdrawal—was a psychotic reaction which could mimic either delirium tremors or a schizophrenic reaction. A similar abstinence syndrome has been described for many of the newer sedative-hypnotics such as meprobomate and glutethimide (Doriden).

In the San Francisco area we are seeing an increasing number of individuals who are physically dependent upon the short-acting and intermediate-acting barbiturates, such as secobarbital (Seconal), pentobarbital (Nembutal), and a mixture of amobarbital and pentobarbital (Tuinal). Several different patterns of barbiturate abuse are prevalent in the San Francisco area, which has frequently been in the vanguard of drug abuse throughout the country.[1] Most of the increase in barbiturate use has been in the younger population, including those of junior-high-school age. There appears to be a social acceptance of drug abuse by the students themselves. Many use barbiturates as an intoxicant, in much the same way as alcohol. But drug use is not confined to extracurricular activities, as evidenced by a recent episode in which 22 high-school students were treated for secobarbital overdoses following a noon "red" frolic (Table 1). Barbiturates are also frequently taken as "downers" following the use of "speed" (methamphetamine). After injecting large doses of methamphetamine, the user may take barbiturates orally or by injection to allow him to sleep or to allay paranoid feelings.

The more classical long-term barbiturate user is similar to the alcoholic; and in many cases there is either a concomitant use of alcohol or a past history of alcohol abuse. These individuals are usually 30 to 50 years of age and they generally obtain their supply of drugs by prescriptions from physicians. They tolerate frustration poorly and take barbiturates to avoid experiencing anxiety.

Dual addictions to heroin and barbiturates are seen on the West Coast because diluted heroin is often supplemented with barbiturates.

When many different psychotropic drugs are available for purchase on the streets, drug-dependence-prone individuals eventually find their "drug of choice." They may become alcoholics, barbiturate abusers, "speed freaks" (intravenous methamphetamine abusers), lysergic acid diethylamide (LSD) or marijuana abusers. Much remains to be learned about the pharmacology and psychodynamics of this drug selection process. Modified psychoanalytic approaches of investigation and interpretation are increasing our insights into this complex psychosocial problem.[2]

Withdrawal From Barbiturates

Although withdrawal from barbiturates is only the first stage of successful rehabilitation of an individual who bases his life-style around the abuse of drugs, this early phase of therapy should be approached with caution since mismanagement can be life-endangering. Classically, barbiturate withdrawal is based on a slow reduction of dosage of the addicting agent, usually a short-acting or intermediate-acting barbiturate, at dosages that produce mild toxic signs.[3]

Experience with heroin withdrawal, using the long-acting synthetic narcotic, methadone (Dolphine), led us to develop a similar technique for barbiturate withdrawal. Using phenobarbital (Luminal), a long-acting barbiturate, as the withdrawal agent, we found that dosages of shorter-acting barbiturates that produce toxic signs are not necessary. Toxic doses frequently produce behavior problems and prolong the disability of the patient. Because of the short duration of action of secobarbital and pentobarbital, a wide range of blood levels would be expected to occur if it is given every six hours as recommended in most withdrawal procedures. Smaller fluctuation in barbiturate blood level will take place when phenobarbital is used as the withdrawal agent, since it has a longer duration of action. We feel that this more constant barbiturate blood level provides added protection against the development of withdrawal symptoms and allows for the safe utilization of a smaller daily dose during the withdrawal. The longer duration of action of phenobarbital does, however, permit accumulation of phenobarbital and can theoretically produce toxic symptoms several days after withdrawal has started. Therefore, the patient should be checked for signs of toxicity before each dose is given. In actual practice we have not found this to be a problem with the dosage schedule recommended below.

Since there is cross-tolerance between barbiturates and nonbarbiturate sedative hypnotics (such as glutethimide and meprobamate), individuals dependent upon nonbarbiturate sedative-hypnotics can also be withdrawn using the phenobarbital technique (Table 2). One agent then, can be used for withdrawing the nonbarbiturate sedative-hypnotics as well as the barbiturates. Toxic signs produced by phenobarbital are more predictable and easier to observe than those produced by the nonbarbiturate sedative-hypnotics. The safety factor for phenobarbital is larger than for the shorter-acting barbiturates, since fatal amounts of phenobarbital are several times greater than the toxic dose. Wikler,[4] who used pentobarbital as the withdrawing agent, reported that some patients convulsed after the stabilization period while being withdrawn from long-acting sedative-hypnotics such as glutethimide or chlordiazepoxide. We have not seen this complication with the use of phenobarbital as the withdrawing agent.

Phenobarbital Technique for Treatment of Barbiturate Dependence

A challenge dose of a short-acting barbiturate is not routinely used, although it may be of some value when the history is unreliable. On the basis of the patient's history, an average daily intake is estimated (usually 0.5 to 3 gm/day). This is converted into sedative doses. From experience we have found taht 32 mg of phenobarbital is an effective withdrawal dosage that can be equated to 100 mg of secobarbital or pentobarbital although recently we have experimented with a 15-mg phenobartibal conversion factor in order to reduce the incidence of phenobarbital side effects. The calculated total daily dose of phenobarbital is divided into four doses, using a larger dose at bedtime. For example, by history the patient alleges that he takes 15 to 20 "reds" (1,500 to 2,000) mg of secobarbital) per day. Assuming the upper dose of 2,000 mg/day, this is equivalent to 600 mg of phenobarbital per day. In the treatment of this patient, two days would be used for stabilization on phenobarbital. The doses of phenobarbital are given every six hours. Before each dose the patient is checked by a nurse, and if slurred speech, ataxia, or nystagmus is present, or if the patient is sleeping soundly, that dose is omitted. At the end of two days the total daily intake of phenobarbital is used as the basis from which to start withdrawal. A typical withdrawal schedule for this hypothetical patient is shown in Table 3.

As long as the withdrawal is proceeding smoothly, the total daily dose is decreased by 30 mg/day. The schedule, however, should remain flexible, and if the patient develops excessive anxiety, tremors, muscular weakness, or postural hypotension, he is then given an injection of 200 mg of phenobarbital and the decrease in dosage stopped until withdrawal symptoms have subsided. The patient should be observed for withdrawal symptoms for at least one week following the last day he receives phenobarbital. Diphenylhydantoin sodium (Dilantin) is not used unless there is a past history of seizure disorder, as studies in animals have failed to provide evidence that diphenylhydantoin sodium will prevent withdrawal seizures.[5] Other psychotropic drugs are avoided during the early withdrawal phase since they can mask withdrawal symptoms.

Mixed Addictions

We are now seeing patients addicted to two classes of drugs, usually heroin and barbiturates. The barbiturate is withdrawn first, and the patient's heroin habit is maintained with methadone, a long-acting narcotic, until barbiturate withdrawal is complete. Since many of the symptoms of withdrawal from narcotics are similar to those from barbiturates, the clinical state is difficult to assess if both drugs are withdrawn together. Following barbiturate withdrawal, the patient is withdrawn from methadone. The following case histories illustrate the phenobarbital technique and some of the problems encountered clinically.

Report of Cases

Case 1. A 38-year old woman was brought to the emergency room by her family because of ataxia, frequent falling, and personality changes over the past month. These personality changes included liable affect, poor personal hygiene, and bursts of slurred, disinhibited speech.

The patient admitted to taking up to 600 mg of phenobarbital each day for the past six months. She obtained her barbiturates by prescription from three physicians for her "nervous condition." The patient was admitted to the hospital and withdrawn starting at 480 mg of phenobarbital per day. The patient became much more pleasant and cooperative with her family, and began long-term supportive group psychotherapy.

Comment. Phenobarbital is not as common an agent of abuse as are the short-acting barbiturates. The above patient was brought to medical attention not because of her addiction but because of personality changes. Addiction was discovered by careful questioning after nystagmus was noted. Withdrawal was uncomplicated and the patient has continued to do well. All patients, however, do not respond well, as illustrated by the next case.

Case 2. A 30-year old woman was admitted to the hospital through the drug-abuse unit for voluntary withdrawal. She was addicted to 3,500 mg of phenobarbital per day and in addition supported a moderate heroin habit. During the stabilization period the patient was started on 1000 mg of phenobarbital per day, and her heroin habit was maintained with 20 mg of methadone per day. No evidence of toxicity was noted during the stabilization period on phenobarbital and withdrawal was started on the third day of hospitalization. On the fourth hospital day, the patient was noted to have an unsteady gait and was observed taking phenobarbital capsules that she apparently had brought with her to the ward.

Patients who are admitted through the drug-abuse unit agree to follow the unit's rules that specifically forbid bringing drugs into the ward. They are automatically discharged if caught breaking these rules. The staff insisted that she be discharged to prevent a wave of illegal drug use on the ward. One month following discharge the unit heard of her death by overdose, presumably of barbiturates.

Comment. This case illustrates many of the practical complications encountered in administering a withdrawal program. The patient was well aware of the consequences of bringing drugs into the ward. The fact that she "allowed herself to be caught" indicated her ambivalence about being in the program, even though she was a voluntary patient and had previously indicated a good degree of motivation. Cases such as the above had led us to question the advisability of modeling a withdrawal program for barbiturates after Bay Area programs for heroin withdrawal. Patients who became introgenically intoxicated exhibit impaired judgement and impulsive behavior to a degree much more marked than with an overdose of methadone. Smuggling drugs into a ward has the potential for disrupting that ward. However, barbiturate withdrawal can be life-threatening whereas heroin withdrawal seldom is. We would favor having the patient voluntarily agree to stay in the hospital for a fixed period, and be more flexible in response to violation of ward rules.

Case 3. A 28-year old woman was admitted to the psychiatric unit, at the insistence of her husband and her social worker, for evaluation of her possible addiction to glutethimide. From her history, it was learned that she has been taking 2,500 to 3,500 mg of glutethimide per day—in addition to several pentobarbital capsules and chloral hydrate.

Although the patient had abused alcohol for many years, she had first begun to use other drugs two years previously while pregnant. At that time she was given dextroamphetamine sulface (Dexedrine) to aid in weight control. She soon began to abuse these, increasing the dose to five to seven tablets per day. She began having difficulty sleeping and started taking meprobamate at night. Following the birth of her child, sedative drugs were substituted for alcohol. The family behavior pattern remained essentially the same. Her husband would hide her pills or flush them down the toilet. He would sometimes severely criticize or beat her when he came home and found her intoxicated on sedatives. The patient apparently preferred her husband's beatings to his ignoring her.

During the month before admission, the patient developed distressing epigastric burning and nausea. On the day of admission she was crying and complaining of numerous somatic symptoms.

Because of her history of drug abuse, we assumed the possibility of withdrawal symptoms; and the patient was started on 400 mg per day of phenobarbital in divided doses. The phenobarbital was rapidly decreased over the next six days without her developing withdrawal signs or symptoms. The patient's epigastric distress disappeared and she was able to adjust her sleeping habits without pills.

After her discharge, family therapy was attempted to break up the established pattern. Soon the patient stopped attending therapy, and thereafter she called her therapist only during an occasional domestic crisis. At present she is using sedatives again.

Comment. This patient's drug habits were intimately woven into the family's dynamics. In addition to the pleasurable pharmacological effect, drug abuse was for her a way of getting attention and manipulating her husband.

The patient in the following case was one of the first addicts with whom we attempted withdrawal with phenobarbital.

Case 4. A 40-year old man was addicted to approximately 2,500 mg per day of pentobarbital and was also moderately dependent on heroin. Over the past 20 years he had been hospitalized many times as a result of complications associated with his addiction.

On admission to the hospital the patient's stabilization on phenobarbital was started, while the patient's narcotic habit was maintained with 35 mg of methadone per day. The starting daily dose of phenobarbital was calculated by equating 64 mg of phenobarbital to 100 mg of pentobarbital.

On the third hospital day the patient was noted to be ataxic and to demonstrate sustained horizontal hystagmus. The next dose of phenobarbital was withheld, and by the following morning the patient was walking and speaking normally. So the calculated phenobarbital dose was decreased 50%. The remainder of the barbiturate withdrawal proceeded smoothly until three days before completion, when the patient left the hospital without authorization to make a "connection" for his girlfriend. Several months later the drug-abuse unit heard that the patient was again using barbiturates.

Comment. When we first tried substituting 64 mg of phenobarbital for each 100 mg of a shorter-acting barbiturate, we found patients generally became intoxicated on the second or third hospital day; thus, a drastic reduction in dose was necessary. Since we have been substituting 32 mg of phenobarbital for each 100 mg of the shorter-acting barbiturate, we have not had any cases of intoxication on the ward.

The final case still leaves us with many unanswered questions, but will be presented because it illustrates several problems.

Case 5. The patient was a 30-year old salesman who apparently had started abusing barbiturates three years previously, when he first began hearing voices and having paranoid ideation. He was brought to the hospital on a mental-illness petition which mentioned a history of drug abuse but did not specify the drug. The patient stated that he took only two or three capsules of a mixture of secobarbital and amobarbital (100 mg of each) at night to aid him in sleeping. No additional history was available at that time. On the morning following his admission, the patient had a major motor seizure. Most unusual in this case was that the patient did not exhibit the characteristic prodromal signs and symptoms associated with withdrawal seizures. Additional history from relatives indicated that the patient was taking 10 to 15 capsules of mixed secobarbital and amobarbital per day, and was frequently intoxicated on barbiturates to the point of staggering. During the three days before his admission the patient had drastically decreased his intake of the secobarbital and amobarbital mixture.

During the 12 hours after his first seizure, the patient had three additional seizures. He received a total of 800 mg of phenobarbital in the 24 hours following the first seizures. For the next two days the patient was given 600 mg of phenobarbital per day. Withdrawal was accomplished smoothly during an additional 15 days. An electroencephalogram done three days after withdrawal was complete showed no seizure activity.

Comment. We have not satisfactorily explained why the patient did not show signs such as tremulousness and hyperreflexia. Although there was no history of a primary seizure disorder, the patient had experienced withdrawal convulsions at a hospital the previous year. Earlier the same year the patient had been given ten electroshock treatments and five flurothyl (Indoklon) treatments at another hospital because of a diagnosis of paranoid schizophrenia.

This case also illustrates the problem of "hidden addictions." For example, 30 tons of barbiturates are manufactured legitimately in the United States each year and it is estimated that 50% of this supply is misused or diverted into illegal channels. The incidence of barbiturate abuse in the United States is unknown, but appears to be much greater than the average physician suspects. The physician who made out the Mental-illness petition could have prevented much of the difficulty had he been more specific about the drug-abuse history. We suspect that with the increase in use of all psychotropic and potentially addicting drugs, more cases will be discovered after the patient has his first withdrawal convulsion. Drug abuse should be considered in the differential diagnosis of any acute brain syndrome in which the cause is not immediately apparent. Appropriate blood and urine samples should be obtained, for toxicological analysis. Since the patient may be unwilling or unable to give an accurate history of drug use, the relative blood level may be useful in establishing the type and magnitude of the addiction.

Table 1. Drugs Commonly Abused in the San Francisco Area

Common Names (Street Names)	Drug Name	Dosages Available (mg)	Common Method of Use
Reds Red devils Downers Seggy	Secobarbital (Seconal)	30, 50, 100	Orally or dissolved and injected intravenously
Yellows Yellow jackets Downers Nembies	Pentobarbital (Nembutal)	30, 50, 100	Orally or dissolved and injected intravenously
Double trouble Rainbows	Equal amts. of amobarbital & secobarbital (Tuinal)	5, 100, 200	Orally
Speed Meth Crystal Crank	Methamphetamine (Methadrine) (Desoxyn)	5, 10, 15; also manufactured on black market	Orally or dissolved and injected intravenously.

Table 2. Common Sedative-Hypnotics With Abuse Potential

Generic Name	Orally Given Hypnotic Dose (mg)	Orally Given Sedative Dose (mg)	Equivalent Phenobarbital Dose (mg)
Chlordiazepoxide	75-100	25	30
Diazepam	20-30	5	30
Meprobamate	800-1200	400	30
Chloral hydrate	1,000	250	30
Glutethimide	500	250	30
Secobarbital	200	100	30
Pentobarbital	200	100	30

Table 3. Sample Withdrawal Schedule*

Day	6 AM (mg)	12 Noon (mg)	6 PM (mg)	12 Midnight (mg)	Total Daily Dose (mg)
1	100	132	132	200	564
2	100	100	132	200	532
3	100	100	100	200	500
4	100	100	100	164	464
5	64	100	100	164	428
6	64	64	100	164	392
7	64	64	64	164	356
8	64	64	64	132	324
9	32	64	64	132	292
10	32	32	64	132	260
11	32	32	32	132	228
12	32	32	32	100	196
13	0	32	32	100	164
14	0	0	32	100	132
15	0	0	0	100	100
16	0	0	0	64	64
17	0	0	0	32	32
18	0	0	0	0	0

*The patient is stabilized at 600 mg of phenobarbital per day for two days. Phenobarbital is available in 16-mg, 32-mg, and 100-mg tablets and capsules.

References

1. Smith D. E., Wesson D. R., Lannon R.: New developments in barbiturate abuse, in *Drug Abuse Papers 1969.* Berkeley, Calif., University of California, 1969.
2. Levy N. J.: Use of drugs by teenagers for sanctuary and illusion. *Amer. J. Psychoanal.* 28: 48-55, 1968.
3. Isbell H.: Treatment of addiction to narcotic drugs. *Med. Clin. N. Amer.* 34:425-438, 1950.

References *(Continued)*

4. Wikler A.: Diagnosis and treatment of drug dependence of the barbiturate type. *Amer. J. Psychiat.* 125: 758-765, 1968.

5. Essig C. F., Carter W. W.: Failure of diphenylhydantoin to prevent barbiturate withdrawal convulsions in dogs. *Neurology* 12: 481-484, 1962.

5 "Speed Freaks" vs. "Acid Heads" A Conflict Between Drug Subcultures

by David E. Smith, M.D., M.S.

In the Haight-Ashbury district of San Francisco, methamphetamine abuse has become the major youthful drug problem. The "speed[a] freak" has replaced or "driven away" the "acid[b] head," and as a result, the Haight-Ashbury has been converted from an "acid subculture" to a "speed subculture." These two drug patterns have very different causes and consequences, and in effect are antithetical. Most segments of the medical community, however, tend to group these 2 drug patterns together thus further increasing their own misinformation about drug use and abuse. The objective of this paper is

---

SOURCE: David E. Smith, M.D., Medical Director, Haight-Ashbury Medical Clinic; Assistant Clinical Professor, University of California San Francisco Medical Center; Lecturer in Criminology, University of California at Berkeley; Editor, *Journal of Psychedelic Drugs.*

to describe and contrast some of the basic characteristics of a "speed subculture" vs. an "acid subculture."

High-Dose Methamphetamine Abuse: The Speed Cycle

To understand a speed subculture, one must, of course, understand the "speed freak."[c] As with any drug, the "speed freak" has certain motivations and expectations for his drug use. A parallel with alcohol use would familiarize this concept for the dominant culture. One may, for example, have a martini during the week and set his expectation for this drug experience as relaxation. On Friday or Saturday, not having to get up the next morning, one sets his expectations as intoxication and has three or four martinis, thus varying the dose to meet his goal. In all cases people have expectations from their drug use. It is important for the physician to attempt to understand these motivations for drug use not only in terms of acute treatment but also in terms of chronic treatment and intervention of a potentially destructive life-style.

The individual who uses high-dose methamphetamine is after the "flash" or the "rush." In other words, he injects the substance and has a very rapid reaction which he describes as a "full body orgasm." The methamphetamine-induced excitation and agitation that follows is, in a "speed freak," a secondary consideration. He is after the initial phenomenon of the injection "flash." Individuals often start on oral methamphetamines and develop a desire for the "high," or the excitation of the oral amphetamines, but for various reasons ranging from group pressure to personality problems they find that the intravenous injection of the substance is even more desirable, leading eventually to a distinctive and destructive pattern of "speed" use.

Methamphetamine interrupts sleep patterns and suppresses appetite. The individual as he becomes more experienced with speed goes on a "speed binge" lasting three or four days in which he "shoots up" from one to ten times per day, always going for the peak experience. He does not eat nor sleep during this time. He is in a continual state of hyperexcitement until for various reasons (exhaustion and fatigue, abnormal psychological circumstances that are frightening to him, or inability to obtain the drug) he decides to terminate this "speed binge."

For whatever reason, the "speed binge" is terminated and we then see the reaction phase of the speed cycle. The reaction phase to the "speed binge" is characteristically the exhaustion syndrome. The individual often lapses into a deep sleep ranging from 24 to 48 hours depending on the duration of the "speed binge," and upon awakening he may eat ravenously. The management of the exhaustion syndrome is relatively easy, and treatment consists primarily of supportive care.

After the speed cycle many of the amphetamine users do not return to a baseline level of personality function. They have a prolonged subacute phase in which profound depression dominates. Very often the "speed freak" shoots methamphetamine again to treat his depression and another cycle begins. The intensity of the post-speed depression cannot be overemphasized. As one 17-year-old girl described to this author, "Without speed I

[a]"Speed" is the street name for methamphetamine hydrochloride.

[b]"Acid" is the street name for L.S.D.

[c]"Speed freak" is the name given to the compulsive high-dose methamphetamine user.

feel so lousy that I'd rather shoot speed and live for one week than live for forty years without it." Very rapidly then a situation of depression develops in which the patient sees no hope for interruption of this pattern of drug use, and the only feasible therapy is to remove the individual from that drug-using subculture. There is a good institutional program at Mendocino State Hospital and a self-help outpatient program in the city of San Francisco directed by the Haight-Ashbury Clinic. So long as the "speed freak" maintains himself in an area where many other individuals are also using the drug, he has a great deal of difficulty resisting the temptation to "go back up" again.

Medical and Psychological Toxicity of High-Dose Methamphetamine Abuse

Last summer we analyzed 310 cases of high-dose methamphetamine abuse seen at the Haight-Ashbury Clinic during a three-month period (June to September 1967). In analyzing these reactions approximately 40 per cent of the patients came to the clinic with physical complaints whereas 60 per cent came in with psychological complaints.

In terms of the physical complaints, we saw an unusually high incidence of hepatitis, a bewildering array of urticarial reactions, abscesses, respiratory complaints, and acute abdominal complaints. In observing the patients, it became apparent that acute gastrointestinal distress or abdominal cramps are part of the high-dose methamphetamine syndrome. I will not go into detail about the physical complaints, however, as I prefer to focus on the types of psychological consequences that these individuals develop. These consequences can be divided into five categories:

(1) Anxiety reaction
(2) Amphetamine psychosis
(3) Exhaustion syndrome
(4) Prolonged depression
(5) Prolonged hallucinosis

The major psychological complaint encountered was the simple acute anxiety reaction. The individual had overdosed and had become acutely anxious, fearful, tremulous, often with tachycardia and somatic concerns. I must emphasize that in talking about dosage, virtually all the methamphetamine now available is black market methamphetamine. It is not therapeutic diet pills diverted into illegal market. It is mainly synthesized by black market laboratories, and therefore it is difficult to obtain an accurate assessment of dosage. Although the average therapeutic dose for appetite suppression is 5 to 15 mg., because of the rapid tolerance that develops with this drug, the "speed freak" shoots between one and five grams per day. The tolerance varies so widely among various users, however, that one questions whether this is a physical or a psychological tolerance.[1,2]

The amphetamine psychosis is less common and is associated with three diagnostic characteristics: (1) Visual hallucinations, (2) auditory hallucinations, and (3) a well-defined system of paranoia including ideas of reference. Paranoia is a characteristic part of the reaction and makes treatment difficult because the individual is very concerned about entering a hospital or encountering the police. He feels comfortable only in a street facility and very often even there questions concerning the police arise. As an example, I saw an 18-year-old white male who had been having an amphetamine psychosis. He had a very well-defined system of paranoia in which he felt that the police were after him and that his roommate and he had come to the Medical Clinic for help. Except for this system of paranoia and distracting hallucinations, he was remarkably lucid. During our interview a staff volunteer of the clinic, wearing a black leather jacket, crossed in front of the door. The patient jumped up and said, "I knew it! You're part of the plot!" and tried to run out the door. While restraining the boy, I called the volunteer and indicated that this was a member of the clinic staff who just happened to wear a black leather jacket. He calmed down immediately. The movement in and out of a paranoia delusional system can be very dramatic, and the physician may suddenly become part of that system. If it happens to be a large or violent individual, the physician may be in some immediate jeopardy.

In the amphetamine psychosis certainly the major psychochemotherapy is antipsychotic drugs of the phenothiazine type. For these psychotic reactions the physician must also give serious consideration to hospitalization if facilities are available, since the psychotic symptoms often persist. For the anxiety reactions long-acting sedatives are enough. However, the acute anxiety reaction is self-limiting, and many times the physician tends to over-treat. Transition from the action to reaction phase can be quite dramatic, and the consequences of the anxiety reaction can be easily handled with a supportive, nonthreatening environment and the cautious use of sedative medication.

I have talked about the exhaustion syndrome and the appearance of a tenacious reactive depression. I would also like to mention the phenomenon of prolonged hallucinosis in which the high-dose amphetamine user experiences persistent auditory and visual hallucinations for days and even weeks after the acute. reaction has passed. Only a few of the individuals who have an amphetamine psychosis manifest this prolonged reaction, and we are not certain if drug factors or personality factors play the major role in this drug-induced thought disorder.[1,2,3]

I want to close my discussion of chronic high-dose methamphetamine use by emphasizing the importance of group factors as a major contributor to amphetamine toxicity. In a series of animal experience we found the LD_{50} of d-amphetamine to be 100 mg per kg when the drug was administered to white mice housed individually. When the animals were grouped together and the environmental conditions remained constant, the LD_{50} decreased to 25 mg per kg. In other words, simple aggregation of the animals increased the toxicity of the drug four fold. In analyzing this phenomenon of aggregate amphetamine toxicity we found a polyphasic mortality curve. The mortality was high at the 25 mg per kg dose and then decreased, so that at 75 mg per kg the drug was less toxic than at 25 mg. It then increased again at 100 mg per kg where a second LD_{50} appeared. In analyzing this polyphasic mortality curve we found that at the 25 mg per kg dosage, the animals were in a hyperexcitable and agitated state in which the mechanism of death was actually that of one animal killing another. As the drug dose was increased the animals became preconvulsive. The dose was not high enough to cause convulsions (the mechanism of death at 100 mg per kg), but the animals were so disorganized that they could not mobilize any directive attack at one another.[4]

The Haight-Ashbury now has some resemblance to a giant mouse cage in that individuals are taking high-doses of central nervous system stimulants and interacting in a violent and often destructive fashion. It has become quite apparent that just taking the drug in a high density population situation increases the toxicity. It is very important for the physician to be aware of the phenomenon of aggregate toxicity. Treatment of any central nervous system stimulant reaction should put great emphasis on a quiet, supportive, nonthreatening environment. A caustic statement by the physician or a nurse bursting into the treatment room would constitute poor treatment in this situation. I hope that the individuals who are treating drug reactions will become aware of the importance of environmental group factors in treating both amphetamine and LSD reactions.

The "Acid Head"

I have discussed a situation in which an individual who is chronically using methamphetamine becomes violent, hostile, and hyperactive. The chronic LSD user or the "acid head," presents an entirely opposite picture. In our clinic population individuals who were using methamphetamine chronically were approximately the same age as the individuals who were using LSD chronically. There were significant differences, however, in personality types and socioeconomic background between the two groups of drug users. Of greater significance, however, is the fact that the chronic LSD user developed a pattern of thought and behavior which was the antithesis of that described above in the chronic methamphetamine user. Rather than seeking a "flash" or a thrill as did the "speed freaks," the chronic LSD user developed a complex set of motivations for his drug use involving self-psychoanalytic, pseudo-religious, and creative aspirations.

To understand the chronic effects of LSD, however, one must understand the psycho-pharmacological effects of the drug.[5] To begin with, the individual under the influence of LSD manifests very marked perceptual changes. Primarily these changes are illusionary phenomena (e.g., objects changing shape and color). On the other hand, one may see the phenomenon of synesthesia in which one sensory phenomenon is translated into another (e.g., a record player gives off colored vibrations or an individual smells purple). Teenagers are well aware of the phenomenon of synesthesia and have immortalized it in songs such as "Good Vibrations." The perceptual changes are the most marked phenomenon that one finds, but hallucinatory activity, that is, the actual perception of an object in one's sensory environment without the physical manifestation of that object, are relatively rare with LSD. One also sees marked alterations in symbolic associations with sensory input. For example, an individual may see a red light and become enamored with the hue of the light rather than make the symbolic association that one stops at the red light. One also sees marked alterations in ideational functioning. Very often individuals who have taken LSD tend to feel that they have had a universal religious experience in which they have found the answer to life. They develop a rather elaborate philosophical position around this sensory pattern and very often, particularly in the young mind, carry this into their non-drug state. In other words, they do not say, "This is just a drug reaction that gave me this subjective or illusionary experience;" they say, "I've found the answer to life!" If LSD is taken in a psychedelic information environment where other individuals have had the same experience, then the interpretation of psychedelic reality is reinforced. Repeated LSD experiences with friends supporting a positive interpretation of the LSD experience produces some very dramatic psychological changes in the "acid head."[6] I have described this characteristic alteration in the chronic LSD user as the "psychedelic syndrome."[7]

The characteristics of this psychedelic syndrome are first, a profound belief in non-violence. The "acid heads" rejection of physical aggression is so profound that very often one sees a change in diet to natural, vegetable foods; his rejection of killing is so great that he refuses to eat meat. There is a great desire to return to nature, adopting the dress and customs of such cultures as the American Indians. There is an emphasis on "natural foods" or foods raised without chemicals, and "natural ways" such as natural childbirth. For example, many young "hippie girls" seek consultation at the Haight-Ashbury for natural childbirth and home delivery, with child-rearing occurring in a tribal or communal setting. Another of the significant characteristics of the individual who uses LSD chronically and develops the "psychedelic syndrome" is a belief in *magic:* mental telepathy, astrology, E.S.P., mysticism, and telekinesia are all parts of his belief system. He believes that his mind can communicate and produce changes in his physical environment because his LSD experiences demonstrated this. The "acid head" develops a life-style based around this particular belief system. An individual may not come to work at the Haight-Ashbury Clinic, for example, because the "stars are wrong," or he says, "It's impossible for me to interact or work with that individual because our signs conflict." Recently there developed a sincere belief that a meteorite was going to hit San Francisco and a large number in the community left for Colorado.

Medical Significance of the "Psychedelic Syndrome"

What medical significance does the "psychedelic syndrome" have? Individuals with "psychedelic syndrom" tend to group together in communal living situations, and it is a combination of chronic LSD usage and the psychedelic community that reinforces this type of behavior. They undergo a profound psychological conversion to belief in an unstructured psychedelic religion.

The medical significance of the "psychedelic syndrome" is vague. In Dr. Kay Blacker's studies[6] at the Langley Porter N.P.I. no classical evidence of organic brain damage was found in chronic LSD users. On the other hand, he found with visually evoked EEG responses an increase in the number of low intensity visual responses. But in another test sensitive to intellectual disorganization or schizophrenia, the auditory two-toned evoked potential, the group of LSD users showed no abnormality. As Dr. Blaker pointed out, an alteration in one type of psychological testing which may be characteristic of a schizophrenic process does not imply an alteration in an entirely different type of psychological testing. His assumption is that the chronic LSD user tends to modulate and organize sensor-input in a different and unique fashion. In other words, he views the world differently from the non or casual LSD user. His subjects had intact and intense interpersonal realtionships and could not, using standard nomenclature, be described as schizophrenic—merely as eccentric. The breakdown in interpersonal relationships occurs between the "Hip" and the straight community or between the non-psychedelic and the individual who is involved in the psychedelic subculture. I believe there is mounting evidence that the young people who regularly use LSD and involve themselves in the psychedelic subculture develop a very profound alteration in psychosocial functioning.

What is the significance of this? Why do I belabor the point? I bring it up because so many people have indicated that young people involving themselves with what can be called the psychedelic movement are going through a "phase" and will easily become "straight" again. Their rationalization is that, these young people are just experimenting like we did when we swallowed gold fish or went to fraternity games, and they will come back." I would submit that at the very least the young people who are deeply and intensely involved in this movement will not easily be able to reenter the dominant American culture because of a profound conflict in value systems. An individual with the "psychedelic syndrome" and committed to non-violence will have great conflict in a society like ours where the ethic is violence and competition. I would submit that the young people participating in the "Hip" movement will not be able to reenter the dominant culture without having some very significant problems. So long as they remain in the psychedelic subculture their "psychedelic syndrome," with its characteristics of nonviolence and magical beliefs, is actually respected. They cannot by standards of that community be called mentally ill—only by the standards of our community can they be called mentally ill. Therefore, so long as the individual remains in the psychedelic subculture, treatment of the "psychedelic syndrome" becomes as beneficial as treating some of our accepted religious institutions. Treatment is indicated and successful only if for various reasons—monetary, parental, or whatever—the individual attempts to reenter the straight society. Reentry can cause severe psychological problems, and as a result "becoming straight" will be a much more difficult process than most adults predict.

On the other hand, the "acid head" community cannot live with the "speed freak" community because of the violent characteristics of the latter. As a result the "hippies" have left the Haight-Ashbury district, moving to the country where they can establish small rural communes which tolerate and reinforce their belief systems. Urban areas such as the Haight-Ashbury can never be a permanent haven for the acid subculture, because in the conflict of "speed freaks" vs. "acid heads," "speed" always drives out "acid" just as in the broader society the philosophy of violence always dominates the higher aspirations of non-violence, peace, and love.

References

1. Smith, D. E., Fischer, C. M., "High-dose methamphetamine abuse in Haight-Ashbury," *J. Psychedelic Drugs*, in press.
2. Smith, D. E., Physical vs. psychological dependence and tolerance in high-dise methamphetamine abuse, *Clinical Toxicology*, in press.
3. Ellinwood, E. R., "Amphetamine psychosis I: Description of the individual and process." *J. Nerv. and Mental Diseases*, 144:273-283, 1967.
4. Smith, D. E., Fischer, C. M., Schoenfeld, E., and Hine, C. H., Behavioral mediators in the polyphasic mortality curve of aggregate amphetamine toxicity, *J. Psychedelic Drugs*, in press.
5. Smith, D. E., "Lysergic Acid Diethylamide: An historical perspective," *J. of Psychedelic Drugs*, 1967, Vol. 1 Issue, pp. 1-5.
6. Blacker, K. H., Jones, R. T., Stone, G. C., and Pfefferbaum, D., *Chronic users of LSD: The acidheads*, presented at the 1966 American Psychiatric Association, in press.
7. Smith, D. E., LSD and the psychedelic syndrome, *Clinical Toxicology*, in press.

Bibliography and Suggested Readings

BIBLIOGRAPHY

Packard, Vance: *The Hidden Persuaders*, Pocket Books of Simon & Schuster, Inc., New York.

Schuessler, Raymond: "How Pure is Our Food," *American Legion Magazine*, May, 1969, New York, pp. 10-58.

SUGGESTED READINGS

Smith, Daniel E.: *Journal of Psychedelic Drugs*, Vol. I, Issue I—Psychedelic Drugs and the Law; Vol. I, Issue II—Psychedelic Drugs and Religion; Vol. II, Issue I—Marijuana Past and Present; Vol. II, Issue II—Patterns of Amphetamine Abuse; Vol. III. Issue I—LSD: The Psychedelic Experience; Vol. III, Issue II—Drug Abuse 1971; Vol. IV, Issue I—The Contemporary Heroin Scene; Vol. IV, Issue II—Drug Abuse 1972, Haight-Ashbury Publications, San Francisco, California.

Smith, Daniel E. and Luce, John: *Love Needs Care: A History of San Francisco's Haight-Ashbury Free Medical Clinic and Its Pioneer Role in Treating Drug-Abuse Problems*, Little, Brown and Company, Boston, Mass., 1971.

Turner, James S.: *The Chemical Feast*, Grossman Publishers, Inc., New York, 1970.

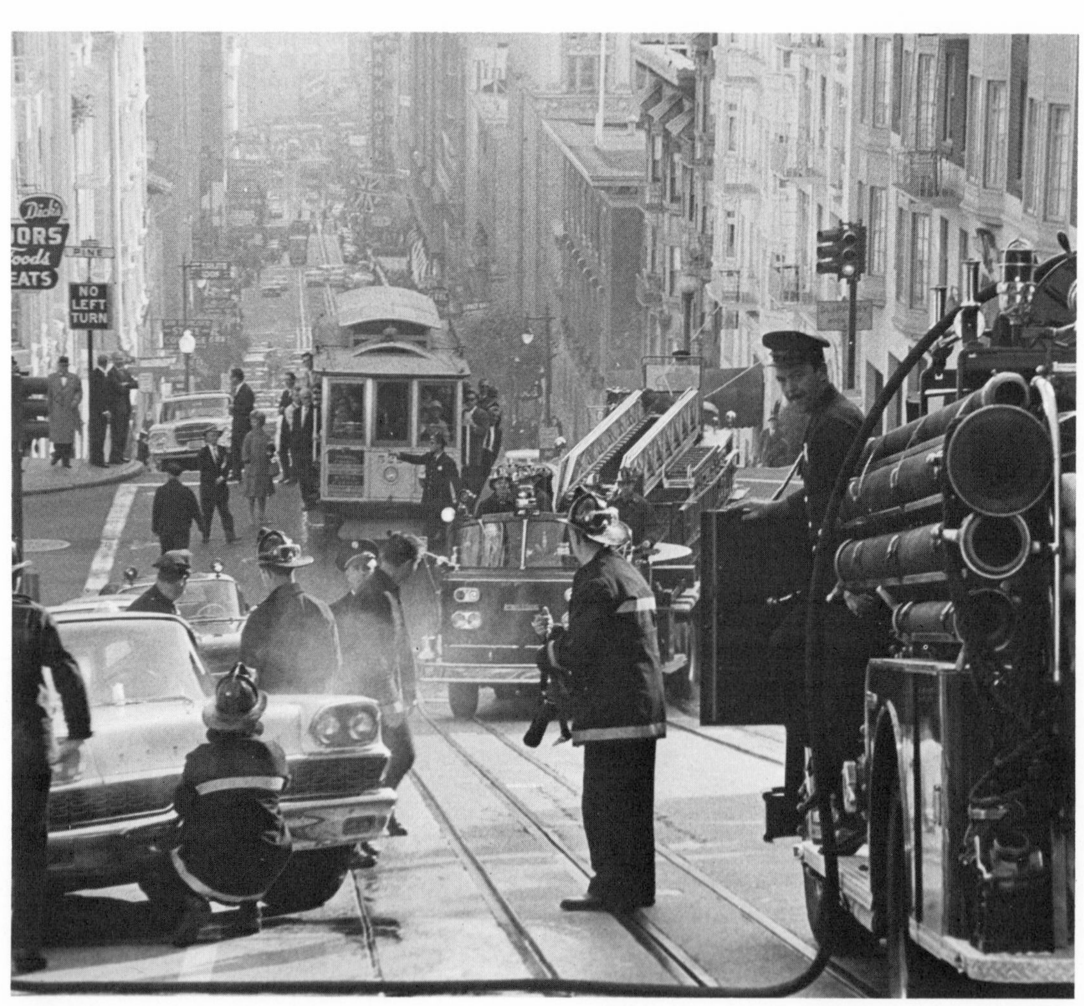
Dick's
PINE
NO LEFT TURN

UNIT 4

Accidents, Suicide and Disease

Ordinarily the greatest immediate cause of death to college age students is automobile accidents which have killed over 7000 youths (mostly males) per year for the last several years. However, this number has been surpassed in the Vietnam conflict in 1968 when a total of 14,592 American men, mostly of college age, were killed. It may possibly have been surpassed in 1967 and 1969 when over 9000 men were killed.

Accidents pose a much greater threat to the lives of the general population than wars, with a total of more than 1,650,000 dying of automobile accidents between 1900 and 1967 and 1,118,000 dying of all wars from the Revolutionary War through 1967.

In recent years there has been a great amount of legitimate concern over lack of automobile safety features for which there is the technology available (Ralph Nader). There is no doubt that many lives could be saved with the incorporation of these devices in the make-up of the automobile. It is also certain that maintaining a car in good condition is important for control of pollution and for driving safety. Scientific studies have found the following relationship between vehicle safety inspections and numbers of auto deaths:

Deaths per 100,000 Population

	States with NO Inspections	States with Yearly Inspections	States with Twice Yearly Inspections
White	38.2	25.1	22.5
Non-white	64.2	37.9	27.5

It was assumed that the increase in deaths in this study was due to decrease in proper maintenance and the racial difference due to a larger percentage of old automobiles.

The most important factor in automobile accidents is the human factor. It is believed that 90 per cent of all accidents could have been prevented by better driver behavior.

Psychological problems ranging from short term emotional disturbances (such as a violent quarrel just prior to the accident) to chronic adjustment problems are involved in a large per cent of accidents. Drunk driving has been the cause of half of all accidents resulting in the death of one or both drivers of the automobiles involved. Drug use, often accompanying a basic psychological problem, has been responsible for many accidents. One study showed that a group of patients who had been receiving tranquilizers for 90 days had 10 times more traffic accidents than the general population. It wasn't determined whether the drug or the psychological problems of the people taking the drug was the major factor. Excessive speed causes 2 out of 5 automobile accidents resulting in death and the ratio is higher for drivers under age 25. Psychologists have evidence that people consider cars as extensions of themselves and use them in attempts to fill their needs. Twenty per cent of all drivers are involved in 80 per cent of all accidents. Life insurance companies particularly are interested in these "accident prone" people. If they could be kept off the roads most accidents could be prevented.

Following well behind accidents as killers of college age people are suicides, homocides and cancer. California Health Department data give the following statistics for Californians between the ages 20-24 in 1967:

Cause of Death	Total Killed
Accidents	1459
Automobile accident	741
Motorcycle accident	75
Suicide	231
Homocide	172
Cancers	143

Dr. Frederick's article gives some philosophy and data on the important topic of suicide. College students suffer, though seldom die, from a number of infectious diseases. This unit contains a general discussion on such diseases and methods of protection against them. The venereal diseases, which are at epidemic proportions and have their highest incidence in the 19 through 24 age group, are discussed in greater detail.

Many young men have infections and other painful problems with their prostate glands. John Lentz, author of the paper entitled A Man's Disease Every Woman Should Know About, believes that women should be aware of these diseases and understand the problems.

Although heart disease is not one of the greatest killers of college age people (43 Californians ages 20-24 died of all diseases of the circulatory system in 1967) behavior during this period in life is preparation for health or disease of the circulatory system for the future. The major causes of both heart attacks and strokes are arteriosclerosis, high blood pressure, and blood clots. Your heredity, diet, exercise, and mental health all through your life are the major determinants of whether you will have a heart attack or stroke in later life. This unit discusses some helpful and little known information on strokes.

1

Ecological Aspects of Self-Destruction: Some Legal, Legislative and Behavioral Implications

by Calvin J. Frederick

If human ecology is the inter-relationship between man and his environment and all behavior is motivated, whether from internal or external sources, then nearly every aspect of human behavior or psychology is ecological. This is virtually unequivocal when other beings

*Dr. Frederick is Assistant Chief, Center for Studies of Suicide Prevention, Division of Special Mental Health Programs, National Institute of Mental Health, Rockville, Maryland; Assistant Professor of Medical Psychology, The Johns Hopkins University School of Medicine, Baltimore, Maryland; and Associate Clinical Professor of Psychiatry (Medical Psychology), George Washington University School of Medicine, Washington, D.C.

are considered part of the environment. A prototype may be found in Newtonian Physics in the Third Law of Motion: for every action force there is an equal and opposite reaction force. Interactions between various stimuli and responses are at the core of modern psychology. Every act man performs has its origin in association with other beings from the time of birth, whether that particular stimulus continues to be present or not. Man can bind time in a way that infra-humans cannot. He remembers much of what happened to him previously and anticipates what will happen in the future. At best, this occurs only in the most rudimentary fashion in the animal world.

To see the results of an individual's surroundings upon him one need only peruse the effects of sensory deprivation on the one hand and overcrowding on the other. Both can lead to aberrant forms of behavior; the former to distorted, psychotic-like experiences and the latter to severe aggression, isolation and pecking order hierarchies (Zubek 1969; Griffitt and Veitch 1971; Robles 1967; Glass, Singer and Friedman 1969). Although he frequently does not use his ability effectively, a potentially hopeful fact is that man has the capacity to choose and avoid responding to destructive factors in his environment. This applies to specific behavior such as smoking too much and to generic acts such as polluting air, rivers and oceans. All too many persons drive autos recklessly, imbibe alcohol heavily, overeat, become overweight, fail to take medication when appropriate, use detergent phosphates and carelessly burn wooded areas. Such acts may be regarded as psychological equivalents of suicide along varying dimensions.

The World Health Organization (1968) has pointed to the need for long-term planning in altering man's social environment in order to solve ecological problems of mental health. The main point is that society should adapt itself to the individual's biological capabilities rather than forcing continuous individual adaptation to an increasingly complex and stressful society. Pushed beyond reasonable limits, man develops mental and psychophysiological disturbances to the point of collapse and death.

One vivid illustration of man's uniqueness is the fact that he is the only organism capable of intentional and voluntary self destruction. Emotionally laden events are readily learned due to their powerful reinforcing qualities. The various means by which suicidal behavior can be learned are discussed at length by Frederick and Resnik (1971). The potent influence of others upon our lives is shown in a number of descriptive studies of suicide such as the work by Paffenbarger et al (1969) with university students, Rieger (1971) in a prison population and Blachley et al (1968) investigating physicians' deaths. "Significant other" persons are almost always involved in suicidal acts, at least psychologically. Suicide notes are written for survivors to read and investigations indicate there is usually some involvement with other persons even when suicide notes do not accompany self destructive acts.

Suicide and dramatic life stresses are a particular problem among young people. The effects of academic stress, per se, are open to some question (Spencer 1958: Davidson and Hutt 1964; Peck and Schrut 1971) but personal and social problems are generally agreed upon sources of difficulty. The writings of Parrish (1956) and Seiden (1969) illustrate the seriousness of the problem among youth. Suicide is the fourth leading cause of death among persons of both sexes between the ages of 15 and 44 years of age (Public Health Service Publication No. 600, 1970).

Legal Aspects of Self-Destruction

The mere fact that laws exist throughout the world penalizing suicidal behavior indicates that it is a public rather than a private problem. Public health and ecological aspects of suicide are discussed by Farberow and Schneidman (1961), Dublin (1967), Breed (1967), Bagley (1968) and Gibbs (1968). Legal and legislative aspects of such behavior are rooted in religious, moral and philosophical proscriptions from early times. Law is related to ecology in the sense that it describes the relationship of man to his fellow man in the environment. It can provide a means for regulating and controlling environmental destruction. The purpose of law is simply to provide rules for living and to regulate man's behavior with appropriate consequences. The law provides a standard method for settling disputes which is intended to be fair, and in civil litigation, involves no physical injury. In criminal judgments the person may be incarcerated or executed where statutes permit. *Civil action* is that occurring between private parties as distinguished from *criminal action*, which is brought by a state or federal government to punish a crime.

While recorded instances of suicidal behavior go as far back as 4,000 years, the early legal indications in Roman Catholic ecclesiastical law go back to 413 A.D., according to Lum (1967) and in English law to 673 A.D., (Stevas 1961). Practices stemming from primitive notions about ghosts returning to earth gave rise to such procedures as burying suicides outside of the graveyard in the center of a highway and driving a stake through the heart. In England only as recently as 1882 were suicides allowed to be buried in daylight hours. They may not be buried with full church rites in either the Anglican or Roman Catholic churches today unless shown to be insane, which is evidence for the clerical existence of present day taboos.

Cases involving suicide are usually settled out of court, and it is sometimes held that it is not criminal because there is no way in which one who commits suicide can be punished directly; only the heirs will suffer. Nevertheless, suicide was always a felonious crime at common law. *Common law* is merely that which was made by judges stemming from custom and ignominious burial are no longer employed as methods of punishment for a suicidal act; nevertheless, in some jurisdictions it is still unlawful and criminal.

To judge one guilty of completed suicide legally, the act must be something more than self destruction. The person must end his own life intentionally and voluntarily while sane, i.e., he must be rational enough to discriminate between right and wrong. Some jurisdictions hold that he must have reached the age of discretion or the age of tender years, which is frequently 12 to 14 years. Below 12 a person is sometimes legally regarded as a child, and between 14 and 18 as a juvenile. A suicide attempt or the completed act is also an indictable offense at common law and under the statutes of several States, yet a person who is guilty of an attempt to kill himself cannot be prosecuted under statutes relating to the crime of assault with intent to commit murder. Separate laws are required. These rubrics underlie the practice of criminal law.

Since American law grew out of English law, the history of the latter is particularly pertinent. It was a breach of God's commandment "Thou Shalt Not Kill" which included the killing of one's self. Because there is no hope of redemption following the killing of the self, it is regarded as a greater religious offense than homocide. There appear to be only about a dozen references to suicidal behavior in the Bible, while there are numerous references to homocide, suggesting the negative feeling about the former, even in Biblical writing.

As a felony under English law, suicide has been viewed as a type of murder. Currently, both Roman and Anglican clergy usually make every effort to be flexible in the matter and permit burial with church rites if at all possible. Suicide attempts are also regarded as a form of attempted murder; yet, it is treated as a common law misdemeanor, despite the fact that the courts haveheld the act to be felonious by statute, especially in England, (Stengal 1964; Williams 1966). *Misdemeanors* are offenses of lesser gravity than felonies and are punishable by fines or jail sentences. *Felonies* are generally punishable by imprisonment in a penitentiary or death. At common law, forfeiture of lands or goods could be accompanied by capital punishment or imprisonment, according to the degree of guilt. Historically, action was taken against a suicide because the community was deprived of a potentially productive, tax paying member; thus, it became a public problem.

United States law has not systematically followed the English tradition since only a few States still clearly regard suicide or attempted suicide as a crime. There are peculiar fine points of the law which may appear puzzling. It might be supposed that if suicide is not a crime, then aiding and abetting should not be a crime either. One cannot depend upon this reasoning, however, because in some jurisdictions aiding and abetting is criminal although a suicide act or attempt is not punishable (Schulman 1968). In States where aiding a suicide is the equivalent of murder, consent to an unlawful act does not alter the nature of the act. In a Michigan case cited by Stevas (1961) a man who placed poison within the reach of his wife was held guilty of murder even though she requested it. In some jurisdictions where suicide is not a felony because of lack of mental capacity, an abettor is not punished, either as an accessory or as a principal. If the distinction between principal and accessory has been abolished by statute, an abettor may be held guilty whether present or absent. The *principal* is one who is the chief actor, perpetrator, aider or abettor and is actively or constructively present at the commission of a crime. An *accessory* is an accomplice who contributes to or aids in the commission of a crime. Without being present he is participating by command, advice, instigation or concealment, either before or after the fact of a crime.

Suicide is an indictable offense only under common law or where statutes exist explicitly stating that it is unlawful and criminal. In the absence of such laws it is not indictable. Unless the act is a crime, an attempt cannot be. The question of mental competence and diminished responsibility have great bearing upon how laws are to be shaped. If an individual is ruled to be competent to stand trial then he can be held accountable for his behavior. This position is implicit in many psychological treatment approaches today. The thought is that unless an individual is helped to take responsibility for his acts he cannot learn new behavior. The consequences of behavior can assist in conditioning subsequent acts.

The law of transferred malice is applied in some cases, making one who accidentally kills another in the process of a suicide attempt guilty of manslaughter or murder. States will differ markedly on these points and it behooves all professionals interested in the helping process to become familiar with local laws.

State and National Legislation

An inherent belief in the value of State's Rights prevails in parts of our country today which is reflected in various statutory differences. Men and women do not attain majority at the same age level throughout the United States. There are differences with respect to consent to donate blood, receive medical and surgical care, treatment for pregnancy, venereal disease, drug addiction and suicidal behavior, whether attempted or committed, as well as aiding and abetting a suicidal act (Lowenstein 1970). There appears to be little relationship between legal sanctions against a third party who aids a completed or attempted suicidal individual and other legal rules pertaining to individual rights such as those noted relating to medical care. In essence, suicidal behavior is in a class by itself. Despite publicity to the contrary, a taboo attitude toward it still exists in the United States, even among professional mental health workers (Frederick 1971).

Most persons in the mental health field believe it would be helpful to have uniform statutes to assist in recording and classifying suicidal behavior. Without a standard nosological procedure there is no reliable baseline which can be obtained nationally. From a statistical point of view it is virtually impossible to compare incidence, frequency or type of behavior from one State to another, and certainly between countries. One can scarcely say that suicide rates have increased or decreased in Norway as compared to those in the United States if the classification methods are not the same, assuming that the raters would be equally adept in making the classification assessments. The vested interests which a State government might have toward a particular position about suicide would likely give way under organized national or professional pressure. Parochial views are less likely to obtain under peer group influence, unless the investment constitutes a serious personal threat.

While laws have been used for both good and evil, under a democratic form of government there has always been a mechanism for change through which current needs of society could be met. Common law sometimes falls short of present needs and the adjudication process is apt to be overly bound by former precedents, while legislation alone can offer a modern State the possibility of adapting quickly to necessary changes (Petris 1969). While the adjudication process is often distressingly time consuming, in some instances the "test case" procedure may prove useful and expedient. Legislators have a mandate to act for the people in questions of mental health but they need the active assistance of professionals.

A traditional problem has been that of equating anything resembling mental disturbance with danger and incompetence. The fallacy of this kind of thinking may be seen by using a medical analogy whereby one might say that if an individual cuts his leg or breaks a finger his whole body is incompetent or unable to function effectively.

What rights does an individual possess over his own mind and body? Presumably the line is drawn when his actions encroach upon the rights of others but the line is fuzzy indeed in the mental health field. To help deal with these problems in institutions the California legislature enacted the Lanterman-Petris-Short Act into law in 1967 (Petris 1969). An exhaustive survey of mental health facilities and professional opinions was conducted by using questionnaires and on-site interviews. The resulting statute provided protection for mentally disordered citizens against inappropriate, involuntary, and indefinite hospitalization. Legal stigma was avoided and provisions made to extract maximal benefit from existing manpower, programs and funding arrangements for mental health services. This Act illustrates how legislation can effect progressive changes in the ecology of mental health.

A classic case of inadequate services occurred in one well known hospital when an individual was still confined at the end of four years for a misdemeanor without having received appropriate treatment, whereas if he had gone directly to jail he would have been free in one year. Anyone who is removed from society and placed in an institution should have the right to the best that modern society can provide in treatment procedures. Yolles (1967) points out that it was not until 1964 that Congress enacted a Statute in the District of Columbia, the heart of the nation's government, establishing a person's right to needed hospital treatment.

Whether an individual's freedom is to be encroached upon legally or not depends upon how the problem is viewed. If suicide is seen as a crime by definition, then restraint of an individual's so called rights are justified, with the use of police power if necessary. Schulman (1968) comments that whenever a relationship has existed between the law and the problem of suicide it has been penal. He suggests that the law can play a more sensible and productive role by aiming for suicide prevention rather than penalization.

Curiously, by calling an individual psychotic and incompetent he may be more likely to receive immediate and needed treatment than if he is not. This is especially true if medical care is necessary through hospitalization. While present laws regarding sanity obtain, one may not be held legally liable for his behavior if found insane. He has some legal protection for aberrant behavior, including the commission of homicidal and suicidal acts while insane. Thus, in the expression of grossly aberrant behavior an insane individual ha more rights, so to speak, than one who is not. However, the mental patient can pay for his acts by long term hospitalization and a greater denial of privileges than if he were incarcerated in prison.

Insurance Problems

In most insurance policies there are restrictive clauses prohibiting payment if suicide occurs within one to two years after its beginning date. Over one third of the states have such limitations prescribed by statute. The hardship to spouse and children from lack of payment is of concern to some mental health workers. Although actuarial data seem to provide some basis for these time periods, the provisions are needlessly restrictive. Inquiry discloses that roughly half of the suicides of insured persons occur within the customary one or two year waiting period. A six month period would be more realistic, since few, if any, persons assume insurance coverage and then deliberately wait a year or more to kill themselves. Companies have been receptive to evaluating the problem and have expressed some willingness to modify their policies if sufficient data warrant a change. In no company surveyed were suicidal persons excluded from receiving insurance five years after an attempt had been made, even though the policies became rated with an increase in premiums.

The suicidal crisis is ephemeral and lasts only for a short period. Because of this, short term treatment with careful follow-up is often appropriate and effective. It is not unlikely that in many cases persons who have received treatment for suicidal ideation or behavior are better insurance risks than many such individuals who have not. Restrictive clauses and social stigma may promote denial and suppression of self destructive feelings and thereby stimulate attitudes and emotions which will explode later in a suicidal act.

Liabilities for Mental Health Personnel

A question often discussed, but arising infrequently, is that of suit for negligence or malpractice on the part of a professional practitioner or a mental health worker. Mere admission to a hospital does not prevent suicides. Once admitted, a suicidally prone person is likely to take his life while in the hospital or shortly after discharge unless careful follow-up procedures are employed. To warrant legal action it must be clearly shown that a suicidal risk was evident and known to the professional staff beyond all reasonable doubt. If a suicidal risk was not apparent, no case will exist. Moreover, the standard of performance by the practitioner is placed against the backdrop of the discipline from which he came. It is likely more would be expected of a psychologist, psychiatrist or experienced suicidologist, for example, than for a volunteer mental health worker on the telephone.

The core aspect of a suit is that proximage cause must be shown. There is a clear distinction between causal connection and proximate cause, as noted by Hepburn (1954). Causal connection may appear, though the negligent act may be the remote rather than the proximate cause. To constitute actionable negligence the plaintiff must not only show causal connection between the negligent act and an ensuing injury, but the negligent act itself must be the proximate cause. In essence, either an act of omission or commission on the part of the hospital, a mental health worker or professional must be clearly shown to have been related to the suicidal act by directly influencing the victim. Usually this is very difficult to prove. Professional service implies reasonable care, which means that which would be performed by the average individual with similar training in that profession in like circumstances. If the hospital, clinic or professional takes proper precautions in the training of workers and acts with ordinary prudence there is litle cause for concern about delivering services to persons in crisis.

Specific Symptoms of Self-Destructive Behavior

Since most books on human ecology and public health issues fail to cover the topic of suicide adequately, if at all, it is deemed advisable to develop the problem here in some detail. Even books aimed at public health administrators do not address themselves to themental health aspects of self destructive behavior (Rogers, 1960; Kilbourne and Smillie, 1969). There are steps which nearly anyone can take to assist with emergency mental or emotional crisis. To this end the ecology of human mental health can be affected positively. For this reason, a description of crisis symptoms and procedures follows.

The term self destructive is used to connote a broader range of behavioral possibilities than is denoted by the term suicide, which is restricted to human beings and usually defined as the willful or intentional taking of one's own life. A continuum of behavioral acts may be described with self assaultive behavior on one hand and suicide at the other with self destructive acts in between (Frederick 1970). One may assault or hurt one's self in many "accident prone" ways without being openly self destructive. Self destructive acts on the other hand, are likely to be more serious in that they include such psychological equivalents of suicide as excessive smoking with a respiratory disorder such as emphysema, reckless driving while drunk, or deliberately overdoing with a serious heart condition. While suicidal behavior is sometimes masked and equivocal, for the purposes of this continuum it can be considered as obvious and easily recognized. Examples would be jumping from a high place, self hanging, ingestion of poison, and the use of firearms and explosives.

With this background let us consider what symptoms one might look for in suicidal behavior. Shneidman (1968) has pointed out that clues may be verbal, behavioral, situational or syndromatic.

(a) *Verbal signs.* Direct verbal comments may be made such as: "I've had it. I think I'll just end it all." or "Everyone would be better off without me." Indirect communications often appear such as "So long, I guess I won't be seeing you anymore." "How does a person go about leaving his eyes or body to a medical school?" Persons not infrequently ask for information about a presumed friend or relative when they are actually inquiring about themselves. Threats should always be taken seriously and never regarded as a gag or joke (Schneidman and Farberow, 1956). It can mean the difference between life and death to talk with someone who threatens to kill himself (Litman, 1966; Schneidman, Farberow and Litman, 1970).

(b) *Behavioral signs.* These clues also may be of a direct or indirect type and of extreme importance, even though many of them may seem subtle. The acquiring of hazardous equipment or materials such as guns, knives, swords, razors, ropes or poison may be direct behavioral indicators of an effort to put others on the alert. Relatively indirect behavioral signs may appear, such as giving away prize possessions, social isolation, a drop in general efficiency, and putting one's affairs in order legally, such as inquiring about insurance or a will. While none of these behavioral events by themselves necessarily indicates a self-destructive potential, the appearance of a number of them together should be cause for concern.

(c) *Situational signs.* Life events comprise situational indicators which can be important in suspecting a self-destructive potential. The loss of a parent or close relative early in life, usually before the age of 16, loss of a job, new divorce, failure in school work, recent death of a "significant other," all comprise situations which can place unusual stress on an individual. External support may provide a bridge between life and death at such times if the person is already in a tenuous emotional state.

(d) *Syndromatic signs.* Although related to life situations, certain factors comprise a grouping of symptoms which are called syndromes. The most common of these would be the clinical depressive syndrome, exemplified by insomnia, anorexia, worry, loss of sex drive, somatic complaints, verbal comments implying guilt, despair or unhappiness, and motor and verbal retardation. Some physical illnesses can bring about a disorder of thinking and feeling which eventuates in suicidal behavior. The dependent - dissatisfied type of individual may or may not be depressed in the traditional, clinical sense at the time. Such persons become increasingly tense and dissatisfied with themselves and others upon whom they feel dependent. As this syndrome grows in intensity, the person becomes more irritable and complaining, which can constitute a warning signal.

Psychological First Aid or Emergency Mental Health Procedures

Knowing some of the general symptoms of behavior is important, but knowing what to do in order to provide first aid until professional assistance becomes available is crucial. A list of appropriate actions for friends or relatives follows.

(1) Listen. Persons in crisis feel they have not really been heard. It is important to convey to them the idea that someone will actually listen to what they are saying. An effort should be made to understand the feelings which are being expressed along with the words.

(2) Take complaints seriously. One should not make the mistake of dismiss-

ing or underrating what is being said. Very profound and seriously disturbed feelings are often presented in a low key, so to speak.

(3) Evaluate the ferality. The deadly quality of the suicidal thoughts and feelings need careful assessment. It is possible that an individual can be more lethal when he is calm than when he is severely disturbed, although this is usually not the case. Once an individual has resolved the conflict in his mind and has decided to take his life, a calm sometimes possesses him which can be deceiving.

(4) Examine the intensity or severity of the emotional disturbance. While it is always cause for alarm when a person is extremely upset, the individual may not be suicidal merely because he is upset. Psychotic persons are often severely disturbed but are not usually suicidal. Other accompanying aspects to suicidal disturbance should be present as well.

(5) Assess the resources available. People have both inner and outer resources to call upon during stress. Basically solid persons who have endured a stressful situation possess inner psychological resources which can be strengthened and supported, such as intellectual accomplishments, job effectiveness, etc. Outer resources refer to those outside the self, such as relatives, ministers and friends whom one can call for assistance.

(6) Do something tangible. Concrete action should be taken such as arranging for the person to see someone else, contacting a hospital or clinic, or whatever appears to be appropriate. It is very frustrating to feel as though nothing has been achieved from talking with another person at a time of crisis. This is apt to heighten despair.

(7) Be affirmative, yet supportive. Strong guideposts are necessary during periods of stress. Give the impression that you know what you are doing and that you intend to do everything possible to prevent the individual from taking his life.

(8) Ask directly about suicidal thoughts and intent. At an appropriate time, harm is rarely done by inquiring directly about self-destructive thoughts. An individual frequently welcomes this question since it gives him a chance to discuss feelings without being veiled. Usually, such questioning should occur later rather than at the beginning of the conversation.

(9) Do not be misled by euphemistic second thoughts. A suicidal person may believe that his disturbed feelings have passed and that he is on firm ground. While this may be so temporarily, suicidal thinking tends to recur and continued monitoring by someone else is of utmost importance.

(10) Do not be afraid to ask for assistance and consultation. Contact whomever is necessary, such as a family doctor, psychologist, school counselor, psychiatrist, minister, school nurse or police. It is a mistake to try to handle everything alone. One should convey the attitude of composure and firmness so that the individual in suicidal crisis will feel that something realistic and appropriate is being done to help him.

It would be valuable to volunteer one's services to obtain an in vivo picture of the functioning of crisis clinics and suicide prevention centers (Frederick and Resnik 1970). The rewards can be of inestimable value. In the final analysis, life is what human ecology is all about.

References

Bagley, C. The evaluation of a suicide prevention scheme by an ecological method. *Social Science and Medicine*, 1968, 2, 1-14

Blachly, P., Disher, D., & Roduner, G. Suicide by physicians. *Bulletin of Suicidology*, U.S. GovernmentPrinting Office, Washington, D.C., December 1968, 1-19

Breed, W. Suicide and loss in social interaction. In E.S. Shneidman (ed.) *Essays in self destruction.* New York: Science House, 1967, 188-202

Davidson M. & Hutt, C. A study of 500 Oxford student psychiatric patients. *British Journal of Social and Clinical Psychology*, 1964, 3, 175-185

Dublin, L. Suicide: A public health problem. In E.S. Schneidman (ed.) *Essays in self destruction.* New York: Science House, 1967, 251-260

Farberow, N. & Schneidman, E. *The cry for help.* New York: McGraw-Hill, 1961

Frederick, C. The school guidance counselor as a prevention agent to self destructive behavior. *New York State Personnel Guidance Association Journal*, 1970, **5**, 1-5

Frederick, C. The present suicide taboo in the United States. *Mental Hygiene*, 1971, **55**, 178-183

Frederick, D. & Resnik, H.L.P. Interventions with suicidal patients. *Contemporary Psychotherapy*, 1970, 2, 103-109

Frederick, C. & Resnik, H.L.P. How suicidal behaviors are learned. *American Journal of Psychotherapy*, 1971, **25**, 37-55

Gibbs, J. (ed). *Suicide.* New York: Harper and Row, 1968

Glass, D., Singer, J. & Friedman, L. Psychiatric cost of adaption to an environmental stressor. *Journal of Personality and Social Psychology*, 1969, 12, 200-210

Griffitt, W. & Veitch, R. Hot and crowded: Influences of population density and temperature on interpersonal affective behavior. *Journal of Personality and Social Psychology*, 1971, 17, 92-98

Hepburn, W. *Cases on the law of torts.* St. Paul, Minnesota: West Publishing Co., 1954

Kilbourne, E. & Smillie, W. *Human ecology and public health.* (4th ed.) New York, Macmillan, 1969.

Litman, R. Police aspects of suicide. *Police*, 1966, **10**, 14-18

Lowenstein, R. Questions and answers: Commumunity mental health centers and the law. Paper prepared for Mental Health Center Training Workshops, Operations Course No. 5, 1970

Lum, D. Suicide: Theological ethics and pastoral counseling. Th.D. thesis Southern California School of Theology, Claremont, California 1967

Paffenbarger, R., King, S. & Wing, A. Chronic disease in former college students: IX. Characteristics in youth that predispose to suicide and accidental death in later life. *American Journal of Public Health*, 1969, **59**, 900-908

Parrish, H. Cause of death among college students: A study of 209 deaths at Yale University, 1920-55. *Public Health Reports*, 1956, **71**, 1081-1085

Peck, M. & Schrut, A. Suicidal behavior among college students. *HSMHA Health Reports*, 1971, **86**, 149-156

Petris, N. New approaches to mental health in the California legislature. In *The future of psychotherapy.* C.J. Frederick (ed.) New York: Little, Brown and Co., 1969

Public Health Service Publication No. 600. *Facts of life and death.* U.S. Government Printing Office, Washington, D.C. 1970

Rieger, W. Suicide attempts in a federal prison. *Archives of General Psychiatry*, 1970, 24, 532-535

Rogers, E. *Human ecology and health.* New York: Macmillan, 1960

Rohles, F. Environmental Psychology: A bucket of worms. *Psychology Today*, 1967, 1, 55-63

Schulman, R. Suicide and suicide prevention: A legal analysis. *American Bar Association Journal*, 1968, 54, 855-962

Seiden, R. *Suicide among youth.* U.S. Government Printing Office, Washington, D.C., 1969

Schneidman, E. Preventing suicide. *Bulletin of Suicidology*, Washington, D.C.: U.S. Government Printing Office, December 1968, 19-25

Schneidman, E. & Farberow, N. Clues to suicide. *Public Health Reports*, 1956, 71, 109-114

Schneidman, E., Farberow, N. & Litman, R. *The psychology of suicide.* New York: Science House, 1970

Spencer, S. Academic revolt and failure among Oxford undergraduates. *The Lancet*, 1958, 2, 438-440

Stengel, E. *Suicide and attempted suicide.* Baltimore: Penguin Books, 1964

Stevas, N.S. *Life, death and the law.* Bloomington: Indiana University Press, 1961

World Health Organization Chronicle, Society, stress and disease, 1971, 25, 168-177

Williams, G. *The sanctity of life and the criminal law.* New York: Alfred Knopf, 1966

Yolles, S.F. The right to treatment. *Psychiatry Digest*, 1967, 28, 7-13

Zubek, J. (ed.) *Sensory deprivation: Fifteen years of research.* New York: Appelton-Century-Crofts, 1969

2 Gonorrhea: California's Major Health Menace

Question: *How serious is the problem of gonorrhea in California?*
Answer: This venereal infection is increasing at an alarming rate. In only a single year—between 1967 and 1968—the number of cases reported in California rose from 61,000 to 76,000. Only ten years before—in 1957—the number of reported cases was relatively low: 15,679. On the basis of the 1968 figures, we can assume that out of every 1,000 persons in the state, at least three are infected with gonorrhea each year. In actual fact, the ratio is probably even higher than that, since it is believed that less than one in ten cases is reported. Gonorrhea can realistically be considered the state's major *public health menace.* It shows up much more frequently than any of the other communicable diseases which are reportable to public health authorities. For example, compared with the 76,000 cases of gonorrhea reported in 1968, there were 18,000 cases of mumps; 11,000 cases of syphilis, the other major venereal disease; and 5,000 cases of German measles (rubella).

Question: *Who are the victims of this widespread disease?*
Answer: Anyone and everyone. It strikes persons of all ages, all classes, all races. Infection is transmitted almost exclusively by sexual contact. A marital partner may be infected by a spouse who is unaware of the infection or has been inadequately treated. More than

SOURCE: Reprinted from Health Tips—A Public Service of the California Medical Association, San Francisco, Calif., July 1969.

half of the reported cases are *young persons under 25 years of age*—and several hundred are actually between the ages of 10 and 14. Health authorities conservatively estimate that one in ten Californians between the ages of 15 and 25 will have gonorrhea this year. The concentration of this disease among young persons is particularly tragic because one of the complications of untreated gonorrhea is sterility. Teenagers with the infection often do not understand the meaning of its symptoms and accordingly do not get treatment; if they do understand that they have gonorrhea, they may be too frightened to consult their parents or other adults who might help.

Question: *What are the symptoms of gonorrhea?*
Answer: In the male patient, the infection is *easy to detect.* There may be a discharge from the penis, or inflammation of the urethra and discomfort during urination. In the female patient, the initial inflammation may be mild and of short duration, without any symptoms. She may or may not have a discharge and often the infection spreads to her entire reproductive system before she becomes aware that she has gonorrhea. In the course of the spread of the disease, she may *unknowingly infect her sexual partners.* Rectal infection rarely presents symptoms and is often undetected.

Question: *How is gonorrhea treated?*
Answer: It is treated by penicillin or, for those strains resistant to penicillin, by some other appropriate antibiotic, either given by injection or taken by mouth. Some strains of gonorrhea are more resistant than others and for these, *increased dosage or longer treatment is required.* Only a doctor can decide what dosage is required for the individual patient and how many times it must be repeated.

Question: *Does this treatment really cure the disease?*
Answer: Yes, without doubt. But the patient must *follow instructions* to the last letter. Inadequate treatment may result in only partial cure and the possibility of chronic disease. In other words, it isn't the medication that fails, but the patient. For example, although the symptoms may clear up within a few days after treatment, the patient may be told to drink no alcohol for a week. If he doesn't follow this instruction, he doesn't get the full benefit of the medication. He will be told not to have sexual intercourse for at least 10 days. If he disobeys, he *may get re-infected* or spread his disease to someone else.

Among patients who are instructed to take their medication orally, there is always added risk of "patient failure." The patient may carelessly skip one dose, may stop before he has taken the full amount prescribed, or may share his medication with friends or with his sexual partner whose infection may not have been reported. In such cases, the patient gets *less medication than he needs* and his infection may reappear.

Question: *What needs to be done to curb this health menace?*
Answer: Fundamentally, what is needed is a drastic change of attitude. The patient must view it not as a private matter but as a matter of public concern. He must realize that his doctor is legally required to report all cases of gonorrhea to public health authorities. He should also be reassured by the knowledge that the record of his infection will be considered *entirely confidential* by these public health officials. Finally, the infected person must cooperate willingly and fully with public health authorities in giving them the names of his contacts—that is, the persons from whom he may have caught the disease. The

purpose of naming the possible sources of infection is to *protect*, not to embarrass nor to punish. Most young people who infect others with gonorrhea *do not know* that they themselves have the disease. Public health workers, who have been given their names, seek them out, tell them they may be infected, and help them to get prompt treatment, which is so necessary for their own health.

The naming of names is often the most difficult step of all, because it reveals information which has traditionally been considered highly personal. But one must remember that this confidential information is used only by trained public health personnel solely for the purpose of stopping this dread disease by getting all infected persons cured. Only by making it possible for public health staff to follow up all sources of gonorrhea can the alarming cycle of infection and re-infection be broken.

Prepared and released as a public service by the California Medical Association. Specific questions on the subject should be directed to your physician.

Man vs. Virus—Why You Got the Flu

3

Health officials officially classify it as "a mild disease." But hundreds of thousands of Americans know better. Their veins seem to be filled with ice water, yet their temperatures hover at 102. Their muscles and bones ache, their heads throb with each raspy cough, and over all is a feeling of lassitude so pervasive that to reach out for aspirin or a glass of water becomes an effort—even while resting in bed.

The cause of all the misery, of course, is the new mutant virus known as A2-Hong Kong-68, a submicroscopic speck of protein and nucleic acid less than a millionth of an inch wide. One of the most contagious viruses known, it travels from victim to victim with the slightest cough or sneeze.

The virus apparently made its initial appearance in China (and in Britain, the disease is known as "Mao flu"). But it was officially named, in accordance with World Health Organization rules, by the place in which the virus was first isolated. "We have," a Hong Kong paper noted truthfully, "acted unwillingly in our role as an entry port for a sneeze by person or persons unknown."

Mobility. The virus erupted in Hong Kong in July and—because it was a new variety of flu virus against which the population was not immune—quickly spread to hundreds of thousands of men, women and children in the Far East during the summer. Then, propelled by jet age mobility—the virus swept into the U.S. last fall before an effective vaccine could be developed. "Man has been running a race against the influenza virus," said Los Angeles County Medical-services officer Benjamin A. Kogan, "and man has lost."

The biggest losers to date live in the nation's crowded cities. The National Communicable Disease Center in Atlanta reported that widespread outbreaks have occurred in all but eleven states; to be sure, some of the sickness was merely fashionable. "You wouldn't tell anybody you had a cold," noted one health officer, "when you could tell them you had Hong Kong flu." But for the healthy ones who haven't yet been hit, the very scope of the epidemic offered some solace. Once a person gets the Hong Kong flu he is not likely to get that variety again for a while. And since so much of the country has been hit simultaneously, there is a lot of immunity around. The NCDC does not expect further epidemic waves in the late winter such as occurred during the flu epidemic of 1957.

Inevitable. In Europe, the worst is yet to come. Mao flu was reported in two crowded Midland cities and British Health Minister David Ennals warned against a panic rush for vaccine. At least a million doses are on hand in Britain, and manufacturers plan to supply another 140,000 a week through the winter. In Germany, the airlifting of 12,000 GI's for military exercises led Health Ministry officials to warn that flu was "inevitable." In Russia, the Health Ministry announced that the flu was expected by the end of January and began a campaign to vaccinate 70 to 80 per cent of the population in major cities.

For most victims in the U.S. and abroad, the flu runs its course in three or four days, with perhaps one or two weeks of lingering lassitude. But for those debilitated by age, heavy cigarette smoking and other illnesses, the A2-Hong Kong-68 virus often turned out to be fatal. These were the people most likely to develop viral pneumonia if the virus attacked their lungs; alternatively their ravaged respiratory tracts were open to "secondary" invasion by bacteria. Directly or indirectly, flu was responsible for the deaths of actress Tallulah Bankhead, 65, and William Calhoun Baggs, 48-year old editor of the Miami News. NCDC surveys of 122 cities showed that deaths from pneumonia and influenza were running three times the expected number for this time of year.

The toll taken by Hong Kong flu is a reminder of the age-old battle between man and the virus enemy within. During the past 30 years, antibiotics, sulfa compounds and other drugs have largely given man mastery over bacteria—the single-celled organisms that cause such diseases as strep throat, certain kinds of pneumonia, diphtheria, tuberculosis, syphilis and whooping cough. Now the virus has emerged as the leading cause of disability and death from infection.

Man is a walking virus target. To date, more than 500 distinct types of viruses have been identified inside the human body. Some 40 to 60 viruses cause the common cold. Others account for the familiar childhood diseases—chicken pox, mumps and measles, both the regular and German variety. Just last week, a measles epidemic brought U.S. physicians to the Dominican Republic to begin a crash program to vaccinate 100,000 youngsters.

Attack. Researchers classify viruses by chemical and physical properties; a more meaningful popular nomenclature uses the site of action or mode of invasion. The so-called enteroviruses invade the intestinal tract; some of them go on to attack the central nervous system and cause polio, but the majority, like the kind that rose with astronaut Frank Borman on Apollo 8, cause the nausea and diarrhea of 24-hour grippe. There are at least twenty varieties of adeno-viruses that attack the adenoids and cause severe sore throats among children and spread disease in military posts. Arboviruses (an acronym for arthropod-borne viruses) are carried by mosquitoes and other insects; they cause such serious diseases as yellow fever and encephalitis. Herpes viruses, a name derived from the Greek word for creeping, cause chicken pox, shingles and fever sores.

At present, in a number of labs, the virologists may be approaching the most important virus identification of all. Since the discovery in 1911 that viruses cause a form of cancer in chickens, the suspicion has grown that they may also be responsible for human cancers as well. Indeed, in the minds of some scientists, this suspicion has turned to a strong conviction. "We used to say we wanted to determine whether viruses cause cancer," says Dr. Frank J. Rauscher Jr. of the U.S. National Cancer Institute. "Now we say we want to find out how many different viruses cause cancer."

Man, and indeed all earth life, has probably always coexisted uneasily with viruses. But no one knows where these viruses come from. The most far out suggestion is that they are strnage life forms that wafted to earth from space. More likely viral ingredients were present in the primal soup that gave rise to earth life. Some virologists suggest that they represent a species of subbacterial particle from which cells later evolved. The majority of virologists believe that the cell came first and that viruses are cells that regressed and lost their ability to reproduce except by becoming parasites.

Contagious. Yet no one ever saw a virus until the late 1930s, though they were known to exist decades earlier. In 1898, Dutch botanist Martinus Beijerinck, looking for the organism that infected and destroyed tobacco plants, ground up a mixture of diseased leaves and pressed the juice through a porcelain filter with pores small enough to trap bacteria. He was amazed to find that the bacteria-free juice itself could spread the disease and concluded that it contained "a contagious living fluid" or visus, the Latin word for poison. In the last two decades, thanks to the super high-magnification of the electron microscope and such techniques for isolating viruses as high-speed centrifuges and tissue-culture flasks, scientists have been able to identify, photograph and measure viruses and learn more about how they cause disease.

Typically, viruses consist of a central core of nucleic acid surrounded by an outer protective coat of protein. The viral nucleic acid is either DNA, the same material that makes up the genes in the nucleus of animal cells, or RNA, the substance that helps the genes regulate the chemistry of the cell and reproduce.

The viruses deposit their nucleic acids inside the cell. Some researchers believe the nucleic acid is absorbed through the cell wall, others believe that the viruses actually bore into the cell through specific "receptor sites" in the cell membrane and then occupy hollow spaces called vacuoles from which they release their nucleic acid (see chart). From this strategic base, the invading viral nucleic acid takes over the chemical assembly line of the cell for its own benefit and survival.

Copies. Soon the cell is turning out new viruses instead of the substances needed for its own well being. After it has produced hundreds or thousands of virus copies, the cell dies. The growing army of viruses then goes on and attacks other cells. The disease—from common colds to (possibly) cancer—has begun. This process raises teleological as well as medical problems. Outside the cell, the virus may lie inert like a crystal or bit of dust. It comes alive only when it invades an intact living cell in order to reproduce. Yet while in the cell, it is no longer a virus since it has become part of the genetic material of the cell. For most virologists, viruses fall between the smallest living organism and the largest inert chemical molecules. According to the late Dr. Thomas Rivers of Rockefeller University, a virus could be appropriately described as a "molechism" or an "organule."

Fortunately, man has evolved a natural defense against viral attacks. Each type of virus contains its own "identification tag" in the form of a specific configuration of one or more molecules in its protein coat called an antigen. Responding to a viral invasion, the body manufactures proteins called antibodies that somehow fit these antigens and prevent the virus from entering the cell. After a viral disease has run its course, the antibodies the body has produced will protect against a further infection by the same virus for months, years or even a lifetime. Similarly, vaccines made from weakened or killed viruses will stimulate the production of antibodies without causing the full-blown disease. Using this principle, virologists have begun producing a steady procession of vaccines to eradicate some of the most important virus diseases.

Vaccines are available against influenza, but their effectiveness is limited by the unique ability of the flu virus to change its antigens periodically. This virus has never been known to live outside the body, and it apparently would die out if it did not mutate. There are two main types of flu antigens, A and B, each with its own subtypes. When a new type appears, such as the A2 variant that caused the Asian flu pandemic of 1957, antibodies which people have acquired through vaccination or their last encounter with flu offer little or no protection. "That," notes Dr. Fred H. Davenport of the University of Michigan School of Public Health, "is why the flu virus is the world's champion spreader."

Damage. At least 30 flu pandemics are on record between 1510 and 1930. By far the worst of the pandemics was the 1918-19 episode that took at least 20 million lives, including half a million in the U.S. The virus of that year appears to have been more virulent than most, causing greater damage to the cells lining the respiratory tract and leading to many cases of viral pneumonia. Moreover, no antibiotics were available at the time to combat the bacterial pneumonias that often follow an attack of flu. Although just as widespread, the Asian pandemic eleven years ago caused a far smaller number of deaths around the world.

Why do some people "resist" a virus and not others? One reason is that even though a virus like the flu bug may be a variant, it sometimes has enough in common with earlier strains so that some persons will have some protective antibodies from exposure to earlier bouts of illness. In 1957, for example, many persons in their 60s and 70s had antibodies against Asian flu, apparently because of antibodies acquired during a serious outbreak in 1889-90. Other people may develop a "subclinical infection" with only mild symptoms—five hours, say, of the 24-hour flu—perhaps because they eat, sleep and exercise regularly. On the other hand, children, who have little acquired immunity, are the most susceptible to flu no matter how healthy they are—but the elderly are more susceptible to its debilitating effects.

Cold Air. The fact that flu seems to hit in the winter suggests to some that cold weather has an effect on the spread of the virus. Indeed, the name influenza comes from the phrase influenza di freddo—an influence of cold. In a typical year, the flu season is in January and February, and there is some evidence that cold air alters the blood supply of the respiratory tract and may make it more vulnerable. Possibly more important is the fact that people are indoors more in winter and in closer contact; most outbreaks of respiratory infection seem to coincide with the beginning of school. There is no place or time to hide, though. It was a warm July when the new flu variant surfaced in Hong Kong. Perhaps the best advice for staying healthy is to be healthy to start with. The problems of public health and vaccine production grow enormously more complicated in the field of cancer virus research.

Since Dr. Peyton Rous of Rockefeller University proved that a form of cancer in chickens was caused by a virus in 1911, more than 70 tumor viruses have been identified in animals. In the 1960s researchers began finding what seemed to be virus-like particles in patients with leukemia. And since 1964, the National Cancer Institute has spent $90 million to support cancer-virus hunters in laboratories throughout the U.S. At present, NCI has contracts with no fewer than 94 universities and private institutions, and less formal arrangements with 50 others.

Wild Genes. In theory, viruses are a logical suspect. Cancer involves a derangement in the genetic material of the cell which causes it to reproduce generations of abnormal, wildly growing tumor cells. And because they contain genetic material it seems logical to conclude that viruses could induce malignant changes in previously normal cells. Researchers suspect that the putative cancer virus would not necessarily replicate inside the cell like the flu virus. Viruses, they note, don't necessarily destroy the cells they invade by forcing them to produce more viruses. Sometimes the genetic material of the virus becomes a part of the genetic material of the cell and lies dormant until some environmental factor brings it back to life. There is a leukemia virus that infects mice, for example, which remains latent and apparently harmless until the mouse is exposed to radiation. Then, the mouse comes down with the disease. In a somewhat similar experiment, Dr. Robert J. Huebner of NCI has found that a latent virus can be "turned on" by infection with another virus.

Huebner, one of NCI's foremost virus experts, is now concentrating on the C-type RNA virus—which seems to be associated with both acute leukemia in young mice as well as the cancer of old age. Huebner regards this as the "only kind of virus that can explain cancer generally" and has given up all other viral studies to investigate it.

The fact that virus particles can't always be found in tumor tissue doesn't mean that a virus didn't cause the cancer. Once the malignant change takes place, the virus may simply become a latent and invisible part of the malignant cell's genetic material. Dr. Maurice Green of St. Louis University has produced malignant tumors in hamsters by innoculating them with adenoviruses. Although he couldn't find virus particles in the cells, he did find the "fingerprints" within the cells—RNA molecules from the virus.

Kissing Bug. The latest direct evidence of a virus in human cancer concerns a member of the herpes virus family. Called the EB virus, it was originally isolated from children with Burkitt's lymphoma. This is a cancer of the lymphatic system suspected of being infectious because it occurs largely among children living in a specific area of Central and East Africa infested with mosquitoes and tsetse flies. About a year ago, Drs. Werner and Gertrude Henle of Philadelphia's Children's Hospital found that many U.S. youngsters had antibodies to EB in their blood; this suggested that they had been exposed to the virus, although they had showed no signs of disease. Later, the Henles found that patients recovering from infectious mononucleosis had high levels of EB antibodies, suggesting that the EB virus is the cause of mono or "kissing disease" (so called because the virus is apparently transmitted by the saliva mingling in soul kisses) that affects so many U.S. college students.

Last fall Dr. James Grace, director of Roswell Park Memorial Hospital in Buffalo, linked the African victims with the U.S. students. Grace reported that patients with several forms of cancer, including Hodgkin's disease and leukemia, also have high levels of EB antibodies. And he also has shown the EB virus causes what look like malignant changes in lymph cells grown in tissue culture. Taking all the evidence together, Grace believes that most people are harmlessly infected with EB during their lives. But in some susceptible persons, the virus causes mono, and in a smaller number of susceptibles, it may cause cancer.

Contact. During the past year, another herpes virus has been implicated in cancer of the cervix, a disease that afflicts some 40,000 women each year in the U.S. Dr. Joseph Melnick of Baylor University School of Medicine found that a high percentage of women with cervical cancer had antibodies to the herpes virus, suggesting that they had been exposed to it sometime in their lives. Few healthy women, on the other hand, proved to have herpes antibodies. The herpes 2 virus is known to cause a blistering disease in the genital tract and because it has been found in smegma it is suspected to being transmitted by sexual intercourse. It could also, Melnick suggests, remain latent in some women who have been infected and cause cancer later in life. This notion of viral transmission may explain why cervical cancer is common in women who have frequent sexual contact and in women whose husbands are uncircumcized.

Implicit in such findings is the possibility of developing vaccines against cancer viruses. In fact, Rauscher notes a vaccine has been developed which will prevent all known types of leukemia in mice. And now, NCI investigators are considering whether to go ahead with a vaccine for EB virus to see if it will prevent Burkitt's lymphoma. "All plans are under way," says Rauscher. "We have the capability for making a vaccine, we have a virus, and good evidence that it causes cancer."

Contaminated. At the same time, the search goes on for vaccines against other common disease viruses that have so far eluded researchers. Among the most important is hepatitis, a disease that produces severe liver damage, jaundice and a lingering debilitating illness in 50,000 to 60,000 Americans a year. Hepatitis is believed to be caused by two viruses. Infectious hepatitis is caused by a virus transmitted in contaminated food or water; serum hepatitis is spread by the transfusion of contaminated blood or dirty hypodermic needles. Development of a vaccine against either type has been blocked by the fact that researchers haven't been able to isolate the virus and study it in experimental animals. But Drs. Friedrich Deinhardt and Albert W. Holmes of Chicago's Presbyterian St. Luke's Hospital may have succeeded in trapping the virus. They have produced what appears to be the classic disease in marmosets by inoculating the animals with blood from hepatitis patients. They are now working with the isolated virus.

New vaccines are also being developed for respiratory diseases. One of them has sharply reduced the spread of adenoviruses among military personnel. NIH researchers are working on a vaccine against respiratory syncytial virus, blamed for about half of the 11,000 pneumonia deaths occurring in children each year. Researchers are also using the current flu epidemic to improve flu vaccines. Most current flu vaccines are only 60 to 70 per cent effective. Using a high-speed zonal centrifuge, workers at the Atomic Energy Commission's Oak Ridge National Laboratory have been able to produce highly purified viruses for vaccine preparation. These specimens are free of the impurities that cause toxic reactions (fever, aching arms) in some vaccine recipients, so vaccines made with purified viruses can be given in larger doses, hopefully boosting effectiveness to 100 per cent. Because they are less likely to produce side effects, the purified vaccines are more suitable than ordinary flu vaccines for children—often the biggest spreaders of flu. Several studies are now going on to see if inoculation of large numbers of youngsters reduces the spread of Hong Kong flu.

Since there are a large number of viruses involved, researchers generally agree that a single vaccine to prevent the common cold is impractical. However, they envision the possibility of combining 20 or 30 killed virus vaccines into a single "vaccine cocktail" to prevent the more serious respiratory infections.

The prospects of developing drugs to fight viruses have become brighter in the last decade. Too often, however, drugs that destroy a virus may damage the cell as well. Five years ago, Burroughs Wellcome Laboratories in England developed a drug called thiosemicarbazone that prevents smallpox, without harming the cell. In the U.S. du Pont has developed a drug that prevents the flu virus from entering cells. It works only in Asian flu, however, and many investigators are not convinced it is the answer.

Another promising approach to curbing virus infection has been opened by the discovery of interferon, a natural substance that the body produces to fight viruses. Interferon was discovered in 1957 by England's Dr. Jean Lindenmann and the late Dr. Alick Isaacs at the National Institute for Medical Research in England. The DNA or RNA of the attacking virus apparently causes the cell to produce this protein which then is carried in the blood stream to other cells and somehow protects them. In fact, many investigators believe that interferon is more important than antibodies in fighting virus infections, although antibodies play the major role in prevention.

Synthetic. Because of the large amounts required, administration of natural interferon is impractical. But now, researchers have shown that administration of natural or synthetic RNA induces interferon production. Dr. Samuel Baron of the National Institute of Allergy and Infectious Diseases (NIAID) reported recently that an interferon-inducer called Poly I:C was effective against a herpes eye infection in rabbits, even when given three days after the disease had begun. And just last week, NIAID's Dr. Hilton Levy reported that Poly I:C even seems to curb cancer in mice. Levy doesn't believe the results were solely due to interferon's antiviral effect, since only two of the cancers studied were of viral origin. Poly I:C, he concludes, may have potential of its own as an anticancer drug and he plans to test it in human beings if toxicity studies show it is safe. Meanwhile, Baron notes, "It is likely that we will see applications of interferon in humans within five years."

The ultimate weapon against the virus enemy may be other viruses. Dr. Sol Spiegelman of the University of Illinois has developed a strain of virus that uses up large quantities of an enzyme that viruses need to make RNA. Perhaps, he suggests, a "good" virus could be raised which, when transmitted to the victim of a virus disease, would rob "bad" viruses of the enzymes needed to reproduce.

This would open an era not only of unprecedented good health but of genetic engineering as well to correct nature's errors. Since viruses contain the stuff of which genes and all of life are made, some researchers predict that good viruses may be used to carry genetic material into cells to correct defective genes. On that millennial day, the hated virus would become transformed into man's best friend.

Fighting the Enemy Within

In 1796 an English country doctor, Edward Jenner, discovered that his patients could be protected against smallpox if he infected them with a related but mild disease called cowpox. He not only turned smallpox into a minor disease but he also discovered the technique of vaccination (though he knew nothing about viruses). Since then, viruses have been discovered and defeated. A list of the conquered diseases and those still to be beaten:

Rabies. Doctors still apply the treatment for rabies first used by Pasteur and his colleagues in 1885. Therapy for the fatal disease, contracted when humans are bitten by infected animals, consists of a series of 14 to 21 injections of a vaccine. Antibodies produced by the vaccine protect against the rabies virus. Sometimes persons exposed to rabies get a horse serum containing antibodies, giving temporary immunity.

Yellow Fever. In 1665, yellow fever reduced a 1,500-man force on the Caribbean island St. Lucia to 89. Some historians believe the disease killed off the crew of the legendary ghost ship, The Flying Dutchman. Yellow fever remained uncontrollable until 1937 when Dr. Max Theiler of Harvard and later the Rockefeller Foundation developed a successful live virus vaccine. The disease, however, still remains endemic in jungle regions.

Polio. Between 1915 and 1955, infantile paralysis struck more than 500,000 U.S. children, killing 57,000 and crippling 300,000. In a recent year there were fewer than 150 victims, thanks to Dr. Jonas Salk, who developed a killed virus vaccine, and Dr. Albert Sabin.

Flu. A vaccine developed in 1957 may offer some protection against prevalent strains of the virus. The new vaccine rushed into production late last year provides protection against Hong Kong flu. Unlike other disease-causing viruses, the flu "bug" can defeat vaccines by proliferating new strains against which no antibodies have been developed.

Measles. At Harvard in 1961, Nobel laureate Dr. John Enders succeeded in growing a benign strain of the measles virus. The resulting vaccine, licensed in 1963, has cut the incidence of measles in the U.S. from 4 million cases a year to 2 million.

Mumps. The case of mumps that afflicted Jeryl Lynn Hilleman five years ago proved to be a milestone. Her father, Maurice, a virologist at Merck Sharp & Dohme, used viruses swabbed from her throat to produce a vaccine that proved 95 per cent effective in trails. The vaccine gives protection for at least four years. The vaccine has recently been approved for everyone over one year of age. Such protection is important, since in adult males mumps can cause sterility.

Rubella. (German Measles) The last U.S. rubella epidemic caused 30,000 still births and miscarriages, and between 20,000 and 40,000 deformed infants. When the next epidemic occurs, most likely in the early 1970's, its toll will probably be significantly reduced by a rubella vaccine developed at Harvard and the National Institutes of Health. NIH recommends giving the vaccine to females when they are between the ages of 1 and 14 in order to assure their protection when they reach adulthood. The vaccine, like rubella itself, can sometimes cause brief, arthritis-like pains in women but the side effect is temporary and harmless.

Common Cold. Strangely, this most prevalent of all virus illnesses has defied efforts to create immunity against it. The reason is that between 40 and 60 separate viruses can cause the familiar symptoms. Each one would require a separate vaccine—an impractically large number to combine in a single dose.

Cancer. At Rockefeller University and other institutions, researchers have found increasing evidence that viruses can cause cancer in man. If human cancer viruses are identified, all-out efforts will be made to produce vaccines against them. Some vaccines have already been developed which are effective against leukemia (cancer of the blood) in mice.

4 Hepatitis

What is Hepatitis?

"Hepatitis" means a swelling and soreness of the liver. Two types caused by viruses, "infectious" and "serum" hepatitis, are most frequent in the United States.

One is called "infectious" because a person with the disease can infect others by contact. This type is also spread by contaminated water and food, including raw clams and oysters harvested from polluted waters.

"Serum" hepatitis was first recognized in people who had been given medicines or vaccines that contained human serum. A person may develop serum hepatitis after receiving a transfusion of infected blood or its derivatives, or after having contaminated needles, syringes, or other skin puncturing instruments (including tattoo needles) used on him.

What is Infectious Hepatitis?

Infectious hepatitis is one of the more common communicable diseases, especially in children. It may be compared to mumps in frequency and seriousness, and in the fact that it is spread from one person to another. The closer the contact, the greater the chance that any susceptible individual will develop the disease. Among children, hepatitis is probably most often spread during play or visits. The risk is small among children who have only classroom contacts; to adults who are exposed to the disease at work, the risk is even smaller.

SOURCE: Department of Health, Education, and Welfare, Public Health Service, Health Information Series, No. 82; Public Health Service Publication No. 446, Revised 1966.

What is a "Susceptible Individual?"

Anyone who has not had infectious hepatitis may get the disease, but people who have once had hepatitis probably will not get it again. Mild in children, usually lasting 1 to 2 weeks, infectious hepatitis is more severe in adults who generally take 4 to 6 weeks for recovery.

What are the Symptoms?

Infectious hepatitis may begin any time 2 to 6 weeks after exposure to the disease. The most common symptoms are tiredness, loss of appetite, upset stomach with or without vomiting, headache, and pain in the abdomen. Fever may occur at first, but it generally stops in a few days. The liver may enlarge and become tender.

The most characteristic sign is a yellowing of the whites of the eyes. The skin may also develop a yellowish or "jaundiced" color, but many people develop hepatitis without this sign. Yellowing of the skin also occurs with other diseases, however, and may not be a sign of hepatitis.

Should the Doctor be Called?

It is advisable to consult your physician, even if the symptoms are very mild. There are several reasons for this:

The jaundice may not be caused by hepatitis, but may be the sign of a more serious disease.

A physician's supervision may help make the illness shorter and reduce the chance of a relapse.

He can advise protective measures to prevent the spread of disease to others.

He can alert the local health department to such conditions as improper sewage disposal, water supply impurity, and substandard food sanitation that could cause an epidemic of the disease.

The treatment for infectious hepatitis usually recommended by physicians is bed rest and an adequate diet. Because recovery is generally slower in adults than in children, some people become unnecessarily concerned, but this depression or "blue" feeling is frequently a part of the disease itself.

How can the Risk be Reduced?

There is no vaccine available to immunize against infectious hepatitis. There are several ways, however, to reduce the risk of contracting the disease.

Community Sanitation. Every home should be connected to a sewer system or properly built septic tank in good operating condition. Safe food and water supplies are also important. Information about proper sewage disposal, water supply purity, and food sanitation can be obtained from the local health department.

Personal Hygiene. Children should be taught to keep dirty objects out of their mouths and to wash their hands thoroughly with soap and water after using a toilet.

Gamma Globulin. This provides temporary protection and may be given by a physician to members of the patient's immediate family. Gamma globulin is the disease-fighting part of human blood. It contains antibodies that hold the infection in check while the body builds up its resistance to disease. This is why an injection of gamma globulin given to a person who has been exposed to the disease will prevent or lessen the severity of infectious hepatitis.

Gamma globulin is made from human blood, much of which may have been donated to the Red Cross or other organizations. Your doctor or health officer can use it as a protection against hepatitis only when exposure is sufficient to make infection very likely.

What is Serum Hepatitis?

Serum hepatitis is caused by a virus that circulates in the blood of some persons for many years. Because it cannot be detected by tests and may not cause any symptoms, infected persons can unwittingly transmit the virus by serving as blood donors.

What are the Symptoms of Serum Hepatitis?

The symptoms of serum hepatitis are similar to those of infectious hepatitis, but come more slowly and are frequently more severe and last longer. Mild cases, however, *do* occur.

An attack of serum hepatitis probably provides immunity against future attacks of the same type, but a person who has had infectious hepatitis is not immune to serum hepatitis; nor is a person who has had serum hepatitis immune to infectious hepatitis.

Should a Doctor be Called?

Yes, for the same reasons listed for infectious hepatitis.

What are the Precautions?

People who have had infectious or serum hepatitis should not donate blood for transfusion purposes. Occasionally, when blood is to be processed and divided into its separate parts, persons with a history of hepatitis may serve as donors, but they should always notify their blood center officials that they have had hepatitis.

Proper sterilization of all instruments used for penetrating the skin is a basic way to prevent the disease. Gamma globulin injections are not known to be effective against serum hepatitis.

What You Should Know About Strokes

5

by Alfred Soffer

Dwight D. Eisenhower recovered from a stroke to return to the presidency, the world's most taxing job. An earlier president, Franklin D. Roosevelt, also suffered a stroke. But in this case, it was catastrophic, and the patient died shortly after.

These two prominent cases underline the confusing facts about strokes: They vary widely in cause, severity, treatment, and degree of recovery.

"Stroke" is an "umbrella" term which means only that interference with normal brain function has occurred; it also is known as "apoplexy" or "cerebral vascular accident." It can strike suddenly and completely, or it can occur in stages. In many cases, it gives its victims warning.

John received his warning during a family Thanksgiving dinner. A 64-year-old plant foreman, he was looking forward to retirement and more time to devote to his garden. A vigorous, self-reliant man, John was surprised and upset to find his arm suddenly so weak that he could not cut the turkey and had to ask for assistance. His speech became slurred, and his family teased him for poor tolerance for beer!

When similar brief episodes appeared several times in the following weeks, John suspected that he should consult his family physician.

SOURCE: Soffer, Alfred, "What You Should Know About Strokes," *Today's Health*, August, 1968. Reprinted by permission of *Today's Health*, published by the American Medical Association.

But he said nothing, perhaps because of an unexpressed fear.

Two days before Christmas, he awakened to find his right hand numb and a little awkward. At breakfast, the coffee pot slipped from his grip. Half an hour later, the clumsiness grew worse and he could not find the right words in conversation. There was no pain, rather, surprise and bewilderment as John noticed that his powerful right arm would no longer obey his commands.

Perhaps it was then that John began to wonder if this was how a stroke happened, particularly as he became aware of his wife's alarm at his garbled speech. An hour later, as he was examined by his physician, he had lost completely the ability to speak, as well as the use of his right arm and hand. Soon, the use of the right leg was lost, too. All this had occurred within a few hours.

It now was evident that John had suffered a clot in one of the major arteries which carries blood to the brain. About 80 per cent of strokes are caused by thrombosis, a closing off or clotting of blood vessels in the brain or in arteries in the neck leading to the brain.

Vivian had been a potential stroke candidate for many years—even though she had not recognized it. A vivacious, active 53-year-old housewife, she felt that she had always been in excellent health. So why should she expect trouble? True, she had been advised to take medication to lower her blood pressure; yet it had appeared so unnecessary to take this advice seriously, particularly since she had no symptoms and her ready smile and ruddy complexion assured friends and family of her physical well-being.

She was doing light housework one afternoon when she explained to a neighbor, "I suddenly have a horrible headache." Seconds later, she slumped to the floor.

Although the family physician was only a few blocks away, Vivian was unconscious when he arrived 20 minutes later. An ambulance was called immediately and the patient was taken to the emergency room of the local hospital. A spinal puncture found blood in the spinal fluid. When the patient began to move restlessly, it was obvious to the intern and the nursing staff that there was paralysis of the right side of her body. Vivian's family was told that a blood vessel within her brain had burst and they were warned that bleeding into the brain, cerebral hemorrhage, is such a serious condition that more than half of its victims die.

Unlike John's stroke, which proceeded by steps, progression of brain hemorrhage is continuous. Commonly, the patient experiences increasing weakness of one side of the body during 10 to 60 minutes until paralysis is complete. If bleeding continues, coma may occur. Unlike thrombosis, there are no warning attacks when apoplexy is caused by cerebral vascular hemorrhage. Events of the morning of April 12, 1945, suggest that President Roosevelt died of massive cerebral hemorrhage.

Jimmy was 14, and more interested in the Monkees than in girls. He was a valued member of his school basketball team and proud of his track prowess.

Catastrophe struck, not during moments of fierce team competition, but during a friendly game of tug-of-war on the school playground. Friends who saw Jimmy sink to the groun could not know of the excruciating pain in the back of his head a few moments before he lost consciousness. Minutes later, Jimmy was alert enough to ask why he was on the ground and what had happened. He knew only that he had a very stiff neck and was terribly confused.

On the way to the hospital, Jimmy felt nauseated and he vomited. A tentative diagnosis of subarachnoid hemorrhage was confirmed by the finding of fresh blood in the spinal fluid.

This type of brain hemorrhage, which can occur at any age, is caused by a weakened spot or blister, like the bulge of a defect in a balloon. This ballooned-out area, called an aneurysm, presumably is present at birth and due to faulty development of the blood vessel. More often, the bulging aneurysm is found in the blood vessels directly beneath the brain. When rupture occurs, blood pours into the space between the brain and its covering membranes and is evidenced by blood found in the cerebrospinal fluid (which bathes the surface of the brain and the spinal cord).

What Causes Stroke? Although many diseases can cause brain damage, the majority of strokes are the work of three villains: arteriosclerosis, high blood pressure, and emboli. Arteriosclerosis is a disease marked by an abnormal thickening and hardening of the walls of the arteries. There are several types of arteriosclerosis but the most frequent and dangerous kind is atherosclerosis—because this can cause a decrease or stoppage of blood flow through arteries.

The process of atherosclerosis which leads to cerebral vascular accidents may also be found in many arteries throughout the body. Thus, in other locations, the disease atherosclerosis can result in coronary heart trouble or serious blood vessel damage in the legs or kidneys.

Recent studies indicate that deposits of the fatty substance, cholesterol, in the walls of the arteries initiate the process of atherosclerosis and that, as a result, progressive narrowing and, finally, closure of the vessel may occur. When these events take place in blood vessels in the neck or brain, blood flow to the brain—which carries crucial oxygen and food—is decreased to a trickle and, not infrequently, stops suddenly and completely.

High blood pressure is intimately related to atherosclerosis and can hasten and aggravate its process. High blood pressure causes thickening of the arteries and this may be followed by a clot, or the vessel may rupture to produce a hemorrhage.

Today, strokes caused by emboli occur less frequently. In this type, a piece of clot, or clots, breaks away from a diseased area in the heart or lungs and is carried to the brain until the blood vessel gets too small for it to travel further. Many of these patients have a history of rheumatic heart disease or are suffering from coronary heart disease. Physicians differ in estimating the exact frequency of different types of strokes, but one widely accepted evaluation indicates that about 80 per cent are due to thrombosis, 15 per cent to hemorrhage, and 5 per cent to emboli.

Stark national statistics show the gravity of the stroke problem. Each year 200,000 Americans die of stroke, making it the third leading killer in this country. A particularly tragic statistic shows almost 40,000 of these victims to be under 65.

Early Recognition Important. Gone are the days when most stroke victims could only resign themselves to bleak futures of custodial care. Dramatic breakthroughs in diagnosis and treatment have drastically altered medical management. But these benefits can be achieved only if an impending stroke is recognized before permanent damage occurs, or if a specific and complete diagnosis is made very early after an attack.

The concept of anticipating a stroke was introduced in 1950, and the early signs and symptoms, which can mean so much to the physician, are graphically described by Dr. Clark Milliken of the Mayo Clinic: (1) impending stroke: patients likely to have a stroke in the near future; (2) advancing stroke: patients who experience stroke symptoms and signs, such as progressive weakness of one side of the body; and (3) completed stroke: victims who have suffered maximal damage.

Fortunately, the obstruction of a blood vessel by a clot is the type of stroke which can be most accurately predicted; a fact of vital importance in treating patients with disease in the large arteries in the neck. The four main arteries to the brain consist of the right and left vertebral arteries and the right and left carotid arteries. The progressive obstruction in these blood vessels now can be identified with considerable accuracy after analysis of laboratory tests and a review of the patient's history.

Frequently, the patient has important warning attacks before a completed clot leads to brain softening. It is believed that these episodes are a result of brief, intermittent decreases in the flow of blood which precede by hours, days, or even months, the complete block.

The patient may experience only numbness and weakness of a hand, a foot, or one side of the face. There may be evidence of forgetfulness or actual confusion. A dramatic warning sign is temporary loss of vision in one eye. Speech may be slurred or mushy and there may be difficulty in understanding the speech of others. A warning attack may include all of these abnormalities—or only one or relatively few signs may appear.

The physician can distinguish an advancing stroke caused by a complete block—even though the signs are similar to those of an intermittent attack—because the patient's appearance gradually worsens over many minutes, or a few hours, and there is persistence of the weakness, speech defect, and other signs. Usually the trouble progresses by steps until all of the particular function is lost.

Three-fourths of patients with advancing thrombosis will have had warning attacks beforehand, the recognition of which is of crucial value in enabling treatment to be started before a potentially lethal clot is formed. And, because "telltale" episodes do not appear before brain embolism or cerebral hemorrhage warning signs are of great importance in establishing the diagnosis of thrombosis.

Watch for "Little Strokes." The medical profession is indebted to Dr. Walter Alvarez for emphasizing the frequency with which "little strokes" occur. The knowledgeable patient, or his family, may be able to identify "little strokes" by changes in the patient's behavior, including degeneration of table manners and the appearance of poor social or business judgment. Dizzy spells and attacks of forgetfulness are common. These and a host of other physical and personality aberrations often can represent repeated episodes of "little strokes" and herald a more ominous occurrence.

Obviously, the patient can greatly assist his physician if he promptly reports details of these warning signs. Doctor Milliken emphasizes that the physician will be able to distinguish between the confusion of speech or manner associated with impending strokes and similar behavior observed in people who have a high fever or are under the effects of drugs or alcohol.

Strokes that aren't! Those who suffer from migraine headaches may experience sensations resembling those which occur in a stroke; a numbness and weakness in one side of the body, trouble with speech and vision. However, these sensations disappear in a few minutes and are followed by the sick headache.

Almost everyone has experienced an arm or leg "going to sleep." This type of numbness or tingling appears after prolonged sitting in a cramped position or following an extended period of pressure, such as that which may happen during sleep. Sustained pressure on a blood vessel or nerve is responsible for these harmless symptoms, and discomfort ordinarily disappears in a few minutes.

Help for Thrombosis Victims. What can modern medicine do for John, our 64-year-old plant foreman with a cerebral vascular thrombosis?

The use of modern vascular surgery in the treatment of strokes was introduced about 15 years ago. If the obstruction appears in a blood vessel inside the brain, surgery is not ordinarily feasible. Fortunately, 30 to 40 per cent of obstructions causing stroke are found in the neck or upper chest. Many of these vessels are neither too difficult to reach nor too small to work upon.

The first problem is to locate the block accurately. In 1927, Portuguese physician Egas Moniz reported that dye injection in arteries could be used to diagnose brain tumors. In subsequent years, development of safe compounds for injecting dye into blood vessels has made it possible to use this profoundly useful technique for the study of diseases of the brain. A few drops of local anesthetic are used to "freeze" the skin in the area of the neck at the injection site.

After the dye has been injected into the artery, a series of x-ray pictures, called angiograms, show the course of dye as it is carried by the bloodstream through the large vessels in the chest, neck, and into the brain.

John, awake and quite alert during this test, experienced only slight, momentary discomfort; indeed, he found the experience not too unpleasant. A neurologist and neurosurgeon reviewed the x-rays—taking account of the typical history (and certain suspicious findings determined by feeling the blood vessels in the neck)—and diagnosed a clot in the internal carotid artery. An operation opened the blocked section of the artery and removed the obstruction.

Called endarterectomy, this technique was quite practical in the case of John. In other patients, the surgeon may find that a longer section of the artery is diseased and will decide to bypass this section by inserting a bypass graft. Human arteries once were used as grafts but, in the last several years, a variety of synthetic substances have been used exclusively.

Regardless of technique, the chances of success are greatly increased if the operation can be performed speedily—within hours, or days, of the attack. John had been taken to a hospital where all these specialized facilities were available and, within 24 hours of the operation had recovered completely from the paralysis and was able to speak quite well. It would, of course, have been far easier for both surgeon and patient if the early warning signs had been recognized before an actual clot had occurred. An operation in these early stages (essentially, the same type just described) might very well have prevented the frightening apoplectic attack.

Recovery from Aneurysms. Newspaper stories recently chronicled the desperate struggle for life of a young actress who had suffered a stroke. It seemed as if all America shared in the family's gratitude when the neurosurgeon found the broken vessel and stopped the bleeding. Intensive rehabilitation and the courageous cooperation of the patient resulted in a nearly complete cure.

As in the case of Jimmy, our young athlete, this stroke was caused by the rupture of an aneurysm at the base of the brain. For both patients, the x-ray dye test made possible an exact pinpointing of the site of rupture. This test must be performed as soon as the patient's physical status permits, because bleeding may recur, particularly within the first two weeks after the acute episode. For Jimmy, these new techniques of diagnosis and surgical intervention permitted a complete cure. There are few more dramatic stories in the history of healing.

Tests that Tell. Complete evaluation of the patient with warning signs or a completed stroke is aided by many other tests, including spinal puncture, brainwave examination, and x-ray films after injection of air into brain cavities. The most recent technique, which promises to be of considerable value, involves injection of small and harmless amounts of radioactive material into brain blood vessels. This test can help a physician decide whether the symptoms suggesting a stroke are due to damage to blood vessels or to brain tumors.

Since there are many types of strokes, different tests may be needed for each patient, depending upon the blood vessels involved, the stage at which the disease is to be treated, and the age and general health of the patient. The angiographic dye test must be understood in this context. It is not ordinarily needed for the basic type of stroke due to thrombosis within the brain itself, and it should not be performed in some types of strokes or hemorrhage.

In some patients with small strokes, or repeated minor attacks due to obstruction within arteries in the neck, the surgeon may decide that it is not feasible to operate at that time. In these situations the physician has another valuable ally. Drugs which prevent clotting, the so-called anticoagulant drugs, often are of great help in preventing recurring attacks of "cerebral insufficiency" caused by narrowing in these blood vessels.

Anticoagulant drugs also are the very cornerstone of therapy when strokes are due to loose particles or clots which plug up brain arteries. Of course, whenever possible, the basic cause for the emboli must be discovered and treated, although at times this is not possible and long-term anticoagulant treatment then is necessary. Obviously, anticlotting drugs should never be used whenever hemorrhage or the suspicion of hemorrhage is present.

Stroke's Warning Signals. More than in most other illnesses, it is vitally important to identify the individual who is susceptible to the ravages of stroke before the disease strikes. In this way, irreversible damage or death often can be avoided.

Physicians who study the "clinical profiles" of thousands of patients insist that it now is possible to identify the potential stroke victim before he becomes ill. The risk factors for stroke are essentially the same as those which are present for disease of the coronary blood vessels and atherosclerosis in other arteries in the body. Significant danger factors include high blood pressure, diabetes mellitus, abnormal electrocardiograms and other signs of heart disease, high blood cholesterol, overweight, and cigarette smoking. High blood pressure (hypertension) has enormously greater importance in strokes than in blood vessel disease anywhere else in the body. Fortunately, treatment now is remarkably successful, thanks to the recent introduction of effective drugs for reducing blood pressure.

Helping Your Physician. The cerebral hemorrhage suffered by Vivian, our 53-year-old housewife, was a double tragedy because: (a) from 50 to 75 per cent of patients with hemorrhage deep within the brain die in the first attack, and those who recover often have a long and arduous convalescent period; and (b) it is entirely possible that this stroke could have been prevented if the patient had heeded medical advice for the treatment of her high blood pressure, by following a careful and comprehensive treatment program during the fateful years when the threat of apoplexy was her constant companion.

Obviously, all of us can do a great deal to reduce many of these risks. The patient who is asked by his doctor to lose weight and the patient who is advised to stop cigarette smoking can be partners with the medical profession in these attempts to prevent stroke. Physicians now can recommend palatable, specific diets for the treatment of patients with high blood fats, and several promising new drugs have been introduced as aids to dietary management.

Better Road to Recovery. What about the individual who has suffered a stroke and is not a candidate for an operation, either because the blood vessel is in an area which cannot be reached or because the hour of maximum benefit has passed? Should these patients be consigned to the waste heap of the totally incapacitated or can they be returned to a relatively active and constructive life?

Skillful and highly motivated teams are returning an increasing number of these patients to society and, not infrequently, to a life of normal longevity. The nurse, the occupational, physical, and speech therapists, the social worker, and the vocational rehabilitation consultant each have an important role. Often, it is not recognized that the patient faces an emotional crisis when discharged from the hospital. In his splendid autobiographical volume, *Episode, A Report on the Accident Inside My Skull*, Eric Hodkins vividly documents the patient's fears and insecurities as he faces the future outside the protective hospital walls.

The family must be instructed about the need for sympathy, but they must also be warned that overindulgence of the patient can delay rehabilitation. They also must recognize that recovery frequently is not total and that many moments of discouragement should be expected. Recovery from the changes wrought by a stroke is a difficult period for both patient and relatives, but there are many positive rewards for those who show persistence and courage.

A stroke is no respecter of age or sex. The misery this disease has caused in ancient and modern times is adequately documented. The crucial lesson for our decade, however, is that "strokes are not unannounced." Telltale signs frequently are there if only patients and their families are alert to their significance. Successful treatment depends upon early diagnosis.

Even more heartening is the promise that the basic causes for strokes often can be attacked by a preventive program of hygiene. Certainly, high blood pressure is a major culprit in so many middle-aged people. The futility of these deaths is evident when we recognize that effective treatment for high blood pressure now is available.

Finally, an optimistic outlook now is justified for the victims of almost all types of strokes, as medicine moves to an ever-increasing position of strength in their prevention and cure.

6 A Man's Disease Every Woman Should Know About

by John Lentz

Many men are ashamed to mention it, even to their wives. Many men delay treatment fearing that it will be a painful ordeal. Many men believe that it signals the end of their sex life.

The disease is "prostate trouble," a catch-all term for a variety of ailments and disorders affecting a gland peculiar to the male anatomy, the prostate. Some parts of this article about it make grim or unpleasant reading. This is quite deliberate—for this article is intended to drive home some lifesaving facts, to remove ungrounded fears and misconceptions and to help wives and husbands—especially men in or nearing middle-age—to act intelligently and promptly.

Normally no larger than a chestnut, the prostate causes trouble all out of proportion to its size. It may swell and disturb or block the vital functions of nearby organs. It may become infected and cause aches and pains in various parts of the body. It may harbor stones large enough to require surgical removal. And, most critical of all, it may become cancerous.

SOURCE: *Today's Health.* Reprinted by permission of *Today's Health*, published by the *American Medical Association.*

Strangely, most men know little about this trouble-making gland. To quote one physician, "When I tell a patient that he has an enlarged prostate, he is likely to ask, "Doctor, what's the prostate?"

The gland is an accessory organ of the male reproductive system. It is located at the base of the bladder and completely surrounds that organ's outlet, the urethra, the tube through which urine passes from the bladder, and the ducts for the ejaculation of sperm cells run through it. The gland's location has been called "one of nature's architectural errors." This is because the prostate, when it enlarges or swells, constricts the urethra and impedes the normal flow of urine. Just what does this gland do? Under the influence of the sex hormone from the testicles, it produces a milky fluid necessary to the survival of the highly active sperm cells during their passage from male to female. This fluid may also have another essential function. When the sperm cells come into the prostate from other parts of the male reproductive system, they are enveloped in mucus. The prostatic fluid apparently does away with the mucus, permitting the sperm cells to swim freely and fulfill their mission of fertilizing the ovum.

The fluid is discharged from the gland through the action of muscle fibers embedded throughout its glandular tissue. At the moment when the fluid is needed—or at the climax of the sexual act—the fibers contract and expel it. The gland is capable of performing its secretory function repeatedly in the course of a night.

Prostatic disease has been popularly and erroneously attributed over the years to a bewildering variety of causes. For instance, "male trouble," as it was once politely called, was ascribed to a man's sexual habits. It was assumed that he either completely abstained from intercourse or that he overindulged.

Masturbation and excessive use of alcoholic beverages also were blamed. Most often, though, the number one cause of "male trouble" was believed to be a venereal infection. To some extent, this false belief persists today and accounts for the reluctance of many men to reveal their condition to their wives.

The fact is that not even the experts agree on the cause of prostate enlargement —although there are several theories, including impaired circulation and hormonal imbalance. There is no generally accepted way to avoid prostate trouble, and it does not seem to affect men in one occupation or category more than another.

Victims of prostatic disease can never brag about the rarity of their trouble. One authority has made the sweeping statement that "very few men escape prostatism in one of its many forms." Another speaks of the enlarged prostate as "the constant companion of the older male." Next to the skin and the lungs, the gland is the commonest site of cancer in the male. Though older men are the main victims of both simple enlargement and serious prostatic maladies, the gland can cause difficulty at any time of life.

To enumerate the symptoms caused by the most common disorder of the gland, picture a 45-year-old man in seemingly fine health. He becomes aware of a sense of fullness or discomfort that sends him to the bathroom more frequently than usual, especially at night. At this point, he procrastinates. He says to himself that it is natural for a man his age to get up during the night (it isn't.)

Later, he finds it increasingly difficult to urinate without straining. Still later, and with increased effort, he voids smaller and smaller amounts of urine. Finally, he feels pain or a burning sensation and notices that his stream is tinged with blood.

Alarmed by the latter symptoms, he goes to his physician. Diagnosis: a greatly enlarged prostate. A course of fairly simple treatments restores his good health, vitality, and peace of mind.

Unfortunately, many cases of prostatic enlargement do not end so happily. In fact, if treatment is delayed too long, the gland may swell until it completely blocks the flow of urine—an agonizing and dangerous condition.

To understand why this is so, consider some facts about the kidneys and the bladder. The main function of the kidneys is to remove waste products from the blood and excrete them in the urine. The bladder receives urine, about four or five pints daily, through two tubes from the kidneys. When filled, the bladder's muscular walls contract and urination occurs.

This process is upset when an enlarged prostate tightly squeezes or blocks the bladder's outlet. In an attempt to expel the urine, the bladder's muscles work harder and harder. As pressure builds up in the bladder, it dilates, like a balloon, to accommodate the increased volume of urine. Indeed, its capacity may expand from the normal pint of urine to as much as two or more quarts.

If the pressure becomes great enough, it also harms the kidneys and their tubes. They, too, dilate and become incapable of filtering and removing waste products. As a result, these products accumulate in the blood and cause uremia, or uremic poisoning. The victim complains of headache, becomes confused, and may have convulsions. Fortunately, this serious, and sometimes fatal, condition can be detected by a blood test.

Another problem stemming from an enlarged prostate is residual urine, or the urine that is always "held back" when the bladder cannot completely empty itself. Like stagnant water, residual urine provides an ideal environment for bacterial growth. If an infection flares up, it results in cystitis, or inflammation of the bladder.

Then there is the problem of prostatitis. This is an infection of the gland found frequently in young men. There is an erroneous impression that it is always brought on by gonorrhea. Sometimes it is; sometimes it isn't. In fact, prostatic infection at any age is often caused by common bacteria, like the streptococcus and staphylococcus, or by a mixture of common microorganisms.

Prostitis may develop secondary to a distant point of infection in the tonsils, teeth, or sinuses. Or the infected prostate may act as a focus of infection and cause pain in the joints or inflammation of the eyes. Many men who go to their physicians with such complaints are amazed when told that an infected prostate is responsible for their vague and recurring complaints.

A less frequent cause of prostatic distress is stone formation within the gland. Generally, the stones are no longer than grains of sand. If they cause no complications, they are left alone. If large stones occur and cause fairly severe discomfort, they must be removed by surgery.

The most dreaded and critical disease of the prostate is cancer. Its incidence, unfortunately, has risen with the increase in the average life span. According to the American Cancer Society, about one in every 10 cancers in men is in the prostate. Actually the disease is more common than statistics indicate. This is borne out by post-mortem examinations of large numbers of elderly men. Although they died of other causes, cancer cells were found in the prostates of many. This poses a baffling medical problem: Why do some prostatic cancers remain more or less dormant, while others grow rapidly and quickly invade other parts of the body?

No one knows why cancer strikes the prostate so frequently. It is generally believed that the body's own hormones are involved since the gland's growth and development are strongly influenced by the male sex hormone, testosterone. This theory is underscored by the fact that prostatic cancer has never been known to occur in men castrated at an early age.

Prostatic cancer is a stealthy thing. In its earliest state, it causes no symptoms at all. But it is usually easy to spot—or at least to suspect—during a periodic health checkup. If the physician finds a hard area, like a foreign body, in a particular part of the gland, he will make diagnostic tests to determine whether it is cancerous. Fortunately, the part of the gland where cancer most often starts is the part most easily examined by the physician. If limited to the gland itself, prostatic cancer can be cured by total removal of the gland. No remnants are left behind to be the site of future trouble.

Treatment for prostatic diseases depends, of course, on the nature and the extent of the trouble. Except for prostatic cancer, surgery is by no means always necessary. For example, in cases of simple enlargement with slight symptoms, the condition can usually be controlled by massage. This involves actual rubbing of the gland either by a gloved finger of the physician within the patient's rectum or by a suitable instrument inserted through the anus. Heat and perhaps gentle dilation of the urinary tube may also be a part of treatment. In fact, most men who get prompt medical care for simple enlargement are spared surgery. It is highly important, however, for men to see their physicians regularly for checks on the results of treatment.

As to infections of the prostate and bladder, they are not the stubborn problems they once were, mainly because of the antibiotic drugs. In treating them, the physician looks for the source of the infection and identifies the bacteria causing the trouble. Then he prescribes the antibiotic drug or drugs most effective against the offending bacteria. During treatment, he may also massage the gland. Surgery is required only when a prostatic infection has been neglected for years.

If an operation is necessary for any type of prostatic disease, the surgeon may choose any one of several very safe ways of removing the entire gland or portions of it.

If the gland is not greatly enlarged and there is no infection, the overgrown portion of the gland may be removed with the aid of a cystoscope. This remarkable instrument is a long, slender, hollow device with an observing lens at one end and a tiny electric light at the other. With it, the surgeon can see exactly what he is doing. After the hollow cytoscope is in place, a slender electrical instrument is pushed up through it until it reaches the prostate. By means of an electrical cutting loop of fine wire, the obstructing part of the gland is removed under the surgeon's direct vision. This approximates bloodless surgery as nearly as anything can.

Another widely used technique, called suprapubic removal, may be a two-stage operation. In the first stage, an incision is made in the abdominal wall, the bladder emptied, and a drainage tube, or catheter, inserted. After drainage has relieved the kidneys and any infection has subsided, the tube is removed.

In the second stage, the prostate is taken out through the same incision. The surgeon peels the tumor out of its surrounding tissue or capsule much as a grape is peeled out of its skin. A catheter is then passed through the urethra into the bladder for urinary drainage.

After a few days, the tube is removed and the wound allowed to heal. Thereafter, the patient soon begins to function normally. Today, this operation is generally performed in one stage if the patient's over-all condition is good.

Still another way of reaching the prostate is through an opening in the perineum, or the area between the rectum and the base of the penis.

To be sure, none of these operations is a pleasant experience. But neither are they the "terrible ordeals" they're often said to be. More important, mortality from the prostatic surgery has been drastically reduced with improved surgical procedures, new drugs, and better nursing care. When fatalities do occur, they are usually among old and almost hopeless men, or in men whose condition makes them poor surgical risks to begin with.

Even in cases of far-advanced prostatic cancer in which surgery would be useless, medical science can often extend life usefully and comfortably. This is accomplished by administering female sex hormones which can control the growth of cancer and relieve severe pain. The hormones are not a cure. But in suppressing the cancer's growth, they prolong life—often for years. Moreover, in some cases which previously would have been inoperable, the female sex hormones cause the cancer to regress sufficiently to permit surgery. Because of the influence of the male hormone on the prostate, the testicles are also sometimes removed.

Currently, several medical centers are evaluating a new technique for removal of the prostate. Surgeons are applying extreme cold, produced by liquid nitrogen, to the gland. This quickly freezes it. Upon thawing, the gland is reduced to a mass of sludge that is passed out with ease through the urethra over a period of six to eight weeks. This new operation has been performed successfully on more than 70 patients. It is an example of the growing use of cryosurgery, of the use of extreme cold, for surgical purposes. This prostatic operation is still in the early experimental stages. Despite its promise, much more study will be required before its value is fully established.

Meantime, the search goes on for a drug that will act upon the prostate and prevent simple enlargement. As yet, no such drug has been found. Men should beware of "injections" or "shots" advertised or promoted by quacks specializing in "men's disease," "bladder trouble," and the like. They are a waste of both time and money.

Finally, it should be clearly understood that removal of the prostate will not "feminize" a man. He will not become beardless, grow fat and lethargic, acquire a high-pitched voice, or lose all sexual drive. Such changes occur only when the testicles are removed. And the truth is that partial removal of prostate usually does not impair a man's potency or ability to have intercourse. Nor does it particularly affect his enjoyment of it.

The only difference that occurs is a diminution in the amount of prostatic fluid ejaculated during orgasm. This may greatly reduce the chances of impregnation since the sperm may not survive long enough to reach and penetrate the female egg. Otherwise, partial prostatectomy usually has no deleterious effect on sexual desire or performance. (Of course, the operation does not restore sexual vigor that has waned.)

From mid-life on, husbands and wives can do a lot to protect their mutual happiness if they will keep in mind these points about prostatic disorders:

1. Don't procrastinate if any symptoms occur. Go to your physician promptly.

2. Don't be ashamed of prostate trouble. Discuss it as fully and frankly as any other threat to life and health.

3. Forget the old wives' tales and the pool-parlor talk about venereal disease as the sole cause of prostatic disease.

4. Remember that surgery is not always required, especially if treatment is begun early.

5. Remember that prostatic operation doesn't mean sexual failure.

6. Have annual checkups. Wives should insist on this, especially after their husbands reach age 50. Between checkups, should prostatic symptoms occur, go to your physician again and follow his advice.

Bibliography and Suggested Readings

BIBLIOGRAPHY

Accident Facts, published by the National Safety Council, Chicago, Illinois.

New Jersey Alcohol Determination Program in Fatal Traffic Accident Cases: Report of Findings—Three Year Study from 1961 through 1963, New Jersey Department of Law and Public Safety, Trenton, N. J., 1964.

Schefferes, Justus J.: "Safety Against Accidents," *Healthier Living*, John Wiley & Sons, Inc., New York, 1965, pp. 353-367.

SUGGESTED READINGS

Nader, Ralph: *Unsafe At Any Speed*, Grossman Publishers, Inc., New York, 1965.

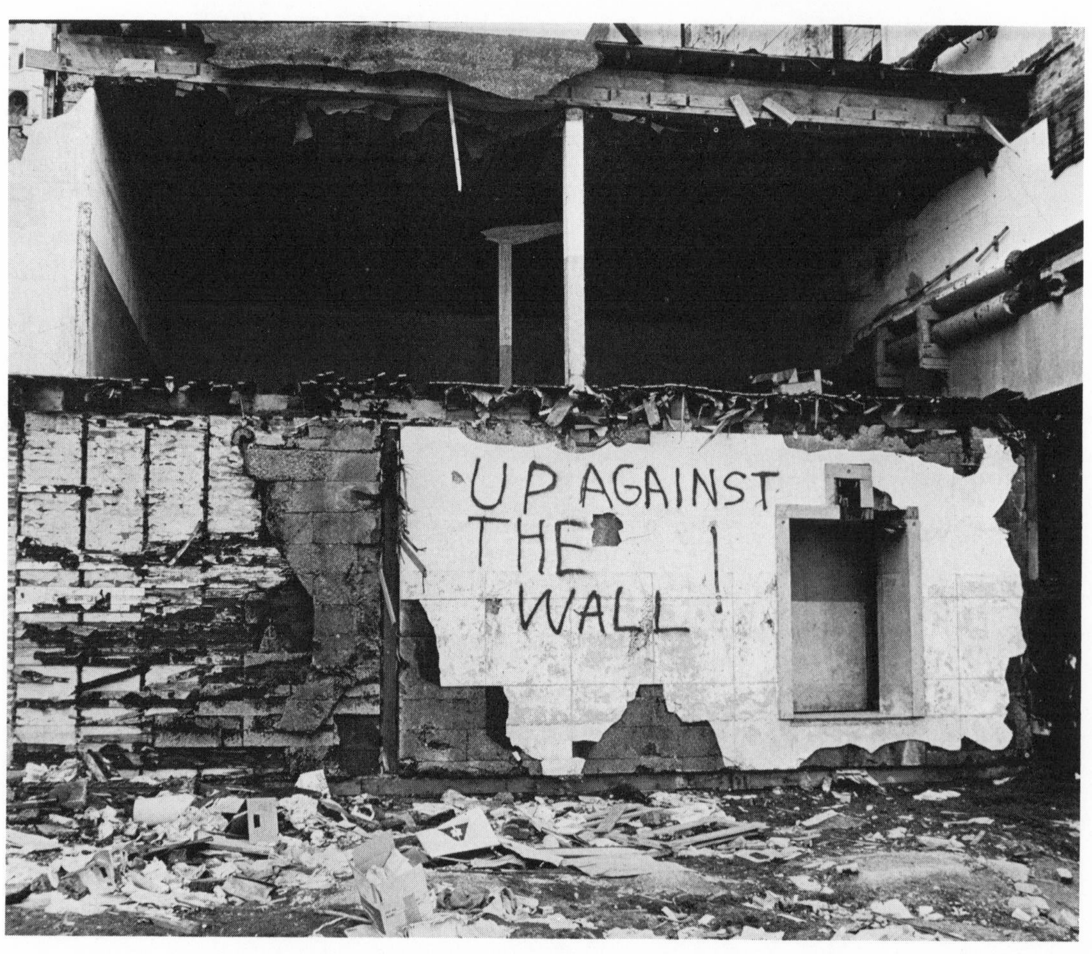
UP AGAINST
THE
WALL !

UNIT 5

Ecological Problems: Their Health Implications

Too many people

A vulnerability to advertisers and promoters caused by our lack of self understanding to a level that we can know our real *needs*

A greed for profit along with a lack of consideration of the effects on the environment and future life by industrialists and promoters who sell us the superfluous commodities

Unless these trends are rapidly reversed, it certainly will result in an end to the quality of life we enjoy in America and could well mean the end of human life on earth through contamination of the environment.

Reliable sources claim that one American uses at least 30 times as much of the world's natural resources as one person living in India uses, that the United States with only 6 per cent of the world's population uses 40 per cent of the total amount of the world's natural resources used yearly and contributes 50 per cent of the annual industrial pollution.

To support one individual in our society 25 tons of materials must be extracted from the earth and processed each year. It is predicted that the United States will have mined outs its natural resources of copper, lead, zinc, tin, aluminum, nickel, chromium, manganese, gold, silver, and platinum by 1980. By 2200 our iron and molybdnum will be gone, too, with the exception of what we recycle. *(Scientific America)*, September, 1970).

The lack of water for anything but the most necessary functions during several summers in New York City has been well publicized. We also are well aware of a number of blackouts and brownouts due to insufficient electrical energy production. We have been warned that the "need" is about to exceed the amount of electrical energy we are able to generate with water or steam-driven generators and are being psychologically prepared for a convertion over to nuclear power plants!

The United States already has 16 operable nuclear power plants with 54 being built and 35 planned for the future. Doctors Gofman and Tamplin of the Livermore Radiation Laboratory warn in their book, *Poisoned Power,* of the danger of creating yet another monster in the environment. They further question our ability to contain the damaging radioactive atoms in the face of accidents and sabotage.

> ..."At the reactor itself, bearing enormous quantities of radioactive poisons, no accidents which can distribute such poisons to the atmosphere, land or water can be tolerated."
>
> ..."Every two years, the fuel carrying this burden of poison should be transported without mishap by rail and truck to the fuel-cleaning plants. Any significant accidental release in this phase of the operation can render sizeable areas of our nation uninhabitable for many years."
>
> ..."At the fuel reprocessing plant absolutely perfect containment must be assured, year in, year out."
>
> ..."The waste radioactivities, dangerous for hundreds of years, must be transported to a final resting place. And this waste must be guarded from any escape into the environment for periods longer than the recorded history of any government."
>
> ..."At no step (reactor, transport, fuel reprocessing, transport, waste burial) can sabotage of the operation conceivably occur without disastrous consequences for human beings. Yet there will be hundreds of plants and transportation vehicles that must be protected against such sabotage perfectly. Senseless, indiscriminate bombings and arson are hardly an unknown occurrence in the United States today."

With full knowledge of a potential shortage of electrical power Pacific Gas & Electric Company, supposedly a service district, is running billboard ads exhorting us to use more electrical appliances. (Our service districts have taken over some of the contrived business of Madison Avenue!) Even now the list of electrical appliances we "need" is ridiculous: electric stoves, dishwashers, freezers, irons, washers, dryers, air conditioners, vacuum cleaners, toasters, blenders, mixers, sewing machines, radios, television, hair dryers, vibrator chairs, blankets, lawn mowers, door bells, clocks, knives, toothbrushes.

Vance Packard in *The Hidden Persuaders* goes into the history and the psychology employed in the creation of "needs" in the American people. His book reviews the rise of many agencies aimed at understanding the psychological needs and fears of people and how to appeal to these emotions through clever advertising, packaging and displaying to sell us absolutely anything! Since the organization of the original two, the Institute for Motivational Research, Inc. and Color Research Institute of America, many others have sprung up, using psychologists, psychiatrists and the scientific method. Their methods have been aired in all the major advertising and business journals and adopted by nearly every industry. Mr. Packard quotes an ad executive as saying, "What makes this country great is the creation of wants and desires, the creation of dissatisfaction with the old and outmoded."

There is a definite attempt on the part of Madison Avenue to create a "psychological obsolescence." Our old stove, though it still cooks well, must be replaced with a new one of modern design and color. We have been effectively programmed by Madison Avenue through appeal to our psychological needs and fears. Not only can we no longer distinguish between our actual "needs" and our "wants" but we feel certain that something is wrong with any American who does not want all the things all "true Americans" want. These "things" include a nice new tract home, filled with new plastic furniture, garbage disposal, television set, telephone, a car for each adult in the family and closets full of the newest I. Magnin clothing. This is the major thing "wrong" with the hippie and the hoards of other people rejecting the "American way of life."

This unit contains papers by specialists from a number of disciplines offering information, warning and some suggestions for remediation in the areas of overpopulation, and various resultant pollutions caused in large degree by that over population (radiation from nuclear power plants, water pollution, noise pollution and a familiar source of air pollution).

Population and Ecology—A Primer 1

by Paul R. Ehrlich

Demography and ecology are two subdisciplines of population biology.

Population biologists deal with all aspects of groupings of organisms and organisms in groups.

Demographers study human population dynamics.

Ecologists study organisms and how they relate to one another and to their surroundings.

Although population biologists and ecologists almost invariably have some knowledge of demography, demographers are often unaware of even the most elementary principles of ecology. As a result, they are often unable to predict the negative ecological consequences of projected demographic changes.

The survival of the human species depends on an accurate evaluation of these potential ecological consequences and prompt action to avoid the worst of them. For the most part, population biologists and ecologists accept for their calculations the current and projected statistics on human population growth provided by the demographers. However, certain critical environmental factors have escaped consideration or else have been dismissed by most demographers as either irrelevant or of minimal importance. In view of the demographers' failure to include these additional inputs, many population biologists and ecologists are convinced that the human population will not continue to grow as predicted. Instead, they agree that it is more likely that this growth will be interrupted by at least one of a number of possible disasters.

Such uncontrolled events would produce an increase in the death rate unforeseen by the demographers and would significantly reduce the overall size of the human population. Virtually all scientists view nature's death-rate solution as an irrational and intolerable answer to the long-range problem of overpopulation. What is at issue are assessments of the magnitude and immediacy of the problem, and thus the urgency of seeking the preferred solution—a reduction of the birth rate. Considering the consequences of a wrong decision, which could conceivably result in the extinction of mankind as we know it, it seems more prudent to protect ourselves and our children from unnecessarily risky experiments on our biosphere. If we adopt a more conservative estimate of the abuse which our ecosystems can withstand, and are wrong, the worst that can happen is that we will have a more pleasant environment in which to live. If we are right, we shall literally "save the world."

In the face of the overwhelming influx of evidence from all sides, only the blindest optimist would deny that we are in the midst of an environmental crisis.

The causes of the present deterioration of the environment are extremely complex and not completely understood, but to a great extent the facts speak for themselves. We would like to present the demographic figures and review some of the fundamental interpretations of the data upon which the conclusions of ecologists and other population biologists are based.

The Facts

At 3.6 billion people, the present human population is the largest in the history of mankind. It is growing at the fastest rate the species has ever experienced: 2% annually, adding 70 million people each year. A demographic transition—the movement from high birth rates and high death rates to relatively low birth rates and low death rates—has failed to take place in the under-developed countries. Birth rates remain high even where industrialization has produced conditions some thought were conducive to lower fertility. Even in the overdeveloped areas—the United States, Japan, Russia, and Europe—which have undergone such a transition, the growth rate remains unacceptably high. It is approximately 1% per year, a doubling time of about 70 years. This pattern cannot continue much longer.

Some History

How did we get into this dire predicament? Perhaps a brief historical review of the growth of the world's population will bring the problem into perspective. It all started about 10,000 years ago when man went through what has come to be known as the Agricultural Revolution. At that time (8000 BC) there were about five million people in the world. However, as man began to domesticate animals and to stay in one spot to grow food for harvest, he made several significant changes in his lifestyle. His agricultural practices began leading to monoculture. Eventually he grew only one crop in a given plot of ground, and; more significantly, he thereby began to simplify the ecosystems upon which his life depended. As man gave up his hunting and gathering existence and stayed in one place, life became more secure and the death rate began to drop. The implications for the future were incalculable.

As a result, over the next six to eight thousand years, the human population grew—to approximately 200 to 300 million at the time of the birth of Christ. It had reached about 500 million by 1650, when improvements in agriculture further reduced death rates and accelerated growth. It reached one billion by 1850. By then the Industrial Revolution was well under way; man began to burn valuable fossil fuels and improve the distribution of food, thereby reducing the impact of local famines on the death rate. Growth surged ahead, helped by the Biomedical Revolution at the end of the 19th century, which reduced the death rate still further through the introduction of public health measures, better distribution of medical care, and improved techniques of disease prevention. The world's population doubled between 1850 and 1930—to a total of two billion people.

Some Projections

Following the introduction of pesticides and "wonder drugs" after World War II, we were well on our way to another doubling—to four billion people projected for 1975. If this rate of growth should continue, there will be approximately 7.2 billion people in the world by the year 2000—barring some sort of worldwide disaster, which will probably occur well before we reach population figures of this magnitude. With a worldwide doubling time of 35 to 37 years and a doubling time in the United States of approximately 70 years, there is little doubt that—lacking a birth control miracle—a massive die-off will occur well before we reach these projected population levels. Most likely it will be sooner rather than later ...

This unpleasant outcome could occur in a number of equally unpalatable ways—all of them related to the incredible rate of human population growth. It is only when compared with the disastrous 3.8% annual growth rate of Costa Rica that the 1% annual growth rate in the United States seem innocuous. We have all seen what a doubling time of 70 years has meant to the United States in terms of the catastrophic deterioration of our environment and the resultant lower quality of life. Our reward for the present frenetic pace of living has been greater affluence—and greater effluence. Foul air and water are but two measures of the declining quality of existence. We have more noise, tasteless advertising, and litter. We have less natural beauty, privacy, and true leisure. If we continue at our present rate of growth, the population of the United States will be 300 million by the year 2000 and 400 million by 2040. This means that if we should, by great effort, reduce by half the negative impact each American has on his environment over that period, the level of our assault on our surroundings will be the same as it is today. The natural systems on which we depend for our very lives cannot survive such an assault for another seven decades.

Our problems are compounded by the age structure of the population—in the United States and the rest of the world. In the United States alone, the World War II "baby boom" babies are just coming of reproductive age. As this group begins to reproduce, we shall experience a secondary baby boom during the 1970's. Of more concern are the statistics on the number of children under the age of 15 who will be coming of reproductive age in the next 10 years. Approximately 30% of our population—or 60 million children—are under 15 years of age. For the world as a whole the figure is 37%; in most of the underdeveloped countries the average is between 40 and 44%; in Costa Rica it is 48%. This means that huge numbers of children—now dependent upon the rest of the population for their livelihood—will be reproducing within the next 15 years.

Economics. Humanistic concerns aside, the economic repercussions of a high proportion of dependent children in a population are a considerable problem. As John Kenneth Galbraith's theory of "social balance" points out, for each person in a society, the greater the expenditure to maintain a constant level of social services. Young people and old people—who are dependent on the productive members of the society for their livelihood—do not pay very much in the form of taxes. Consequently, the burden of taxation is shifted to those in the middle age brackets. The result of producing more children is either a massive tax increase, or a reduction in the social services and quality of life, or both. Certainly, there is a significant decrease in the number of options available to the society concerning what to do with public funds. All of these financial burdens cause further alienation and antagonism and serve to divide various groups along age and socio-economic lines.

Hunger. Perhaps the most obvious phenomenon associated with overpopulation is hunger. Today, more than 1.5 billion human beings are either undernourished or malnourished. There are more hungry people today than comprised the total population of the world at the turn of this century. According to Michael Harrington, author of *The Other America*, there are approximately 30 to 50 million impoverished people who are slowly starving in the United States alone. They may not starve to death in the technical sense; but many, especially children, will die from ailments which would not have killed them if they had been properly fed.

Taking into account our own inadequate system of distribution, this means that perhaps 10% of all the people in the United States are lacking sufficient protein or other nutrients, or are hungry. Possibly another third of the people are on the borderline of malnutrition by virtue of their dietary habits, due to lack of information and to the quality of foods available in American retail food stores.

In most cases, they are not getting enough protein, but in many instances they are also not getting enough calories. The brains of infants on such a diet may never develop properly. Hungry people will, of course, suffer from a variety of deficiency diseases—and many lack the energy to sustain them during even an ordinarily active day of work or school. The average person in India gets about 1800 calories per day, while the average American gets about 3200 calories.

Medical care. In addition, these same people are not getting the medical care they need. There simply are not enough physicians to take care of all the people who need medical attention. Predictably enough, it is the citizens in the lower income groups who need the most and get the least. California has just begun to recognize the acute shortage of trained medical personnel to take care of its growing population. The specific figures are rather revealing.

In 1950, California had a population of 10.6 million people. It now has a population of 20 million—an increase of almost 10 million in 20 years. The projected figures show an increase of 3.6 million, to 23.6 million, by 1975 and an increase of 6.8 million, to 26.8 million, by 1980. At the present time, there are 33,000 practicing doctors in the state, or 165 doctors for every 100,000 patients. To maintain even that discouraging ratio, California will need a total of 39,000 doctors by 1975 and 44,000 by 1980: more than 1000 additional doctors per year for at least the next 10 years.

Unfortunately, California's medical schools turn out only 570 doctors per year—fewer than the number of doctors who retire or die each year! In other words, California is in serious trouble if it does not begin to limit its population gorwth or double the number of doctors who migrate from other parts of the country or graduate from California medical schools.

California voters recently rejected a proposed measure which would have provided for more medical training facilities. It seems unlikely, then, that conditions will improve significantly in the near future. In several California counties there has already been a decrease in the number of doctors. Immigration of doctors has fallen off because of California's deteriorating environment and the high cost of malpractice insurance. Similar shortages are developing in other states. This means that millions of people are not getting satisfactory medical care right here in the United States. Moreover, the situation is likely to worsen in the next few years.

Regrettably, this is not the worst of our dilemmas. In fact, irrespective of our empathy with starving people as fellow human beings, the problem of hunger is merely symptomatic of a potentially more lethal environmental disorder. With a billion and a half hungry people and grossly insufficient medical facilities, *Homo sapiens* has the weakest population—the most susceptible to disease—in its history. We are ripe for an epidemic of horrendous proportions. It is well known that the larger the host population, the greater is the possibility of mutations in viruses and bacteria which are lethal to the host.

With our modern high-speed transportation systems, which can move us from continent to continent in less than 10 hours, we could have a mutant viral plague which could kill or disable half the world's people.

As a matter of fact, we have already had several close calls. In 1967, some African velvet monkeys were being used in Marburg, Germany for experimental purposes. In the laboratory, a deadly virus never before seen in man was transferred from these lab animals to the experimenters. This so-called Marburgvirus infected 30 people. In a well-fed population which was neither very young nor very old—with medically sophisticated care—seven of these people died. It takes little imagination to envision what might have happened if this virus had been transferred to food handlers in the London airport while the monkeys were on their way to Marburg.

Just this past spring another virus was brought back to the United States from Nigeria. The Lassa virus, which causes Lassa fever, was being studied at Yale University, where two of the investigators contracted the disease. One was not known to have had contact with the disease; when this victim died, the experimenters decided that the virus was a little too hot to handle. The other scientist was saved by serum from a survivor of a previous African outbreak. A pandemic caused by just such a virus might well reduce the overpopulation problem. Since human beings presumably have other choices besides death-rate solutions, one would hope that man will opt for the rational answer and begin to practice wide-scale birth control.

Who's to Blame?

The most serious overpopulation problem and the worst environmental deterioration are caused by affluent white Americans. At the present level of 205 million people, the population of the United States constitutes approximately 6% of the world's population of 3.6 billion. Nevertheless, Americans account for 30 to 40% of the annual consumption of the world's natural resources, and it is projected that this will increase to 50 to 80% by 1980. From these figures it appears that the United States is the most disproportionately greedy consumer in the world.

In terms of per capita consumption of electric power—which is a good index of the magnitude of our demand for the worldwide supplies of fossil fuels—the average American puts 50 times more stress on the environment than does the average citizen of India. In terms of per capita consumption of steel—which is a good index of how we are using much more than our fair share of the world's supply of nonrenewable natural resources —the birth of an American baby puts 300 times more strain on the environment than does an average Indonesian birth.

To document further the consumption patterns of Americans, one needs only to review the data on per capita production of solid wastes. Today, the average American produces 5.3 pounds of solid waste per day. By 1975, that figure is expected to increase to approximately 7 pounds per day. By 1980, it will be nearly 10 pounds per day per person. Not only are our present levels of affluence and consumption producing a culture of acquisitive consumers, but the accompanying pollution is also killing us and other species. The sole reason we can maintain the present level of consumption is that we are using up not only resources needed by other humans today, but also our descendants' share of the resources. At projected rates of consumption, the United States alone would "need" all the known reserves of certain valuable resources, such as petroleum and tungsten, within 100 years.

Furthermore, when one considers our present inefficient and inequitable system of distribution, it is clear that an even smaller percentage of the American 6% of the world's population is doing most of the destructive consuming. Contrary to the belief of many affluent Americans, it is not population growth among ghetto dwellers or those on welfare which is exerting the most dangerous pressures on our environment. In fact, for self-evident economic reasons, poor people cannot afford to buy many things—it is precisely these people who consume the least and are the worst victims of the pollution created to maintain the affluence of the upper-income groups.

For all practical purposes we can forget about the birth rates of the lower income groups. These groups simply do not have the opportunity to destroy our ecological systems. Besides, as soon as they have the same social, economic, and educational opportunities as the more affluent segments of our society, their birth rates will undoubtedly converge with those of the affluent members of society. When that happens, we can begin to deal with the problems of their overconsumption.

Environmental Deterioration

Until then, we must concentrate our attention on the real environmental despoilers who are breeding and consuming us to the brink of eco-catastrophe. At any level of affluence and technology, a greater number of people causes a greater amount of environmental deterioration.

The greater the amount of per capita affluence, the more deterioration results. We cannot consider the problem simply in terms of pollution—we must think of the more serious overall question of environmental deterioration. Unfortunately, many people still think "pollution" is merely an esthetic inconvenience or a health threat. What they fail to recognize is that contaminants and irritants are a major cause of ongoing destruction of our life-support systems. And they also fail to recognize that the very acts of farming and paving destroy complex ecosystems and degrade our environment.

Carrying Capacity. Environmental deterioration is a direct threat to the earth's carrying capacity. The carrying capacity of a finite environment can be measured by the maximum population which can be sustained on a long-term basis by the resources of that environment. Obviously the capacity will vary according to whether the population is to be sustained in luxury ... reasonable comfort ... or bare subsistence. As studies of animal populations illustrate, if a population becomes too large to be supported in its environment without additional food or space, the result is a massive die-off or "population crash." When this occurs, the population will be decimated or extinguished entirely.

By over-reproducing and overconsuming, we are putting stress on the ecosystems which determine the carrying capacity of our country and of the world as a whole. The ultimate result, of course, will be a human population crash. But worse yet, as we try to expand the carrying capacity of the earth by interfering with complex, stable, natural ecosystems, we are destroying the worldwide life-support systems upon which our lives depend. In other words, we may so damage these systems before the eventual population crash that few humans—if any—will be able to survive in the hostile postcrash environment.

In the United States. Even if man is clever enough to circumvent mass die-offs from starvation or disease, it is becoming increasingly clear that other dysfunctions in society are generated by overpopulation

Certainly the side effects of crowding and high-density urban populations have not escaped public notice. In the United States, we are experiencing the acute ill effects which seem related to crowding and tension. Violence and crime are rising meteorically on a national scale, especially in urban areas. Sexual deviance seems to be increasing, perhaps as a natural adaptive syndrome in an overpopulated environment. American psychiatrists have all they can do to treat the increasing number of neurotic and psychotic victims of our society.

Moreover, there can be no doubt that a rapidly growing population does not work toward the best national interest when considered in the context of our domestic political situation. How can we expect a democratic form of government—which was developed in ancient Greece for tiny city-states—to function on an optimum basis in a country as huge as ours at a time of extremely rapid change? With a total of 535 members, Congress must legislate for a nation of over 200 million people. This means that each member of the House of Representatives represents a constituency of over 450,000 people. In other words, each citizen has less than 1/450,000th of a vote in the House. Obviously, for the most part, our senators must represent even larger groups of constituents. This makes it extremely difficult to have a representative democracy which is truly responsive to the wishes of the people. Finally, there is no doubt that as overpopulation increases we can expect greater governmental control of individual freedoms. Socialized medicine will look like unbridled liberty compared to its replacement.

Internationally. On the international level, the problem is even more acute. As each nation's population increases, it exerts more pressure upon its own limited natural resources and on the finite natural resources of the world as a whole. This competition for resources, in turn, exacerbates international tensions. The foreign policy of the United States provides an excellent example of this process.

The United States depends on cheap raw materials which it imports from the underdeveloped countries. At the present time, we are involved in conflicts in the Middle East and the Far East to maintain our access to the resources of these two areas. The result is a highly volatile international situation which could erupt without warning into a thermonuclear war. Because of the far-reaching effects of the subsequent radioactive contamination, very few people, if any would survive. Any survivors would probably have mutational changes which would affect their offspring, if not themselves. As the human population continues to grow, the likelihood of a thermonuclear holocaust also grows.

Several other unsavory alternatives are also available. With the advent of modern chemical-biological warfare (CBW) any nation can have its own doomsday device. Why should any Third-World nation refrain from developing its CBW capability? The overdeveloped nations still speak of "nuclear deterrence" and "overkill" while continuing to pursue their politics of global thievery. Hunger-crazed nations are unlikely to be overly rational once they are pressed against the wall in the population-resource crunch.

Dr. H.R. Marshall, of the Department of Political Science at Stanford University, describes the resulting irrational decision-making under acute pressure as "psychological jamming." At the point when the pressure becomes too great, leaders may cease to consider rational alternatives and may resort to suicidal measures. Given our modern technology, conventional limited warfare—such as we have practiced in Vietnam—is no longer environmentally feasible because of the enormous depletion of valuable nonrenewable resources expended for war material. Through defoliation and massive bombing we are not just killing Vietnamese, we are also reducing the ability of their country to support human life for an exceedingly long period of time.

Where Do We Go?

The direction in which we must move is clear. We must limit our population growth rate to zero as rapidly as possible. Concentrating on the upper and middle income brackets, we must exert maximum social pressure on couples to have no more than two chilren. Simultaneously, we must begin to turn down the growth rate of our economy and move toward, a spaceship economy. We must greatly reduce the enormous pressure we put on world resources.

In short, we must *de-develop.*

An essential step is to control our military-industrial complex, while we assist those in the lower income levels to achieve a decent level of material comfort. We must deemphasize consumption and move to a philosophy in which quality of life, quality of products, and recycling of materials are the goals. We must abandon the production-consumption-waste ethic which has caused the quality of life in the United States to deteriorate so precipitiously during the past 20 years.

We must maximize the capabilities of our human resources by giving everyone the same social, economic, and educational opportunities. This will have the secondary effect of reducing the birth rate of oppressed minority groups to the same level as the birth rate of the privileged classes. We must help all Americans to achieve an inner security and a psychologically healthy leisure ethic to replace the neurotic attitude of overwork, acquisition, and consumption of material things.

We must make life worth living again.

The Physician's Role

There is no doubt that technological innovations will help—but technology will not provide the entire answer. Technology must complement a new lifestyle which will be essential if man is to survive for as long as we would like. The medical profession can be extremely influential in this endeavor. As students of community medicine are learning, modern medicine is capable of providing better distribution of medical services in which the quality of life is improved for everyone, rather than for only a privileged few. Instead of concentrating on techniques such as organ transplants and genetic surgery, the medical profession must concentrate its efforts and its research funds on socially more important areas—such as nutrition, public health and, especially, the production of safer, more effective birth control techniques.

At the present time, the United States ranks 22nd in the world in terms of its infant mortality. It should be unacceptable to us that the richest, most developed, and the most powerful nation in the world should allow its young to die this way. If the United States can have a gross national product of a trillion dollars and spend on the order of $3.5 billion a year to send men to the moon, then why can't we see to it that our expectant mothers receive adequate food and medical care? Every newborn child should have the human right of sufficient medical attention to guarantee him an equal start.

The medical profession and the American Medical Association should be spearheading the movements for reform. Medicare and Medicaid are a result—as much as anything else—of the reluctance of the medical profession to initiate a viable program to make certain that every American citizen gets decent medical care. Most doctors would agree that good health is a right—not a privilege. If the medical profession is slow to regulate itself and does not institute its own reforms on a timely basis, it will continue to find—as big business is learning—that there are far too many people who want to preempt that responsibility. We all know who they are: the agencies of the United States government. Certainly, a federally subsidized health insurance plan would be preferable to programs administered by the government. Hopefully, this type of system would retain the benefits of private enterprise while providing good medical care to everyone at a reasonable cost.

Abortion Reform. Right now, a critical issue is abortion reform. Without it millions of women are sentenced to compulsory pregnancies . . . children are born unwanted . . . women are subjected to the foulest practices of criminal abortions . . . and 500 to 1000 women die each year from illegal abortions. The right of any woman to have an abortion should be guaranteed by the federal government. Her decision to terminate a pregnancy or not is one which should be based on consultation between her and her physician. The advocates of the reform of present medieval abortion legislation do not urge compulsory abortion—only legislation to protect the individual's right not to be subjected to compulsory pregnancy. The medical profession should be in the vanguard of the fight for abortion law reform.

Perhaps even more important is the need for legal provisions for an organized sex education program for our schools. Free information on contraception should be advertised by the government and made readily available upon request to members of all socioeconomic groups. Free contraceptive devices should be made available to anyone who requests them, and they should be advertised by the government on the same basis as the information on contraception. Finally, free, subsidized terminations of pregnancy should be provided by the government for those who want them. To avoid coercion in such programs, they should be administered at the local level by people drawn from the communities they serve.

Another major area in which the medical profession could be immensely influential is in the changing of the public's attitudes toward the male-female roles in the process of contraception. As most doctors will readily tell their male patients, a vasectomy is a perfectly safe, minor operation which offers a much less hazardous means of effective contraception than either the pill or a tubal ligation for a woman. However, one major obstacle is the attitude of the average American male and the luctance on his part to recognize his reciprocal responsibility in contraception. Another is the assumption on the part of many doctors that it is their business to decide when it is appropriate for an adult man to be sterilized. Clearly, except for explaining the operation and its consequences, the physician should not intrude into the decision if the patient is over 21.

These are areas in which the medical profession as a whole should be taking an active humanitarian stand. As soon as the majority of the members of the medical profession have a solid understanding of the gravity of the present population-environment crisis, they can be of immense help in directing the nation toward environmental sanity and leading the way toward significant changes in the way we live. The prestige of the medical profession is enormous—and the potential for using this prestige to benefit mankind has never been higher.

We have dealt briefly with a series of individual problems, but, of course, they are all interrelated. We no longer have the luxury of dealing with problems one at a time. Improving the quality of the urban environment is as important as restoring the purity of our air and water. Eradicating racism, exploitation, and war must accompany attempts at population limitation and environmental cleanup; otherwise, the necessary cooperation of all people will never be obtained. All phases of the program to limit population and to improve the quality of life must proceed simultaneously, or else we may well be distracted by individual symptoms and fail to treat the causes of the syndrome. Our deteriorating environment does not need bandages and aspirin for its cancer—it needs major surgery. And we must act now.

Conclusion

There are two ways that we can terminate our random experimentation with the human race. Either we shall act rationally in a humane fashion to limit reproduction and stabilize our population at a level that the earth can support comfortably over a long period of time, or else, we will undergo a massive die-off. The implication is clear: It is gross irresponsibility to meddle with the death rate without making a compensatory adjustment in the birth rate.

Physicians have long been hard at work on the death rate. They must now work equally hard on the birth rate—or see the loss of all the gain they have made for humanity.

Confronting the A.E.C.

2

by John W. Gofman

In 1940, I came to the University of California to work for a Ph.D. For my thesis I chose a problem suggested by Glen Seaborg. That work became part of what was the Manhattan Project. I stayed with it until 1944, when I left to complete medical school, which I had begun before going to Berkeley. So I know something about the early developments of the modern atomic era.

In 1947, after medical school, I returned to the University of California at Berkeley. I was teaching medical physics and doing research, in part under Atomic Energy Commission auspices, and was involved in studying the origins of heart disease. In many of these research projects, I collaborated with Dr. Arthur R. Tamplin. We were associates both in teaching and in carrying out research on the problems of atomic energy and its hazards.

In 1953, the Lawrence Radiation Laboratory was divided into two labs. To the Berkeley laboratory was added a new branch at Livermore. For the most part, Livermore was created for Edward Teller to devise hydrogen bombs with the approval and blessing of its director, Ernest Lawrence. Because I was a close friend of Ernest Lawrence's and because he thought there were several hazardous features connected with the weapons work being done at Livermore he asked me to come

SOURCE: Reprinted from *OMEGA*, "Murder of the Ecosystem and Suicide of Man," Paul K. Anderson, with the permission of the author.

to Livermore two days a week to watch over the people involved. They were handling radioactive hydrogen, tritium, and plutonium in very large amounts, and doing so under rather urgent schedules, preparing for tests in the Pacific. So for two days a week I went to Livermore to observe the people there. I continued my observations for four years. In 1957, I asked to be relieved of the responsibility.

Some six years later, I received a call from Dr. John Foster, whom I had come to know at Livermore. He asked me to see him at the lab. Dr. Foster said that he had an interesting request from the Atomic Energy Commission. The A.E.C. wanted to know if the Livermore laboratory would undertake a long-range program to evaluate the impact of its activities—weapons testing, the peaceful uses of nuclear explosives; in fact, every aspect of atomic energy—on man and the biosphere. I thought it was strange that in 1963, something like eighteen years after the A.E.C. had been formed, with some eighteen or twenty laboratories around the country involved in biomedical aspects of radiation and radioactivity, it wanted to set up still another laboratory to consider the impact of radiation on man.

But there was a definite need for it. The background for it was set in 1961, after the voluntary moratorium, when the Russians resumed testing. Then, during the 1961-62 period, President Kennedy ordered a resumption of American testing to take place in the Pacific and in Nevada. As a result of some tests made above ground in Nevada in 1962, the state of Utah was hit hard with radioactivity—the levels of radio-iodine found in milk were quite high, for instance, and that of course has an effect on children's thyroids. The tests had been smaller than some conducted in the nineteen-fifties and the actual dose to thyroids was not as great in the 1962 tests as those that resulted from earlier ones. Even so, the A.E.C. found itself in trouble. The agency decided that by setting up a biomedical laboratory at Livermore—with biologists working closely with the people who were making nuclear explosives and firing them off—it might in some way be able to avoid a recurrence of the Utah incident.

It was obvious that research was needed. In spite of all the other laboratories in the country under A.E.C. auspices that were investigating one or another aspect of the hazards of radioactivity, no one in any one of those laboratories and no one in the A.E.C. ever asked the question: If we do this weapons test, what will it mean? How will it affect health? If we use nuclear explosives for making harbors or canals or getting at underground resources, what will be the cost to society?

Dr. Tamplin and I and a few others decided we would consider going into this job of evaluating the impact of radioactivity on man and the various activities within the atomic energy field—provided that we were able to conduct the research in our own way, had long-term support, and were given professional independence. We said, in effect, that we would investigate the problems, but whether the results were favorable or unfavorable to atomic energy programs, we would make the results available on an open, unclassified basis to both the scientific community and the public, because these are matters of vital concern to everyone. This was agreed to and the program was scheduled. Three months later, however, the Nuclear Test Ban Treaty, calling off tests in the atmosphere, was signed. Thereupon the A.E.C. seemed to think the problem of fallout was solved. We had already committed ourselves to doing the research and went to work, even though our budget was cut to a third of what was originally planned.

Our problem, as we saw it, was clear enough. We set out to develop an integrated system of calculating the extent over space and time of radiation and radioactivity from any kind of nuclear source—an explosion, a reactor, any radio-isotope source. Dr. Tamplin took it upon himself to develop a thoroughgoing system to enable us to make exactly this kind of prediction, tracing and measuring the effect of, say the radioactivity from an underground nuclear explosion traveling through food chains to man. The other half of the problem was crucial; we wanted to know, after we had knowledge of the measure of radiation man would receive, what its effects would be.

Dr. Tamplin's findings showed that the standards established by the Federal Radiation Council, detailing the allowable levels of human exposure to radiation, were useless. The regulations which state how much a nuclear reactor could release do not take into consideration the increased concentration of radioactivity as it works through the food chains; the radioactivity in water, for instance, might become five thousand times as concentrated in a fish.

The A.E.C. was extremely disturbed by the airing of these facts. It contended that the Commission could rely on the fact that there was a primary standard, not on how much radiation a reactor could release, but on how much was tolerable for humans. Even if the standards establishing what level of radiation reactor or power companies may release are wrong, the people are protected from exposure to any more than a certain amount set by Federal Radiation Council. Though there is no scientific basis for accepting the Council's guidelines as safe, the A.E.C. consistently, whenever questioned about those standards, claims that the standards represent a harmless amount of radiation, or an amount of radiation to the individual so small it would hardly be noted when detected. If pushed a little harder, the Commission retreats to the position that everything one does in life entails a risk. The view that the benefits the atom can bring far outweigh the risks was taken into account in setting the standards of tolerance. Indeed, one of the most grievous errors of government management was placing in the hands of the Federal Radiation Council the authority not only to evaluate the risks but to evaluate the benefits and set standards accordingly.

One such risk-benefit ratio involves the question of ventilating the Colorado Plateau uranium mines a little more in order to bring a halt to the current epidemic of lung cancer among the miners. It is estimated that over a hundred miners are already dead of lung cancer from radiation, and that out of a few thousand miners the ultimate toll will be a thousand.

When this problem first came up, the A.E.C. and the Joint Committee on Atomic Energy disavowed all responsibility for setting standards for mines; it was traditionallypart of the Labor Department, the Bureau of Mines. Nevertheless, hearings were held and Willard Wirtz, then Secretary of Labor, recommended lower levels. Before he left office, Secretary Wirtz directed that the levels in those mines must go down; the directive is supposed to take effect later this year. Just recently, the Federal Radiation Council and the A.E.C. awarded a two-hundred-thousand-dollar contract to the Arthur D. Little Corporation to evaluate the economic impact on the uranium industry if the levels are pushed down to those required in the directive. So, having once abdicated from responsibility, they now want to assume it, because it is compromising the industry they are trying to promote.

Even when it was pointed out that the conditions in the mines may bring about a repetition of the European experience in Joachimsthal, Czechoslovakia (where, over a period of years, seventy per cent of the miners—five thousand men—died of lung cancer), the Federal Radiation Council said we must remember that the mines are important to the economy of Colorado, the national defense needs uranium, and the country is going to need atomic electricity.

All are non sequiturs with respect to why the miners should be dying, but comprise the strange ways of risk-benefit calculations. The benefit to the electric power industry is cheap uranium. The risk is death to the miners.

Sooner or later we have to come to grips with a reliable estimate of what the tolerance levels of the Federal Radiation Council has set actually mean. Evidence concerning the effects of radiation continues to come in from Hiroshima and Nagasaki, and the follow-up period is getting longer. In the early period, leukemia showed up, but as the years passed a series of new cancers began to appear in excessive numbers.

From Britain have come reports on some fourteen thousand men who had radiation treatment for arthritis of the spine, and what the effects were after five, ten, and fifteen years. An analysis of the data from a Nova Scotia tuberculosis sanatarium showed that women who have received repeated fluoroscopic examinations to the chest (averaging a hundred and fifty examinations in the course of their treatment), had, in the fifteen years following, twenty-four times as much breast cancer as the women who had not been fluoroscoped. Dr. Karl Morgan, an eminent health physicist at Oak Ridge, Tennessee, and a member of the International Commission on Radiological Protection, estimates that the current use of fluoroscopy and x-ray in the United States, giving only a third or a tenth as good medical information as one would want, is responsible for somewhere between twenty-five and a hundred thousand deaths each year.

All the evidence that we have examined has led us to believe, with as good assurance as most laws of biology or chemistry provide, that all forms of cancer can be induced by radiation. (Spontaneous cancer, of course, occurs for reasons no one knows, but our studies concentrated on those induced by radiation exposure.) Not only are all forms of cancer induced by radiation, but the dose that it takes to double the incidence of a particular cancer remains, within a factor or two, the same for other types of cancer. That is, if there is one cancer that is very rare—maybe only one case per year in a million people—the dose necessary to double it to two cases turns out to be about the same dose it takes to double a cancer that is a hundred cases a year to two hundred.

From data on pregnant women who had been irradiated in utero for diagnostic purposes, it was found that even one diagnostic x-ray, or a couple, can give a fifty-per cent increase in the incidence of childhood cancers and leukemia in the first ten years of the child's life. Another of our conclusions (from these data and some others), was that a child is roughly ten times as sensitive as an adult to induction of cancer by radiation.

So, too, with animals. Doses given all at once to young animals result in a great incidence of cancer. If an animal receives the same dosage spread out over a longer period,when the animal is older and therefore less sensitive, the result is less cancer. On that erroneous basis, the A.E.C. has contended that fractionating the dose over an interval provides the necessary protection; since the effects of all peaceful nuclear energy activity will be spread out in this way, there will be no danger to human beings.

Our own estimation was that if everyone in the United States were to get the dose that the Federal Radiation Council allows, it would mean at least one extra cancer or leukemia for every twenty that occur normally. Put another way, it would mean sixteen thousand additional, unnecessary cancers per year in the United States. That was a conservative estimate. We knew it was conservative when we presented testimony before the Joint Committee on Atomic Energy last January; we raised it to thirty-two thousand because we had evidence to support it.

The A.E.C. said our data were wrong—even after we pointed out that our data were in agreement with the highly respected International Commission on Radiological Protection—and said that much of the data concerning cancers came from people who have had appreciable dosages. Somewhat below that dose, they said, there must be a dose that is safe.

The International Commission and all responsible biologists, however, have long pointed out that that attitude shows no real regard for public health. A safe threshold can never be assumed unless there is proof for it. All the evidence shows no suggestion whatever for a threshold.

In spite of the claims the A.E.C. makes for the safety of the standards currently in force, there may now be some hope that the standards will be revised. Earlier this year, at the request of Senator Edmund Muskie, we submitted our findings to the attention of Robert Finch, Secretary of Health, Education and Welfare, who is also chairman of the Federal Radiation Council. The Council, while not agreeing with every premise and conclusion of our findings, did agree that no safe threshold of radiation exists, that every amount of radiation produces its commensurate amount of cancer. Mr. Finch has ordered a complete review of the standards, with a view to resetting them if needed, for the exposure of the population at large.

3 The Noise is Killing Us

by Henry Lexaus

Industry tries to keep factory noise below 85 decibels, but a kitchen blender registers 93 and a rock 'n' roll band as high as 138. Edison predicted that eventually all civilized men would be deaf.

Visited a boiler factory lately? You'd be surprised: it might be quieter inside than it is out on the street. Ever since 1948, when a drop-forge worker named Matthew Slawinski won a $1,661 lawsuit for job-caused deafness, American businessmen have been steadily muffling industrial noise.

Inside the factory, the rule of thumb has been to try to keep noise below 85 decibels, if possible. This is the level at which prolonged exposure can cause partial deafness in some persons.

But pity the poor workman who goes home. Maybe he takes an hour's ride on the subway at 95 decibels, and then decides to mow his lawn with his 107-decibel power mower. Or maybe he just loafs, listening to his wife preparing dinner with her 93-decibel food blender. "The noise level in the modern kitchen," says one acoustical expert, "is just below that of a DC-3 cabin."

And pity the poor fellow who lives near an airport. At rush hours several years ago, people of suburban Park Ridge, Illinois, used to hear a take-off roar or landing whine every 40 seconds from runway 9-27 of Chicago's O'Hare Field. The residents were able to have the noise diverted elsewhere, but only after collecting conclusive evidence. A police truck from the suffering suburb parked with a noise meter three miles away from the end of the runway. This procedure delivered proof that 75 per cent of the flights on runway 9-27 registered over 90 decibels. That's the amount of noise you hear from a freight train at a distance of 500 feet and more noise than you hear from a motorcycle 300 feet away.

"Many noise levels encountered in the community exceed standards found in industry," says Dr. Oliver I. Welsh, a Boston hearing expert. That is so because thousands of people are professionally concerned about the standards for industrial noise. However, few people are working on the everyday noises in our homes and cities.

Millions of people are outraged by the SST and the sonic boom that threatens us in the 1970's. But surprisingly few people worry about the greatest sonic problem of all, the background noise in our cities. It affects all of us; it is here now; it has been increasing at the rate of one decibel a year for the last 30 years; and it is going to get worse.

In anticipation of an expected gigantic increase of air traffic in the 1970's, almost every major city in the country is talking about building another airport. Smaller towns, too. In a few years, 400 airports, twice as many as serve jets today, will be handling the new short-range jets. The end of the Vietnam war will probably see an explosion of the helicopter taxi business. There will be more and more people, therefore more and more motorcycles, more and more outboard motors, more and more household gadgets to make living easier and the place in which we live noisier.

If the present noise level is intolerable, what do the experts say about even more noise?

One theme prevails. The World Health Organization calls the rising tide of noise in our cities one of the earth's major health problems. "It is rapidly becoming more pernicious than air or water pollution."

Physicist Vern O. Knudsen, former UCLA chancellor, says, "Noise, like smog, is a slow agent of death. If it continues to increase for the next 30 years as it has for the past 30, it could become lethal."

The New Dutch Catechism gets to the heart of the problem. The Commandment "does not just forbid murder. It also condemns everything thatmakes life less agreeable for ourselves and others: pollution of the air, dirt, breaches of traffic laws.

"Noise has ruined many people's nerves," the Catechism continues. Then its tone suddenly becoming more impassioned: "There is no protection. One can shut one's eyes, but not one's ears."

Noise is murderous. By deafening us, it deprives us of the use of part of our bodies.

This physical effect of noise has been known ever since the 1830's when a British investigator started looking into the question of why blacksmiths paid so little attention to the noise they made.

Why do so few city dwellers object to the rising tide of noise? Perhaps for the very same reason that few blacksmiths did. They are partially deaf. Thomas Alva Edison, a long time ago, noted that noise seemed to be an inevitable side effect of the machine age, and predicted that eventually all civilized men would be deaf.

We have already, for example, grown quite accustomed to the idea that old people should be deaf. At 50, the average person has lost 20 decibels of sound perception. But how much of this is caused by aging and how much by prolonged exposure to the sounds of civilization?

Dr. Samuel Rosen, the pioneer of stapes surgery, has taken the trouble to investigate this question. On a field expedition to the Sudan, he discovered that among the Mabaan people, who live a quiet pastoral existence near the upper Nile, tribesmen hear as well at 75 as they do at 25.

Dr. Rosen does not advocate a quiet pastoral existence for Americans; some noise is inevitable in our lives. It is that phrase "prolonged exposure" which is the key to a solution of the noise problem.

Our bodies have a partial defense against loudness; in a sense we can close our ears. Sound that vibrates your eardrum is transmitted through three articulated earbones (the hammer, anvil, and stirrup) to the cochlea of the inner ear. There it is transformed from mechanical energy into electrical energy for transmission to the brain through the auditory nerve.

If you are prepared for loud noise, the muscle from the eardrum to the hammer is tightened, decreasing the vibration, and another muscle pulls the stirrup bone away from the cochlea to protect the nerve endings.

The tightening muscles are not strong, however. Steady protracted noise or frequently repeated noise causes fatigue to set in. The muscles relax and your inner ear takes a greater pounding. As time goes on you start to hear a ringing in your ears when the noise is gone (a "tin ear"), and you will have lost permanently a tiny bit of your hearing. Further exposure to loud noise may cause total deafness.

The first sounds to go are the high frequency ones: your ear starts to miss consonant sounds like f, s, th, ch, and sh. This is the condition older people complain of when they say that they "can hear the sound, but can't make out the words."

It is not only older people who are being deafened. Recently, Dr. David M. Lipscomb of the University of Tennessee studied his university freshmen. "We were shocked to find that the hearing of many of these students had already deteriorated to a level of the average 65-year-old."

Dr. Lipscomb went on to study 3,000 Knoxville teenagers, and became even more shocked. Five per cent of 1,000 6th-graders, 14 per cent of 1,000 9th-graders, and 20 per cent of 1,000 high-school seniors had suffered a measurable hearing loss.

The most likely culprit, Dr. Lipscomb thinks, is rock 'n' roll, commonly played in closed reverberating rooms at the loudest possible amplification. "We have measured sound in discotheques at 138 decibels, only two decibels below the pain threshold," he says.

To test his thesis, he engaged in an unusual experiment. He exposed a guinea pig to "rock" in a typical teenager's pattern. After a total of 88-1/2 hours of 120-decibel rock music had been applied to the animal in an off-and-on pattern over a three-month period, he took microphotographs of the pig's inner ear. Many of the cells of the cochlea had "shriveled up like peas."

Dr. George T. Singleton of the University of Florida has come to the same conclusion. Driving his daughter Marsha home from a dance one night, he noticed that she couldn't hear what he said. So, for the next dance, he tested the hearing of 10 of the 9th-graders immediately before and after. The boys all showed temporary hearing loss—an average 11 decibels—while one boy's hearing dropped 35 decibels.

Temporary partial hearing loss is usually not dangerous. It happens to all of us on occasion. But it is a sign that you are in a noisy environment. Protracted or repeated exposure to that noise level will cause permanent impairment of hearing.

Dr. Aram Glorig, director of the Callier Hearing and Speech Center in Dallas, suggests three rules of thumb for people who wish to preserve their hearing intact. Start worrying if: (1) noise is loud enough to make people shout into each other's ears; (2) noise causes a slight temporary hearing loss; (3) noise brings on a ringing in the ears.

The physical effects of noise, partial or total deafening, are bad enough. But the psychic effects, which are still nebulous and little studied, may be even closer to the traditional definition of murder.

"I believe," says Dr. Rosen, "that we will one day recognize a chronic noise syndrome. At an unexpected or unwanted noise, the pupils dilate, skin pales, mucous membranes dry, there are intestinal spasms, and the adrenals explode secretions. The biological organism, in a word, is disturbed."

These reactions were once a useful defense mechanism for primitive man. When noise alerted him to danger, his heart beat jumped, his blood pressure shot up, his muscles contracted, and he was instantly ready for a superhuman burst of effort.

It made sense in the real jungle, but now we are living in effect in city jungles, under conditions of incessant alarm, and it can't be good for us.

"Noise in the city usually contributes to the health problem by an erosion of emotional well-being," says Dr. Lee E. Farr of the University of Texas School of Public Health. He suggests that noise might be a triggering agent for physical ailments such as ulcers and hives as well as mental illness. Tests by the Stanford Research Institute show that a sleeper's brain-wave patterns are radically changed by noise that is insufficient to awaken him. So is the flow of blood in his capillaries.

What can you do to protect yourself against noise? You can't very well walk around with earplugs. (Or can you? With men who know noise best, it's earplugs two to one. "I wear earplugs when I mow the lawn," says Dr. Glorig.)

Dr. John D. Dougherty of the Harvard School of Public Health says that the average person should "seriously consider the amount of time he spends each day in a noisy environment.P'

The best thing you can do is to build a quiet refuge for yourself away from the noise of the city jungle. A great deal can be done to make the average home quieter, though it must be admitted that this is against the temper of the times.

Modern interior decorating styles have done much to make homes noisier. The emphasis on sweeping uninterrupted spaces permits noise to radiate farther. What you want are barriers in the sound's path.

The disappearance of overstuffed Victorian furniture has decreased the cushioning effect of many soft surfaces. Clean lines make hard surfaces which reflect rather than trap sound. You can't very well bring back the Victorian sofa, but you can keep in mind when you decorate that you need plenty of substitute absorbing surfaces, drapes, acoustic ceiling tiles, carpets.

Modern construction methods also encourage noise: dry-wall partitions that reverberate in place of lath-and-plaster that muffles; light, hollow doors; back-to-back plumbing fixtures in high-rise apartments.

Next time you rent an apartment you might ask how thick the walls are. New York rental agents say that noise is the cause of 25 per cent of failures to renew lease. A frequent complaint in new buildings is that you can't tell whose phone is ringing, yours or your neighbor's

Builders could do more to soundproof homes and apartments but they seldom do because it costs more money—from two to 10 per cent are the common estimates—and there is little demand. It is an easy item to skimp on when you are trying to cut costs.

Soundproofing only limits the transmission of sound from one place to another. The best solution, of course, is to eliminate the noise at its source. You can't do much as an individual about this, but you can help to create a demand so that those who can will take action.

Harvard's Dr. Dougherty says that the citizen "should consider the noise levels of the appliances he buys for his home, as well as making his weight felt with his legislators about community noise not under his control."

Next time you buy an appliance ask how much noise it makes. Better yet, next time you're in a department store ask how much noise an appliance makes, and don't buy it. Feedback from merchants will stimulate manufacturers to consider the noise problem.

U.S. Public Health Service engineer Herbert H. Jones says, "Although refrigerators and, to a lesser extent, individual air-conditioning units are quieter than models of 20 years ago, there is still room for improvement in washers, dryers, dishwashers, garbage disposals, and commodes."

Complain, complain, complain! Most Americans are too easygoing, too ready to see the other fellow's point of view. We need more and bigger airports; airports have to be built somewhere; somebody's got to suffer. Agreed. But if an airport commission has to fight every inch of the way to enlarge its field, if an airline has to fight to fly over somebody's house, somebody is going to give airplane manufacturers a motive to build quieter planes.

The most important thing the average man can do about noise is to develop a fine sense of outrage. Make what the lawmakers call "noise." Legislation to provide federal funds to help states and cities set up noise control programs is bottled up in Congressional committees. Nobody has made enough "noise" to stimulate Congressmen to do anything about real noise.

Decibels

The decibel scale is logorithmic. A 10-decibel sound is twice as loud as 1 decibel, 20 decibels is four times as loud, and 100 decibels is 1,000 times as loud.

1 — softest audible sound
10 — leaves rustling
20 — whisper
30 — tick of a watch
40 — quiet room
50 — quiet street, quiet restaurant
70 — automobile at 30 mph
80 — motorcycle, average factory, noisy office, busy stream, automobile at 70 mph
90 — truck at 50 mph
100 — subway train
110 — rock 'n' roll
120 — propeller plane taking off, thunderclap
130 — riveting, machine gun
140 — jet take off, threshold of pain
150 — flight deck of an aircraft carrier during launching
160 — wind tunnel
170 — rocket launch
175 — kills mice

America's Shame: Water Pollution

4

by Louis Clapper

A crow drifts slowly down the Missouri River riding a raft of solidified grease and animal tissue held together by a binder of hog hair. Only a carrion bird could stand the smell, yet many downstream cities take their drinking water from this river.

Live viruses, dumped into our coastal waters from sewers and dirty bilge tanks, have caused hepatitis in persons who ate clams harvested from sewage-laden waters on the Atlantic Coast, and oysters from the polluted Gulf.

Nitrochlorbenzene, an extremely poisonous organic chemical, is detected in the Mississippi at New Orleans—and followed a thousand miles upstream past many city water intakes to an industrial waste discharge in St. Louis. No one can yet guess the damage this might do to man and wildlife.

This is only a sampling of what is happening in many parts of this country. The detailed story is much longer, equally appalling, and adds up to America's Shame—the pollution of our waters.

"Water pollution in the United States is a menace to our health and an economic burden which is robbing us of water we need," asserts G. E. McCallum, Chief of Water Supply and Pollution Control in the U. S. Public Health Service. "It is a destroyer of fish and wildlife habitat, a threat to outdoor recreation, and in many communities, an aesthetic horror."

SOURCE: Reprinted with permission of the author.

Words, at least words that can be used in mixed company, cannot describe the filth we pour into many of our streams, lakes and oceans. Sewage, slaughterhouse offal, thousands of lethal chemicals, radioactive matter—these and other of man's wastes combine to form what sanitary engineers, for lack of a better term, call "gunk." Gunk defies analysis and perplexes health authorities who are desperately trying to keep up with its harmful effects on man and other living creatures.

We are faced with some inescapably gruesome facts:

Sewage treatment plants are, at best, only 90 per cent efficient with organic material—and some inorganic wastes defy treatment.

The Public Health Service has isolated polio, infectious hepatitis and more than 30 other live viruses which may carry disease from treated sewage effluent.

Because we increasingly re-use water, chances are four out of ten that the water you drink has passed through someone's household plumbing or an industrial plant sewer.

Then what prevents us all from being sick?

"The fact our water treatment plants are the best in the world," answers McCallum. So we have some of the worst pollution, but the safest drinking water—thanks to its being disinfected by chlorine and other chemicals which kill most bacteria, even though the water sometimes has a disagreeable taste and odor. But we are riding a thin edge.

The effects of water pollution are much broader than health. Industrial plants are rejecting water as unfit for their uses. Swimmers are finding beaches posted "UNSAFE FOR SWIMMING." Water skiing? Not when the coliform bacterial count per drop of water has reached 80 at the Detroit waterfronts; 65 in the Androscoggin River; 20 in the Mississippi at St. Louis, (A count of five per drop is considered unsafe for swimming.)

Bad news for fishermen! Last year pollution killed 50 million fish in rivers and coastal waters. These are only the reported kills.

Radioactive wastes have been found in the Colorado River drainage, danger signals of more trouble to come as we enter the atomic age. Floating garbage and other filth clogs water supply intakes of many cities which take their water from open streams. Potent fumes from New Hampshire's Androscoggin River have peeled the paint from the walls of nearby buildings.

Detergent foam runs from water faucets in several states—you brush your teeth in someone else's dishwater. Acids, seeping from mines in Pennsylvania and West Virginia, have polluted streams and poisoned wildlife. Chemical pesticide sprays are lining lake and stream banks with dead fish. Unsewered septic tanks drain into underground waters, and farm chemicals are finding their way into subterranean streams. Oil spills have killed countless birds and spoiled many beaches.

Since time immemorial, water has been known as the natural purifier. Nearly all religions in one way or another use water as the symbol of purity. Yet two presidents of allegedly the most advanced nation on earth have called the pollution of American waters "a national disgrace." Why?

The problem hit with run-away speed. We were using only 160 billion gallons of water daily in 1945. Today, we use 355 billion gallons. The average home uses 60 gallons daily. It takes only three gallons of water to wash dinner dishes by hand, twice that amount by machine. It takes two gallons to flush garbage down the drain, five gallons a minute to take a shower.

The big jump in water usage has come with industrial growth. It takes 500 gallons of water to manufacture one yard of woolen cloth; 320,000 gallons to make a ton of aluminum; 500,000 to make a ton of synthetic rubber.

With a fixed supply of 315 billion gallons of fresh water available today, *we must re-use our water.* The Public Health Service estimates that the total flow of the Ohio River is being used 3.7 times before it reaches the Mississippi. By the time the water in the Mahoning River reaches Youngstown, Ohio, it has been re-used more than eight times. That's why water pollution is so dangerous to us all.

But most citizens are blissfully unaware of where their water comes from, and unconcerned about where it goes. As a result, both cities and industry have dragged their feet. "Of all our public works projects, waste treatment facilities are the least glamorous and the hardest to sell," says McCallum.

A few industries have exerted political pressure to evade anti-pollution laws. One popular claim is that "the plant will have to shut down" if forced to comply with the law, thereby throwing local people (who are also voters) out of work. "To the best of my knowledge, we have yet to shut down an industry or defeat a mayor," says James M. Quigley, assistant secretary of Health, Education, and Welfare.

All 50 states have water pollution laws, but enforcement is sometimes indifferent. You are more likely to be fined for throwing a candy wrapper out the car window in some states, than for dumping poisons and ruining a stream.

The Federal Water Pollution Control Act passed in 1956 started the ball rolling with its powerful one-two punch: (1) construction grants to cities, and (2) threat of court action. Cities were spending less than $300 million annually on sewage treatment plants before the act was passed. But with the help of federal grants—first $50 million annually and then nearly double that figure—cities are now building at the $600 million rate per year.

The Division of Water Supply and Pollution Control has had 25 cases since it got more enforcement teeth. Fifteen were initiated by the Secretary of Health, Education and Welfare, and the rest by state governors. In none of these cases was a court injunction necessary. Mere threat of federal action caused offenders to clean up.

Dramatic progress has been made along the Missouri River where ten years ago not one major city treated its sewage. Today, Sioux City, Omaha, Kansas City and St. Joseph all have treatment plants in operation or under construction, and meat packing plants have really cleaned up. St. Louis recently voted a $95 million bond issue for waste treatment.

Many industries have invested millions and gone to much trouble to reduce water pollution. Through the National Technical Task Committee on Industrial Wastes, organized in 1950, major industries work with the federal government in task groups with mutual problems.

As a direct result, the Shell Oil Company at Anacortes, Washington, has installed a complete treatment system to avoid polluting the area's waters and to protect the local commercial and sport fisheries. Kaiser Steel at Fontana, California, reclaims integrated mill wastes with a settling and recycling system which keeps its water requirements at a minimum. The Allegheny County Sanitary Authority at Pittsburgh has a joint treatment operation in 68 communities and more than 10 industrial plants.

But despite all of these efforts, the pollution of our waters is the worst in history, most experts agree. We're making gains in some areas; in others, we appear to be losing. Our water, when doctored with chlorine and up to a half dozen other chemicals, has been about as safe as any in the world. But some responsible scientists are beginning to question: Is this safe enough?

As population skyrockets and industry expands, water intakes and sewage outlets are jammed closer and closer together. Sewage treatment plants are not the cure-all that most of us blissfully assume. A third of our cities use only primary treatment (screens and settling basins) which at best remove only 35 per cent of the organic wastes. More efficient plants use a secondary treatment (bacterial action to eat up the dissolved organic matter) which removes up to 90 per cent of this material, but leaves many other pollutants untouched.

Chicago, for example, has the best treatment available. Yet they pour an effluent into the Illinois River daily that is equal to the raw sewage from a city of a million people, containing 3,435 tons of solid wastes.

Moreover, our treatment processes are out of date. They cannot remove the complex wastes resulting from manufacture of such substances as plastics, detergents, synthetic fibers, pesticides, and medicines. Some synthetic chemical waste causes tastes and odors. A large number are highly toxic to fish and aquatic life. Many do not respond to biological treatment and persist in streams for great distances. "We do not know how to detect most of these compounds in water, or how to treat or remove them in waste effluents. Nor do we know of their long range toxic effects on man," the Public Health Service warns.

Each year increasing amounts of these wastes come into our water supply intakes. Obviously, even with the chlorine cocktails to kill bacteria, we are subjecting ourselves to increased exposure to harmful wastes, including radioactive substances and lethal pesticide chemicals.

Our future water needs are staggering. By 1980—just 11 years from now—we will be using 600 billion gallons of water daily. By the year 2,000 a trillion gallons. It would take a tank car train 600,000 miles long to haul it. Unless we can find a cheap way to convert salt water to fresh, hydrologists estimate our maximum fresh water supply will be only 650 billion gallons a day. So re-use is a must. We'll need to re-use our water six times by 1980, according to some authorities.

These are the increased demands of the immediate future, yet we are barely holding our own today. "Even those states doing the best job on water pollution are doing an inadequate job," Assistant Secretary of Health, Education and Welfare Quigley told a Congressional committee. Last year, for the first time, we started gaining on municipal pollution, although we have a backlog of 5,831 projects which will cost $2.2 billion for treatment plants and sewers. Industry needs to build 6,000 plants. Federal institutions, too, need to clean up.

Some industrial groups have opposed the federal program of grants to cities on the grounds that pollution is a local and state problem. The reason for this attitude, it is suspected, is that once cities clean up pollution, the finger of guilt will inevitably point to the other polluters—mostly industrial plants. Organic wastes from industrial sources are *double* that from cities.

Water pollution is not an impossible problem. We know that the Ruhr River, which drains the heavily industrialized, heavily populated Ruhr Valley of western Germany, is managed so well it is still safe for boating and swimming. One possible reason—there's a tax on industrial wastes.

We have three big needs in the pollution fight: More money invested in city and industrial water treatment plants. More research to develop more efficient techniques of water treatment. And better enforcement of strong pollution laws—federal, state and local.

How clean and pure we attempt to maintain our streams is a matter of economics and realities, and of values, both tangible and intangible. But of these things we can be certain: Pollution *must* be kept below the levels of significant personal healt damage. Pollution must not destroy recreational and wildlife values. Users of water do not have an inherent right to pollute—they must return it as nearly clean as possible.

What can *you* do to help correct this shameful situation?

First, investigate personally to learn how community and industrial wastes are handled in your community. Second, let elected officials at local, state and federal levels know you want strong anti-pollution laws, and want them enforced. Third, through your conservation club, garden club, women's club or civic group, join in converted actions to improve controls. Only through a wave of expressed public disgust can we clean up our polluted waters and insurea safe, continuing supply for the many jobs water does for us.

5 There Are Two Kinds of Mercury: Environmental, and Man-Made Pollutant

by Emerson Daggett

State and federal scientists went to work last July to find out how little is known and how much there is to learn about the dangers to human and wildlife populations from mercury, a ubiquitous metal 17 times heavier than water which has been found in California's streams, lakes, bays, and the ocean for a century or more.

Both an industrial waste and a natural phenomenon, mercury is found worldwide, varying in concentrations as dangerous as those near Minamata, Japan, which killed or maimed 111 persons between

SOURCE: Reprinted from the April 1971 issue of *California's Health.*

1953 and 1960, and in Sweden where it almost wiped out several species of wildfowl before it was identified and controlled.

First Report

Headed by Ephraim Kahn MD of the State department of public health, the interagency committee on environmental mercury wrote its first report in January 1971.

In addition to department of health staff, the committee is comprised of scientists from State departments of fish and game, agriculture, water resources, water resources control board, and the University of California at Berkeley school of public health; the federal food and drug administration, water quality administration, and public health service.

"We've only learned in recent weeks that the livers of Alaska seals and Pacific Coast sea lions contain large amounts of mercury," Dr. Kahn said, "and that some batches of canned tuna fish have a significant mercury content. The federal food and drug administration has just discovered, too, that swordfish is heavily contaminated with mercury residues far above what has been set as permissible levels."

"It appears," he dryly added, "that we have unwittingly permitted widespread environmental mercury contamination to develop. Now we've got to find out what its ecological and human health consequences mean."

Recent tests of other species of fresh and salt water fish in California waters and the Great Lakes and throughout the country have resulted in the banning of some fish—fresh, frozen and canned—from the lockers and shelves of supermarkets across the nation.

Controls in Effect

This is not to infer that Californians are in imminent danger of dying or becoming brain-damaged from the effects of innocently ingested mercury. Controls are already in effect across the State and nation; and an international exchange of knowledge about mercury's effects, and new, sophisticated testing methods is being activated.

Symptoms of mercury poisoning have been tricky to diagnose, until quite recently. It had been supposed that this heavy metal, discharged in industrial wastes into streams, lakes and bays from factories ("natural" pollution of course!) would sink to the bottom and remain there inert.

But mercury, scientists now know, doesn't necessarily stay in the glistening columns found in thermometers, barometer tubes, and sphygmodynamometers as metallic (inorganic or phenyl) mercury. Once deposited in the bottom muds of lakes, streams or bays, various forms of anaerobic (non-oxygen requiring) bacteria go to work on the metal, transforming it into methyl mercury.

Then it becomes an active compound, easily absorbed into aquatic or marine food chains where it goes upward and onward, concentrating in the flesh of larger predatory fish and water birds until it eventually enters man, the most predacious of all animals.

Attacks Brain Cells

Methyl mercury, once in the human system, has a peculiar affinity for brain cells. Even the tiniest amount may be able to destroy brain cells before any identifiable clinical symptoms appear at all.

Methyl mercury also attacks the fetus of mammals, including man, easily crossing the placenta which is nature's fortress against most such incursions.

Among the 111 persons killed or brain-damaged in the Minamata Bay incident, congenitally defective babies were born to mothers who had eaten the contaminated fish and shellfish.

The interagency committee headed by Dr. Kahn, and its laboratory sub-committee, chaired by the health department's Joseph Thom, began its work by collecting all of the literature on mercury from all sources, worldwide. It was sketchy. No experience had been recorded as to how much methyl mercury could be ingested by humans without harm, or how long it stayed in the system or how soon excreted, or what was the danger point in its cumulative buildup.

Found in Nature

Mercury is found everywhere in nature. Its presence in seawater was demonstrated as early as 1799. It is considered part of our evolutionary heritage, and necessary to life. Dr. Kahn's committee faced the problem of insuring that industry and agriculture didn't make too much of an originally small, good thing.

Swedish scientists had stumbled quite accidentally on the reason why nearly a whole generation of game birds had died, in the 1950s. They had been feeding on methyl mercury-treated seed grain which the Swedes had developed during World War II, and had kept using in larger quantities afterwards. In 1965, the Swedes drastically reduced the use of the poisoned grain, and in one year the birds came back to normal populations. The Swedish scientists also found that their fish and shellfish were heavily contaminated.

Economic Decision

For a nation of fish-eaters and fish and shellfish exporters this was bad news. The government set an acceptable tolerance limit of 1 part per million; their scientists proposed a maximum of 0.2 ppm, but they weren't listened to. "It was an economic decision," Dr. Kahn said, "rather than a 'people' decision."

In California, a family of Mexican farm workers came by a sack of the pink, poisoned seed grain in Imperial County. The mercury-coated seed grain has been planted here by the millions of pounds.

The state's giant agricultural firms have been using mercury-coated seed grain to stave off mildew until the seeds have a chance to germinate. The grain was dyed pink, the internationally-recognized color code for "POISON—DANGER!" Unfortunately, farm hands don't have access to the literature.

Danger Eliminated

Nobody knows how many farm families have been permanently brain damaged, or killed, by eating the grain themselves or using it as cattle or hog feed, and then eating the animals. The danger is now known and is being eliminated in this country. But hundreds have died from the same poison sources in Iraq, Pakistan and Guatemala. The Imperical County workers used it as food for themselves and their chickens. Several of them died.

Fortunately, Dr. Kahn reports, the agricultural commissioner in another county, San Diego, learned of seed leaking from freight car shipments en route, and alerted farm communities along the tracks to the danger, and no more deaths were reported.

The pink seed grain, trade-named "Panogen," has been ordered off the California market at the end of 1971 by the State Department of Agriculture, on the interagency committee's recommendation. Stopping the incursion of this lethal weaponry was only one of the committee's jobs.

It also sampled commercial fish, sport fish, pheasants and wild ducks, and inland fresh and bay and sea water for mercury levels.

The federal food and drug administration has set a tolerance level of 0.5 ppm—for fish. All other foods must maintain a "zero" level, and the World Health Organization recommends that mercury in anybody's entire diet shouldn't exceed 0.05 ppm—one-tenth the level set for fish by the FDA.

Numbers Game

"But this is a numbers-game," Dr. Kahn warns. "The FDA's 0.5 figure is only a yardstick. People who eat more fish may be loading up on higher mercury levels, if the fish re contaminated. Two meals a week of 0.25 ppm-contaminated fish equals an intake of one meal at 0.5 ppm. And the effect is cumulative!"

Where and how do fish take on methyl mercury? Largemouth bass in Clear Lake and the lower Feather River were found to be significantly contaminated, but not those in the Colorado River. Salmon, coastwise, tested low. Some tuna and swordfish were found to be high enough to ban them from the market.

Where would tuna and swordfish, which range over thousands of miles of ocean, pick up such significant contamination? It would be easier to trace an infestation source of fleas on a Boeing 737.

"Mercury has been known as an industrial poison for centuries," Dr. Kahn said. "But nailing it down as an environmental poison too, is quite recent."

Seven Years

"In the 1953 Minimata incident, it took seven years to pinpoint the poisoning to methyl mercury," he continued, "and it was only after another outbreak in 1965, at Niigata several hundred miles away, that this type of poisoning was finally confirmed and fully accepted by scientists and the managers of polluting industries."

A major problem in running down methyl mercury as a new, deadly environmental pollutant has been its effects, when they finally surface—after the irreversible damage is well under way—because they mimic encephalitis, cerebral palsy, or even "Lou Gehrig" disease. The symptoms aren't typical of central nervous system degeneration, but pop up spottily. "Actually, only an autopsy can prove methyl mercury poisoning, sometimes," Dr. Kahn added.

Forty-niners

"California just naturally has a built-in environmental mercury contamination," Dr. Kahn said. "The Coastal Mountain Range is rich in mercury deposits, and more is mined here than in any other region on the continent. Cinnabar, the ore from which mercury is extracted, is deposited naturally all over the region. It leaches out into streams, and contaminates lakes even in such non-industrial areas as Clear Lake and Lake Berryessa."

"Then also," he continued, "the Forty-niners used plenty of mercury in gold-mining operations in the Sierra Nevada foothills. It's been estimated that a million flakes—each holding 76 pounds of mercury—have been used here since 1849, and most of it eventually drained into the San Joaquin and Sacramento river delta."

So mercury is with us, both in the natural environment as trace elements in the air, water, and earth, and as industrial pollution discharged into the handiest body of water by factories. It also was used to process felt in East Coast, English and European hat factories where it poisoned the hat-workers and inspired Lewis Carroll's famous "Mad Hatter."

Until recently mercury was used to prevent sliming in pulp and paper mills, in air-conditioning towers, and as an anti-mildew agent in swimming pools, paints, and some types of chlorine-alkylide manufacturing.

Silting

Mercury is hard to get rid of. The only known way of muffling its toxicity is the natural silting action that occurs in mud beds under bodies of water. A two-inch layer of silt over the metal will render it harmless. But some lakes in Sweden, heavily contaminated, have retained their danger for decades because they have no silt input

The Stauffer Co. and Dow Chemical Co., two large-scale manufacturers of chlorine gas and caustic soda—both of high value to many industries—stopped its use a year ago in their California plants, after the Dow Middle West plant's discharge of 50 to 100 pounds of mercury a day into Lake Erie was discovered to be poisoning fish at a highly dangerous rate.

"We've just now got a fingertip hold on this environmental phase of mercury," Dr. Kahn said. "So far as our information goes, no one has died in California from the environmental aspect."

"But the committee would like to keep on the track. We feel that epidemiological and toxicological studies are urgently required. We hope we get the tools to continue."

A Damaging Source of Air Pollution

6

by Philip H. Abelson

Public concern about air pollution has grown rapidly during the past few years. In a recent poll, 80 per cent of respondents felt that additional measures should be taken to minimize this problem. Most people, when they consider air pollution, think of the automobile, the smokestack, or the trash burner. Few point to a most damaging source of air pollution—the cigarette.

One of the toxic products of the automobile is carbon monoxide. Exposure for 1 hour to a concentration of this gas of 120 parts per million causes inactivation of about 5 per cent of the body's hemoglobin and commonly leads to dizziness, headache, and lassitude. Concentrations of carbon monoxide as high as 100 ppm often occur in garages, in tunnels, and behind automobiles. Such concentrations are tiny in comparison with those (42,000 ppm) found in cigarette smoke. The smoker survives because most of the time he breathes air not so heavily polluted. However, in a poorly ventilated, smoke-filled room, concentrations of carbon monoxide can easily reach several hundred parts per million, thus exposing smokers and nonsmokers to a toxic hazard.

Another air pollutant issuing from automobiles is nitrogen dioxide. Nitrogen dioxide is an acutely irritating gas; also, it gives rise to nitrite, a potential mutagenic agent. Concentrations of NO_2 as high as 3 ppm have been noted in Los Angeles, and levels of 5 ppm are considered dangerous. Cigarette smoke contains 250 parts of NO_2 per million.

Many of the toxic agents in cigarette smoke do not have counterparts in ordinary air pollution. One of these, hydrogen cyanide, is particularly noteworthy. It is highly active against respiratory enzymes. Long-term exposure to levels above 10 ppm is dangerous. The concentration in cigarette smoke is 1600 ppm.

These inorganic pollutants are three of many noxious substances that have been found in tobacco smoke. Among others are acrolein, aldehydes, phenols, and carcinogens, an important one of which is benzo(a)pyrene. Evidence points to synergistic effects among the toxic agents. The phenols, though not themselves notably carcinogenic, increase markedly the carcinogenic potency of benzo(a)pyrene.

The toxic effects of cigarette smoke are also enhanced by other environmental factors. A recent study of asbestos workers showed a very high incidence of lung cancer among smokers, in contrast to a low incidence among nonsmokers. In a group of 283 asbestos workers who had a history of cigarette smoking, 24 of 78 deaths were due to bronchogenic carcinoma. Of 87 asbestos workers, who were nonsmokers, none died of lung cancer during a comparable period. A study of the uranium miners stricken with lung cancer has also revealed an effect related to smoking. The rate of fatalities was much higher among smokers than among nonsmokers.

Another example of a synergistic effect is seen in the smoker who breathes polluted urban air. The incidence of lung cancer among smokers is higher in the city than in rural areas.

The principal effects of smoking are borne by the smokers themselves. They pay for their habit with chronic disease and shortened life. Involved are the individual's decision and his life. However, when the individual smokes in a poorly ventilated space in the presence of others, he infringes the rights of others and becomes a serious contributor to air pollution.

7 Conservation And Environmental Organizations

General Conservation

Conservative Foundation
1250 Connecticut Avenue N.W.
Washington, D.C. 20036

Friends of the Earth
30 East 42nd Street
New York, N. Y. 10017

National Audubon Society
1130 Fifth Avenue
New York, N. Y. 10028

National Parks Association
1701 18th Street, N.W.
Washington, D.C. 20009

Nature Conservancy
1522 K Street, N.W.
Washington, D.C. 20005

SOURCE: Adapted from a list which has been compiled by the Sierra Club, 1050 Mills Tower, 220 Bush Street, San Francisco, Ca. 94104.

Open Space Institute
145 East 52nd Street
New York, N.Y. 10022

Wilderness Society
729 15th Street, N.W.
Washington, D.C. 20005

Wildlife

Defenders of Wildlife
1346 Connecticut Avenue, N.W.
Washington, D.C. 20036

National Wildlife Federation
1412 16th Street, N.W.
Washington, D.C. 20036

Environmental Problems

Committee for Environmental Information
438 N. Skinker Boulevard
St. Louis, Mo. 63130

Committee of Two Million
760 Market Street, Rm. 1032
San Francisco, Calif. 94102

Environmental Defense Fund
P.O. Drawer 740
Stony Brook, N.Y. 11790

Ecology Action
3029 Benvenue
Berkeley, Ca. 94709

Water Pollution Control Federation
3900 Wisconsin Avenue, N.W.
Washington, D.C. 20016

Soil Conservation Society of America
7517 N.E. Ankeny Road
Ankeny, Ia. 50021

Citizens for Clean Air
40 West 57th Street
New York, N.Y. 10019

Citizens League Against Sonic Boom
19 Appleton Street
Cambridge, Ma. 02138

Town-Village Aircraft Safety and Noise Abatement Committee
196 Central Avenue
Lawrence, N.Y. 11559

Population

Planned Parenthood-World Population
515 Madison Avenue
New York, N.Y. 10022

Zero Population Growth
3545 El Camino Real
Palo Alto, Calif. 94306

Professional

American Association for the Advancement of Science
1515 Massachusetts Avenue N.W.
Washington, D.C. 20005

Ecological Society of America
c/o Biology Department
Duke University
Durham, N. C.

League of Women Voters
1730 M Street, N.W.
Washington, D.C. 20036

California

Northern California Committee for Environmental Information
1811 Francisco Street
Berkeley, Ca. 94703

Planning and Conservation League
909 12th Street
Sacramento, Ca. 95814

San Francisco Bay Region

Ecology Center
2179 Allston Way
Berkeley, Ca. 94701

Bibliography and Suggested Readings

BIBLIOGRAPHY

Brown, Harrison: "Human Materials Production as a Process in the Biosphere," *Scientific American*, September, 1970, New York, New York, pp. 195-208.

Cottam, Clarence; "The Ecologist's Role in Problems of Pesticide Pollution," *Bio. Science*, July, 1965.

Ehrlich, Paul R.; *The Population Bomb*, Ballantine Books, New York, 1968.

Jones, Kenneth L.; Dhainberg, Louis W., and Byer, Curtis O.; *Environmental Health*, Harper & Row Publishers, New York, 1971.

"How Today's Noise Hurts Body and Mind," *Medical World News*, **10**, No. 24, June 13, 1969.

SUGGESTED READINGS

Ehrlich, Paul R. and Ehrlich, Anne H.; *Population/Resources/Environment;* W. H. Freeman and Co. Publishers; San Francisco, California; 1970.

Gofman, John W. and Tamplin, Arthur R.; *Poisoned Power;* David McKay Co., Inc.; New York; 1971.

Tofler, Alvin; *Future Shock;* Random House, Inc.; New York; 1970.

Index